Advanced Materials for Biomechanical Applications

Mathematical Engineering, Manufacturing, and Management Sciences

Series Editor:

Mangey Ram

Professor, Assistant Dean (International Affairs), Department of Mathematics, Graphic Era University, Dehradun, India

The aim of this new book series is to publish the research studies and articles that bring up the latest development and research applied to mathematics and its applications in the manufacturing and management science areas. Mathematical tools and techniques are the strength of engineering sciences. They form the common foundation of all novel disciplines as engineering evolves and develops. The series will include a comprehensive range of applied mathematics and its applications in engineering areas such as optimization techniques, mathematical modeling and simulation, stochastic processes and systems engineering, safety-critical system performance, system safety, system security, high-assurance software architecture and design, mathematical modeling in environmental safety sciences, finite element methods, differential equations, and reliability engineering.

Swarm Intelligence: Foundation, Principles, and Engineering Applications
Abhishek Sharma, Abhinav Sharma,
Jitendra Kumar Pandey, and Mangey Ram

Advances in Sustainable Machining and Manufacturing Processes
Kishor Kumar Gajrani, Arbind Prasad, and Ashwani Kumar

Advanced Materials for Biomechanical Applications
Edited by Ashwani Kumar, Mangey Ram, and Yogesh Kumar Singla

Biodegradable Composites for Packaging Applications
Edited by Arbind Prasad, Ashwani Kumar, and Kishor Kumar Gajrani

Computing and Stimulation for Engineers
Edited by Ziya Uddin, Mukesh Kumar Awasthi,
Rishi Asthana, and Mangey Ram

For more information about this series, please visit: https://www.routledge.com/Mathematical-Engineering-Manufacturing-and-Management-Sciences/book-series/CRCMEMMS

Advanced Materials for Biomechanical Applications

Edited by
Ashwani Kumar
Mangey Ram
Yogesh Kumar Singla

CRC Press
Taylor & Francis Group
Boca Raton London New York

CRC Press is an imprint of the
Taylor & Francis Group, an **informa** business

First edition published 2022
by CRC Press
6000 Broken Sound Parkway NW, Suite 300, Boca Raton, FL 33487-2742

and by CRC Press
4 Park Square, Milton Park, Abingdon, Oxon, OX14 4RN

CRC Press is an imprint of Taylor & Francis Group, LLC

Library of Congress Cataloging-in-Publication Data
Names: Kumar, Ashwani, 1989- editor. | Ram, Mangey, editor. | Singla,
Yogesh Kumar, editor.
Title: Advanced materials for biomechanical applications / edited by
Ashwani Kumar, Mangey Ram, Yogesh Kumar Singla.
Description: First edition. | Boca Raton : CRC Press, 2022. | Series: MEMMS
series | Includes bibliographical references and index.
Identifiers: LCCN 2021058010 (print) | LCCN 2021058011 (ebook) |
ISBN 9781032054490 (hardback) | ISBN 9781032261515 (paperback) |
ISBN 9781003286806 (ebook)
Subjects: LCSH: Biomedical materials.
Classification: LCC R857.M3 A378 2022 (print) | LCC R857.M3 (ebook) |
DDC 610.28—dc23/eng/20220222
LC record available at https://lccn.loc.gov/2021058010
LC ebook record available at https://lccn.loc.gov/2021058011

ISBN: 9781032054490 (hbk)
ISBN: 9781032261515 (pbk)
ISBN: 9781003286806 (ebk)

DOI: 10.1201/9781003286806

Typeset in Times
by codeMantra

Contents

Aim and Scope

The modern era of advanced materials, the latest manufacturing techniques, product modeling and analysis, complex geometry analysis, and nonlinear analysis have been shifted from traditional methods to advanced techniques that provide precise solutions. *Advanced Materials for Biomechanical Applications* provides in-depth knowledge to readers about easier, fast, efficient, and reliable methods for understanding orthopedic and dental implant problems with the help of advanced techniques using simulation and experiments.

The book *Advanced Materials for Biomechanical Applications* consists of details about advanced materials like titanium, titanium alloys, cobalt–chromium alloys, stainless steel, and composite materials for biomechanical applications like joint replacements, bone plates, bone cement, artificial ligaments and tendons, hip implants, and dental implants for tooth fixation. The book consists of 15 chapters dedicated to biomechanical and biomedical applications of advanced materials. Modern medicine takes advantage of the progress in engineering, physical, and chemical sciences. One of the best examples of such a combination is biomaterials used for biomedical applications. The basic requirement of a biomaterial is that it should be compatible with the body, and problems with biocompatibility must be resolved before a product can be used in a clinical setting. Production and synthesis of biomaterials require various technologies and methods. These methods produce the best-suited materials. The book presents the inventory of the latest achievements in the development and production of modern biomaterials that are used in modern medicine and dentistry application.

The content of the book is focused on orthopedic and dental implants. The authors covered two key topics in 15 chapters, which are quite interesting and with the potential for further research. The book covers basic and advanced research, which makes it useful for researchers, postgraduate students, and working professionals in the field of orthopedics and dentistry. With lucidity presenting the book *Advanced Materials for Biomechanical Applications* to all readers.

Editors
Dr. Ashwani Kumar
Prof. Mangey Ram
Dr. Yogesh Kumar Singla

Preface

The book *Advanced Materials for Biomechanical Applications* consists of the design, simulation, and manufacturing of advanced materials and their characterization for medicine and dentistry applications. Materials for orthopedic and dentistry applications are the central theme of the book. These two key topics have been explained in 15 chapters. All chapters are well organized and easy to follow. The above could help to ensure the completeness of the book and to satisfy the needs of the potential researchers and postgraduate students (MSc, PhD) in areas having biomaterial applications.

In origin, biomaterials can be obtained from nature or be synthesized in the laboratory with a variety of approaches that use metals, polymers, ceramics, or composite materials. They are often used or adapted for medical applications. Biomaterials are commonly used in orthopedic and dental applications such as joint replacements, bone plates, bone cement, surgical sutures, clips, and staples to close wounds, pins and screws to stabilize fractures, surgical mesh, breast implants, artificial ligaments and tendons, dental implants for teeth stabilization, blood vessel prostheses, heart valves, vascular grafts, stents, nerve conduits, skin repair devices, intraocular lenses in eye surgery, contact lenses and drug delivery systems.

Chapter 1 provides details about the influence of technology under the umbrella of bio-mechanical engineering on the health of humans in the society. Different types of implants, instruments used in surgery, development of prosthetics, etc. are also explained in this chapter. It creates an environment of biomechanics and provides a push for further reading of chapters. *Chapter 2* deals with the biocompatibility of materials. In this chapter, the processing of biomedical alloys through cross rolling (CR), a rolling process where the strain path is changed by 90° in between two passes, is discussed. The earlier reported works indicate that CR can serve as an effective technique to obtain the desired microstructure, texture, and mechanical properties, which promotes the biocompatibility of the processed material. In continuation, *Chapter 3* deals with additive manufacturing in the context of biomedical materials. At present, additively manufactured biomedical materials find extensive applications in a wide range of avenues ranging from orthopedics to urology. Additive manufacturing (AM) techniques based on layer-wise deposition of materials allow for fabrication of complex-shaped biomedical components with a high level of accuracy.

Chapter 4 highlights the use of cellulose for biomedical applications. Cellulose is the most abundantly available organic resource. As a result of its promising features such as high mechanical strength, renewability, biocompatibility, biodegradability, and low toxicity, it has been widely explored as an ideal substitute for synthetic polymers especially in biomedical applications such as the development of drug delivery systems, production of wound dressing materials, construction of tissue engineering scaffolds, fabrication of wearable electronic biosensors, etc. Like cellulose, magnetic iron oxide nanoparticles are promising materials in the biomedical field due to their superparamagnetic behavior. *Chapter 5* deals with the use of magnetic iron oxide nanoparticles for biomedical applications. *Chapters 6 and 7* highlight the use of magnesium and its nanocomposites for biomedical applications. Nowadays, the popularity of magnesium alloys in biomedical applications is increasing as they have excellent mechanical properties and the capacity for precipitation of a bone-like apatite layer on their outer layer. Also, after clinical use, magnesium totally degrades in the human body as it is a biodegradable material, which makes magnesium alloys most suitable for many biomedical applications.

Chapter 8 puts a focus on the investigation of titanium lattice structures for biomedical implants. In this study, three different types of AM-manufactured metal lattice/porous structures (Gyroid, Diamond, and Schwarz W) and their three different pore sizes (0.4, 0.5, and 0.6 mm) are investigated for tailoring the elastic modulus of a Ti6Al4V ELI material to match that of cancellous bone. *Chapter 9* deals with the economic analysis of biomaterials. In this chapter, cost estimation of polymer materials has been done for biomedical application of human knee implants. *Chapter 10* highlights improvement methods in the mechanical properties of biomaterials. The chapter describes various SPD techniques characterization and the process parameters to achieve ultra-fine grains. In continuation to Chapter 10, *Chapter 11* describes an improved biodegradable material for orthopedic implant applications. The chapter provides a rigorous insight into the various possible strategies to develop improved biodegradable implant materials for futuristic orthopedic applications.

In *Chapter 12*, the stress shielding effect, i.e. premature failure of the implant material for orthopedic applications, has been investigated. The extended finite element method (XFEM) is utilized to numerically investigate the performance against a ductile fracture from crack nucleation till fracture during tensile loading. Further, elasto-plastic crack growth simulations are accomplished by XFEM through enriching the standard approximation for an SLM-processed TNTZ alloy. *Chapter 13* deals with important aspects of this book where the design of a low-cost prosthetic leg is described. It deals with the design and modeling of a prosthetic leg for above-knee amputees using MR fluid. MR fluids are smart materials, which change their rheological properties according to the magnetic field around them. *Chapter 14* deals with the analysis of humerus bone fracture and healing. A hairline fracture is investigated using FEA. In this chapter, hand vibration and whole-body vibration are explained. *Chapter 15* proposes a new design for energy harvesting. A new configuration is proposed, which is oriented vertically and excited in the transverse direction at its base, and attempts to find out the motion parameters to maximize the energy harvesting capability. The model of a low-cost shaker is developed and analyzed.

Having a high quality of content, this book will serve as a reference book for understanding orthopedic and dentistry problems with literature review, solution, methodology, experimental setup, results, validation, and future scope. Lucidly presenting the book *Advanced Materials for Biomechanical Applications* provides a foundational link to more specialized research work in biomechanical engineering.

Editors
Dr. Ashwani Kumar
Prof. Mangey Ram
Dr. Yogesh Kumar Singla

MATLAB® is a registered trademark of The MathWorks, Inc. For product information, please contact:
The MathWorks, Inc.
3 Apple Hill Drive
Natick, MA 01760-2098 USA
Tel: 508-647-7000
Fax: 508-647-7001
E-mail: info@mathworks.com
Web: www.mathworks.com

Editors

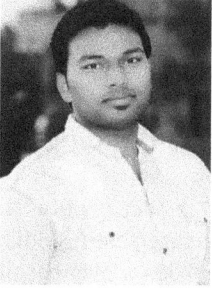

Dr. Ashwani Kumar received a Ph.D. (Mechanical Engineering) in the area of Mechanical Vibration and Design. He is currently working as Senior Lecturer, Mechanical Engineering (Gazetted Officer Class II) at Technical Education Department, Uttar Pradesh (Government of Uttar Pradesh), India since December 2013. He has worked as an Assistant Professor in the Department of Mechanical Engineering, Graphic Era University, Dehradun, India from July 2010 to November 2013. He has more than 12 years of research and academic experience in mechanical and materials engineering. He is Series Editor of the book series *Advances in Manufacturing, Design and Computational Intelligence Techniques* published by CRC Press (Taylor & Francis) USA. He is Associate Editor for the *International Journal of Mathematical, Engineering and Management Sciences* (IJMEMS) Indexed in ESCI/Scopus and DOAJ. He is an editorial board member of four international journals and acts as a review board member of 20 prestigious (Indexed in SCI/SCIE/Scopus) international journals with high impact factors, i.e. *Applied Acoustics, Measurement, JESTEC, AJSE, SV-JME,* and *LAJSS.* In addition, he has published 90 research articles in journals, book chapters, and conferences. He has authored/co-authored and edited 17 books of Mechanical and Materials Engineering. He is associated with international conferences as Invited Speaker/Advisory Board/Review Board member. He has delivered many invited talks in webinars, FDP, and workshops. He has been awarded as the Best Teacher for excellence in academics and research. He has successfully guided 12 B.Tech., M.Tech., and Ph.D. theses. In administration, he is working as a coordinator for AICTE, E.O.A., Nodal officer for the PMKVY-TI Scheme (Government of India), and an internal coordinator for the CDTP scheme (Government of Uttar Pradesh). He is currently involved in the research area of Machine Learning, Advanced Materials, Machining & Manufacturing Techniques, Biodegradable Composites, Heavy Vehicle Dynamics, and Coriolis Mass Flow Sensor.

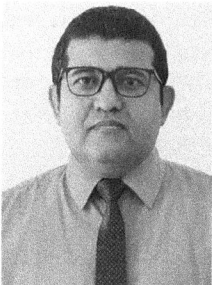

Prof. Mangey Ram received a Ph.D. degree major in Mathematics and minor in Computer Science from G. B. Pant University of Agriculture and Technology, Pantnagar, India. He has been a Faculty Member for around 13 years and has taught several core courses in pure and applied mathematics at undergraduate, postgraduate, and doctorate levels. He is currently the Research Professor at Graphic Era (Deemed to be University), Dehradun, India and Visiting Professor at Peter the Great St. Petersburg Polytechnic University, Saint Petersburg, Russia. Before joining Graphic Era, he was a Deputy Manager (Probationary Officer) with Syndicate Bank for a short period. He is Editor-in-Chief of *International Journal of Mathematical,*

Engineering and Management Sciences; *Journal of Reliability and Statistical Studies*; *Journal of Graphic Era University*; Series Editor of six Book Series with Elsevier, CRC Press-A Taylor and Francis Group, Walter De Gruyter Publisher Germany, and River Publisher, and a Guest Editor and Associate Editor with various journals. He has published 250 plus publications (journal articles/books/book chapters/conference articles) in IEEE, Taylor & Francis, Springer Nature, Elsevier, Emerald, World Scientific, and many other national and international journals and conferences. Also, he has published more than 50 books (authored/edited) with international publishers like Elsevier, Springer Nature, CRC Press Taylor & Francis Group, Walter De Gruyter Publisher Germany, and River Publisher. His fields of research are Reliability Theory and Applied Mathematics. Dr. Ram is a Senior Member of the IEEE, Senior Life Member of Operational Research Society of India, Society for Reliability Engineering, Quality and Operations Management in India, Indian Society of Industrial and Applied Mathematics, He has been a member of the organizing committee of many international and national conferences, seminars, and workshops. He has been conferred with the "Young Scientist Award" by the Uttarakhand State Council for Science and Technology, Dehradun, in 2009. He has been awarded the "Best Faculty Award" in 2011; "Research Excellence Award" in 2015; and "Outstanding Researcher Award" in 2018 for his significant contribution in academics and research at Graphic Era Deemed to be University, Dehradun, India. Recently, he has received the "Excellence in Research of the Year-2021 Award" from the Honorable Chief Minister of Uttarakhand State, India.

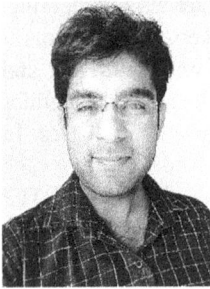

Dr. Yogesh Kumar Singla associated with Case Western Reserve University, USA has done his Ph.D. from IIT Roorkee. He has more than 6 years of research and teaching experience. He is working in the area of Manufacturing, Welding, Surface Engineering, Tribology, Materials Characterization, Welding Metallurgy, and Mechanical Behavior of Metals. He has ten SCI publications and five Scopus Indexed publications. Apart from this, four SCI papers are in-process. In his career, he has successfully guided one Ph.D. and four M.E. theses. He is a reviewer of many SCI journals of Elsevier and Springer having impact factors ranging from 0.7 to 5.289. He is about to submit one patent on a solar dryer. He has given many expert talks at state- and central-level institutes/universities. He also has the experience of conducting a 10-day Faculty Development Program. In addition to this, he is an Editor of two international books entitled *Advanced Computational Methods in Mechanical and Materials Engineering* and *Advanced Materials for Bio-Mechanical Applications* to be published by CRC Press (Taylor & Francis Group, https://taylorandfrancis.com/books/) in 2021.

Acknowledgments

We express our heartfelt gratitude to **CRC Press (Taylor & Francis Group)** and the editorial team for their guidance and support during the completion of this book. We are grateful to all chapter authors and reviewers for their suggestions and illuminating views on each book chapter presented in the book *Advanced Materials for Biomechanical Applications.*

This book is dedicated to all budding researchers....

Contributors

Suya Prem Anand
Department of Mechanical Engineering
(CBCMT)
VIT
Vellore, India

Suresh Bandi
Department of Metallurgical &
Materials Engineering
Visvesvaraya National Institute of
Technology
Nagpur, India

Shivprakash Barve
School of Mechanical Engineering
MIT World Peace University
Pune, India

K. Chandraraj
Department of Biotechnology
Indian Institute of Technology Madras
Chennai, India

Seung-Bok Choi
Department of Mechanical Engineering
The State University of New York
Korea (SUNY Korea)
Songdo, South Korea

Ashish Das
Department of Production and
Industrial Engineering
National Institute of Technology
Jamshedpur, India

Abel Eldho Jose
Department of Mechanical Engineering
(CBCMT)
VIT
Vellore, India

Moumita Ghosh
Department of Biotechnology and
Medical Engineering
National Institute of
Technology
Rourkela, India

Yatika Gori
Department of Mechanical
Engineering
Graphic Era University
Dehradun, India

Vikram Hastak
Department of Metallurgical &
Materials Engineering
Visvesvaraya National Institute of
Technology
Nagpur, India

T. Jagadeesha
Department of Mechanical
Engineering
National Institute of Technology
Calicut, India

Parveen Kalra
Department of Production & Industrial
Engineering
Punjab Engineering College
Chandigarh, India

Vikram G. Kamble
Institute of Materials Science
Technical University Dresden
Dresden, Germany

Vishwanath Karad
MIT World Peace University
Pune, India

Ashwani Kumar
Technical Education Department Uttar
    Pradesh
Kanpur, India

Ashwin Sunil Kumar
Department of Mechanical Engineering
    (CBCMT)
VIT
Vellore, India

Kundan Kumar
Department of Production and
    Industrial Engineering
National Institute of Technology
Jamshedpur, India

Pankaj Kumar
Department of Mechanical Engineering
National Institute of Technology
Goa, India

Prashant Kumar
Manufacturing Science &
    Instrumentation
CSIR-CSIO
Chandigarh, India

Manab Mallik
Department of Metallurgical and
    Materials Engineering
Centre of Biomedical Engineering &
    Assistive Technology (BEAT)
National Institute of Technology
Durgapur, India

Ankit Meena
Department of Mechanical Engineering
National Institute of Technology
Calicut, India

Vijay Kumar Meena
Manufacturing Science &
    Instrumentation
CSIR-CSIO
Chandigarh, India

Shashank Mishra
Department of Mechanical Engineering
Maulana Azad National Institute of
    Technology
Bhopal, India

V. Murugabalaji
Department of Production Engineering
National Institute of Technology
Tiruchirappalli, India

Chitresh Nayak
Department of Mechanical Engineering
Medi-Caps University
Indore, India

Manoj Nikam
Department of Mechanical Engineering
BV College of Engineering
Navi Mumbai, India

Tarun Panchal
Manufacturing Science &
    Instrumentation
CSIR-CSIO
Chandigarh, India

Vishal Parashar
Department of Mechanical Engineering
Maulana Azad National Institute of
    Technology
Bhopal, India

Pralhad Pesode
School of Mechanical Engineering
MIT World Peace University
Pune, India

Shashi Bhushan Prasad
Department of Production and
    Industrial Engineering
National Institute of Technology
Jamshedpur, India

Grreshan Ramesh
Department of Mechanical Engineering
(CBCMT)
VIT
Vellore, India

Sachin Rana
Department of Mechanical
Engineering
ABES Institute of Technology
Ghaziabad, India

Matruprasad Rout
Department of Production
Engineering
National Institute of Technology
Tiruchirappalli, India

Mainak Saha
Department of Metallurgical and
Materials Engineering
Indian Institute of Technology Madras
Chennai, India

R. Selvakumar
Department of Nanobiotechnology
PSG Institute of Advanced Studies
Coimbatore
Coimbatore, India

Neelesh Kumar Sharma
Department of Mechanical
Engineering
Indian Institute of Technology
Patna, India

Ganapati Shastry
Department of Mechanical
Engineering
National Institute of Technology
Calicut, India

Mukul Shukla
Department of Mechanical
Engineering
Motilal Nehru National Institute of
Technology
Allahabad, India

Ravindra Kumar Sinha
Department of Applied Physics
Delhi Technological University
New Delhi, India

Ajeet K. Srivastav
Department of Metallurgical &
Materials Engineering
Visvesvaraya National Institute of
Technology
Nagpur, India

S.P. Suriyaraj
PSG-STEP: Nanotech Research
Innovation and Incubation Centre
(NRIIC)
PSG College of Technology Coimbatore
Coimbatore, India

Bhaskar Thakur
School of Mechanical Engineering
MIT World Peace University
Pune, India

A. Thirugnanam
Department of Biotechnology and
Medical Engineering
National Institute of Technology
Rourkela, India

Manvendra Tiwari
Department of Mechanical
Engineering
National Institute of Technology
Goa, India

Ashish Toby
Department of Mechanical
  Engineering
National Institute of Technology
Calicut, India

N. Vignesh
Department of Biotechnology
Indian Institute of Technology Madras
Chennai, India

Brijesh Yadav
Department of Mechanical
  Engineering
Graphic Era University
Dehradun, India

1 Bio-Mechanical Engineering and Health

Vishal Parashar and Shashank Mishra
Maulana Azad National Institute of Technology Bhopal

Chitresh Nayak
Medi-Caps University Indore

CONTENTS

1.1 INTRODUCTION

Bio-mechanical engineering has gained importance in the latter half of the twentieth century. There are now dedicated researchers and scientists working on the design and development of bio-mechanical types of equipment. Universities across the world offer courses in this domain. The overall objective of learning and progress in this sector is to employ technology in the area of medical science for the betterment of public health. One can observe the involvement of technology in the aforesaid domain. To get a deeper insight, researchers have subdivided bio-mechanical engineering into the following categories [1]:

- Artificial Organs and Prostheses
- Monitoring, Controls, and Health Care Engineering
- Bio-Mechanics
- Bio-Materials

DOI: 10.1201/9781003286806-1

1

With the development in the field of engineering and technology, monitoring and diagnosis of health-related matters are getting simple to use more precisely. The reason is that the course of treatment and proper monitoring of health is getting much more effective than earlier it was. For example, we observe that the development of sensors and actuators has encouraged the fabrication of a digital sphygmomanometer that can be used directly by the patient to keep a track record of the blood pressure and observe the abnormality if any. Similarly, blood sugar tests and pregnancy tests can be performed at home saving time and making the user alert of any type of minor abnormality. This trend is also visible in the field of surgery planning, surgical procedure, and artificial implants. There are different types of digital instruments which are developed in recent times that can effectively and rapidly diagnose the medical condition of patients by employing advanced sensors. Progress in materials science and medicines has produced a healthy, friendly, and biologically compatible environment for the treatment and recovery of patients. The requirement for an effective medical procedure is now served with reduced allergic side effects from medicines and producing superior performance against the conventional counterpart. Accompanied by the aforesaid advancement, more efficient materials like polymer matrix composites and ceramics are now used for implants and prosthetics, providing lighter weight, less corrosive materials with reduced toxicity. In this chapter, recent developments in different parts under the discipline of bio-mechanical engineering and its influence on the public health sector are discussed. Figure 1.1 shows some applications of engineering in the biomedical domain.

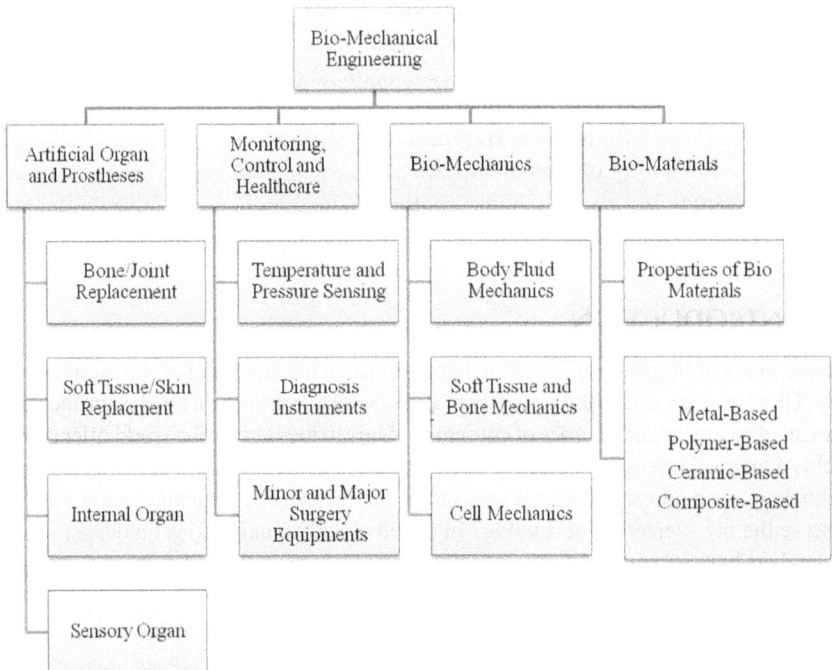

FIGURE 1.1 Bio-mechanical engineering with sub-sections.

1.2 ARTIFICIAL ORGANS AND PROSTHESES

The development of artificial organs has always been a matter of attention in medical science. Various body organs perform different functions for the survival of the human body. An artificial replacement of the same must do all the functions as the natural organ and should also be developed from a biocompatible material with utmost accuracy. Replacement of an organ is a complex task in surgery. Surgeons are always looking for alternative artificial implants. Charles G. Gebelein has further divided the artificial organ replacement into four subcategories [2].

1.2.1 BONE/JOINT REPLACEMENT

The injury caused by any severe accident or maybe a result of some disfigured structure in the body since birth may demand replacement of a particular bone or joint. The substitution must be capable of serving the following enlisted purposes [2]:

   a. Ready lubrication
   b. Stress and erosion resistance
   c. Natural motion
   d. Biocompatibility
   e. Firm and permanent fixation
   f. Maintenance of normal joint space

1.2.2 PROSTHESES

Prostheses are provided to those patients having one or both lower limbs missing. The design requirement for the fabrication of a prosthetic socket varies from patient to patient. The shape is complex and differs every time. In addition, it requires a high level of precision so that the patients feel comfortable while wearing the prosthetic. There are several types of prosthetics depending upon the needs of the patients. The nomenclature used by the doctors is provided in Figure 1.2. Lower limb orthotic sockets and lower limb prosthetic sockets are shown in Figures 1.3 and 1.4, respectively [3]. Chitresh et al. developed a prosthetic socket using a novel approach and compared the performance and comfort of the same against the one developed using the conventional method. A prosthetic socket is the interface between the amputee limb and the prosthetic. This novel approach used in the aforementioned study integrates the concept of reverse engineering (RE) with that of additive manufacturing. A pictorial demonstration has been shown in Figure 1.5 [4]. The modern approach of socket development that utilizes 3D scanning and digitization for the design and development of a prosthetic socket also provides provision for topology optimization of the drafted socket model by employing modern simulation software. The optimized socket design removes the material from the location, where the stress magnitude is lower, eliminating the chance of material wastage. The optimized design is complex in shape, making it difficult to fabricate. However, employing advanced manufacturing processes like 3D printing makes it feasible and effective. Nayak et al. [5] provided a detailed review on the mimicking human ankle. Ankle

Prostheses

AK Above knee prosthesis
BK Below knee prosthesis
TT Trans-tibial prosthesis
TF Trans-femoral prosthesis

Orthoses

FO Foot orthosis prosthesis
AFO Ankle-foot orthosis
KO Knee orthosis
KAFO Knee-ankle-foot orthosis
HpO Hip orthosis
HKO Hip–knee orthosis
HKAFO Hip–knee-ankle-foot orthosis
SIO Sacro-iliac orthosis

FIGURE 1.2 Nomenclature used for prostheses and orthoses.

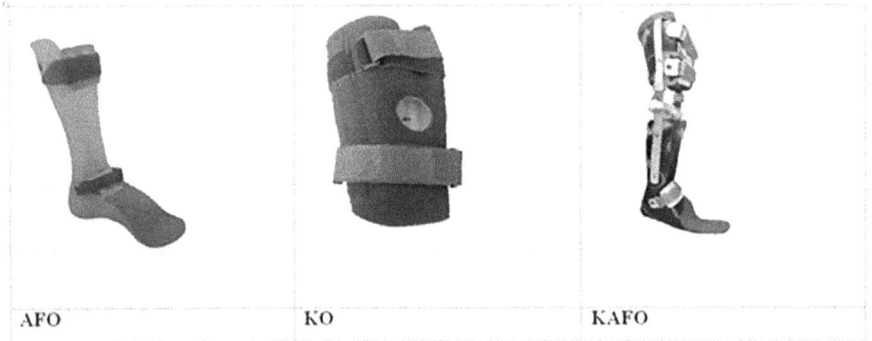

AFO   KO   KAFO

FIGURE 1.3 Lower limb orthotic sockets [3].

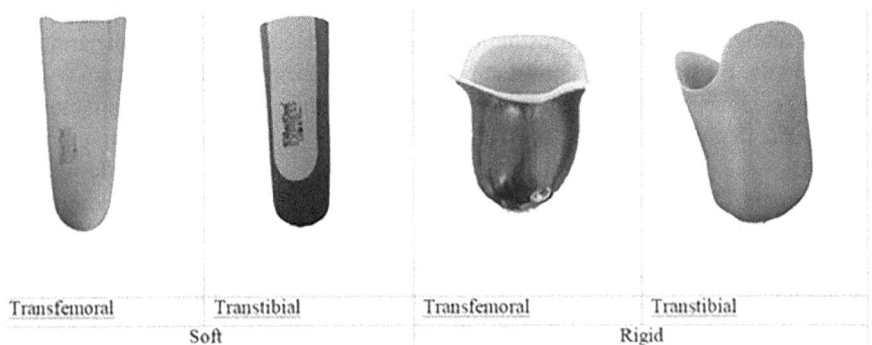

Transfemoral   Transtibial   Transfemoral   Transtibial
Soft   Rigid

FIGURE 1.4 Lower limb prosthetic socket [3].

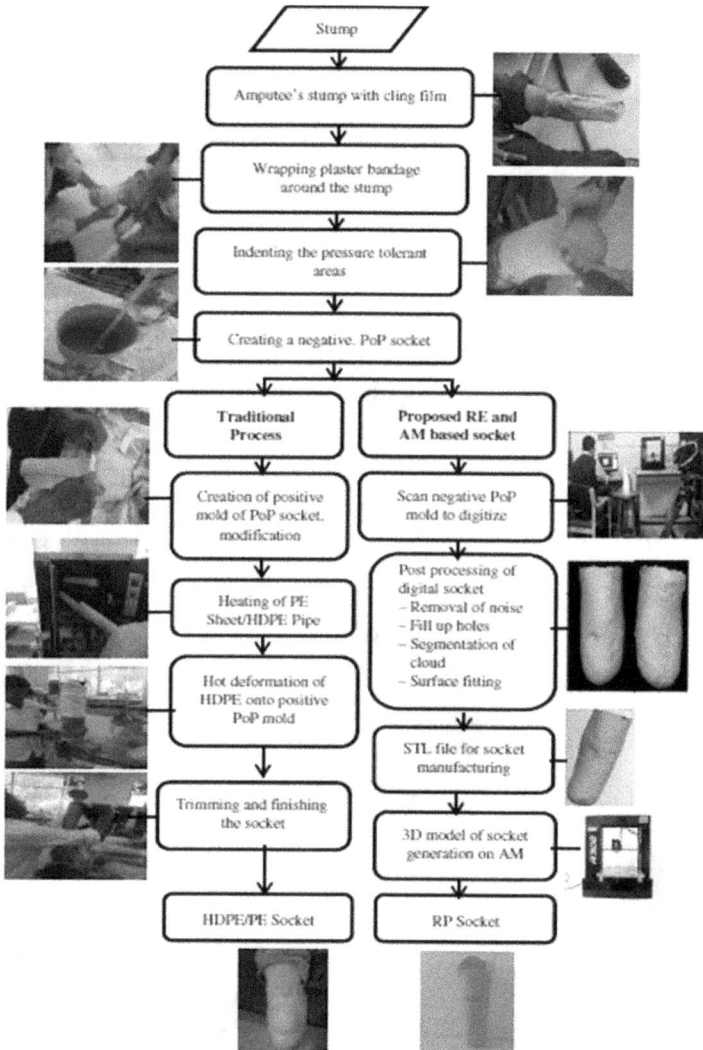

FIGURE 1.5 Comparison of conventional prosthetic socket manufacturing against a novel approach [4].

mobility is a complex mechanism, and hence, it is difficult to replicate. The author has provided a detailed description of the mechanism of ankle mobility, along with the different types of artificial ankle replacements. Some replacements do not mimic the motion as performed by the ankle but serve the purpose of walking. These types of ankles are shown in Figure 1.6. The motion and the mechanics of the ankle are studied, and researchers have attempted to replicate this mechanism. Prostheses that perform motions similar to natural ankle are developed. Different types of such ankles are shown in Figure 1.7 [6].

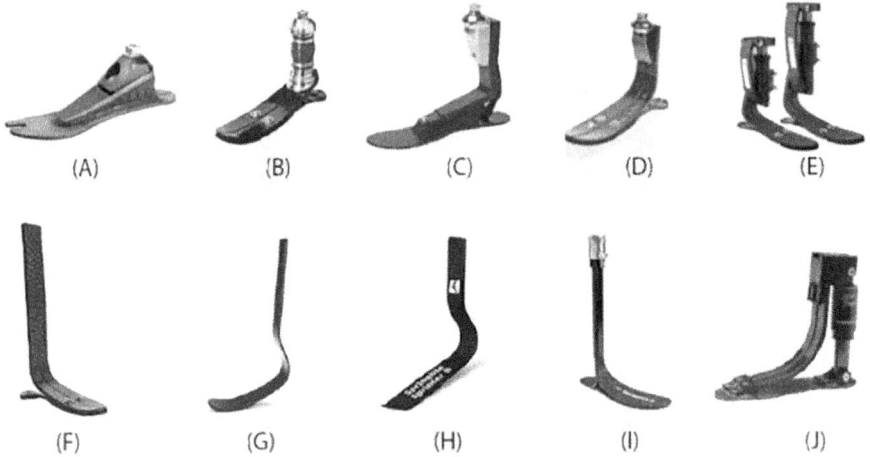

FIGURE 1.6 Advanced ESR feet. (a) Flex-Foot Axia. (b) LP-Ceterus. (c) Talux foot. (d) VariFlex. (e) Re-Flex VSP. (f) Modular III. (g) Flex-Sprint. (h) Sprinter. (i) Springlite foot. (j) Pathfinder [6].

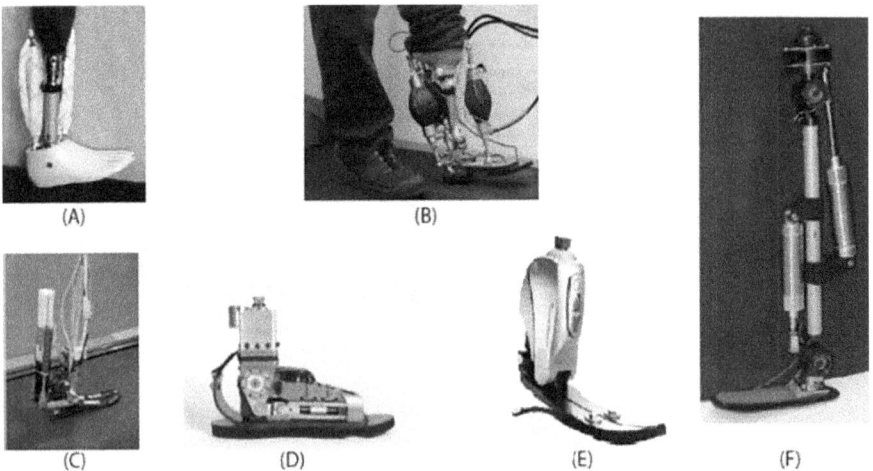

FIGURE 1.7 Bionic feet. (a) TT prosthesis powered by McKibben artificial muscles. (b) TT prosthesis powered by PPAMs. (c) SPARKy. (d) Electrically driven foot of MIT. (e) Proprio foot. (f) Powered transfemoral prosthesis of Vanderbilt University [6].

1.2.3 SOFT TISSUE/SKIN REPLACEMENT

Skin covers a large volume of the human body. Skin types vary for different body parts. Injuries are caused by burns and accidents, and these events are reported throughout the year. Soft tissues are protected by skin; damaged skin may result in infection and lead to the loss of body fluids and electrolytes. Substitution of damaged skin with an artificial material is one of the most complex tasks from the surgical point of view. In addition, finding a suitable biocompatible material is a challenge. Tissues below the skin are known as soft tissues. These soft tissues cover a large portion of the human body. Every year there are surgeries dedicated for the replacement of soft tissues with artificial implants, which include facial plastic surgery, breast implant, and hernia repair. Challenges associated with soft tissue implants are the increment in the rigidity of the implant material with the growth of tissues over the period.

1.2.4 INTERNAL ORGANS

Heart, heart valves, liver, pancreas, gastrointestinal tracts, and blood vessels are the internal organs considered for artificial implants. These are vital organs for survival; implants associated with these organs are supposed to replicate certain functions as served by natural organs. Obtaining the same purpose from an artificial material is almost impossible. The pacemaker is a device frequently employed in heart patients to regulate heartbeat. Almost all the four valves present in the human heart are replaceable by surgery. Artificial arteries in bypass surgery are frequently employed.

One of the most vital organs is the human heart. Heart attack accounts for a lot of unfortunate events annually. Research is going on for the design and development of total artificial heart (TAH). There are examples where patients were provided with TAH for a few weeks until any heart donor was available. For obvious reasons, heart donors are not readily available. However, heart problems are very persistent in society, and TAH is highly needed. It is needless to mention that the operation performed by TAH is achieved by external means. The challenge associated with the development of biocompatible materials needed for the fabrication of TAH is the focus area of contemporary researchers. Intra-aortic balloon pump (IABP) is a device frequently used to assist heart surgery. The device contains a balloon developed from polyether polyurethane urea (PEUU). It is inserted into the aorta and performs expansion and contraction matching the heartbeats [2]. It has been observed that the integration of LVADs (left ventricle assist devices) with a rotatory pump is comparatively more effective than the other substitutes [7]. The other crucial and frequently used system is dialysis, informally known as an artificial kidney. The dialysis unit consists of tubing, regulatory equipment, and a pumping system; all are employed to remove waste materials from the blood. The primary poisonous material removed from the blood is urea. The system available in the concurrent scenario weighs as heavy as 100 kg. The mobility of patients, while dialysis is going on, is not possible. The requirement of dialysis is frequent, almost three times a week, and patients going through dialysis feel exhausted after the procedure. When focusing on the efficiency of the system, the results are barely satisfactory, and the patients in severe cases hardly make it up to 5 years, which is lower than many types of cancers. Much development is observed in the display and control system of the dialysis systems, but the system itself has not advanced since 1950. Some physicians believe that the dialysis system brings lots of money and such a development will only reduce the profit of the company. However, companies challenge this statement arguing that they are working constantly for the improvement of the system incorporated in hemodialysis. Brad Puffer, from Fresenius Medical Care in Waltham, Massachusetts, USA, has mentioned that his company is working to develop a more biocompatible dialysis system to prevent the development of blood clots, which is a common side effect. Recently developed prototypes are marketed as portable systems. These systems weigh 34 kg and provide a certain amount of mobility to the patients. Still, the water requirement for this is around 120–180 L used in a 4-hour session. It can be used in homes avoiding regular visits to hospitals for dialysis, provided that the water supply maintains certain quality standards. CDI researchers at Seattle have introduced a technique that pushes the dialysis solution through a cartridge where the key toxic substance, i.e., urea is converted into carbon dioxide and nitrogen making the dialysis solution suitable for recycling. The setup is capable of converting 15 g of urea in 24 hours sufficient enough for most kidney patients. This method requires 750 mL of solution, but the value is low compared to other systems. The device weighs around 9 kg and should be used on a daily basis. Another device has been developed by Lausanne, Switzerland, based Dutch Kidney Foundation. It weighs 10 kg and requires 6 L of solution, suitable to be used at homes. It contains an absorbent material that soaks up the toxins putting a limitation on the quantity of the solution used. A Singapore-based research team belonging to AWAK, a medical-technology-based company, has successfully tested a device weighing 3 kg or even less. The tests were conducted on 15 adults with no adverse effects. Minor discomfort and bloating were reported by some. This technique is designed for peritoneal dialysis. It makes use of a catheter to send the dialysis solution into the abdominal cavity where the peritoneum filters out the toxin from the blood into the solution and the solution is then drained into an empty bag. Other important organs that do not have any artificial substitutions and are a matter of concern from the perspective of medical science are the pancreas, liver, gastrointestinal tract, and tube. There are rare examples of transplants and artificial implants related to these organs, and they require immediate attention of researchers [7].

1.2.5 SENSORY ORGANS

Implants of sensory organs are made for restoring the sense of hearing, speaking, and vision. There are devices developed to serve these purposes. Examples include hearing aid, electrodes that are implanted in the cochlea, and lenses developed for eyes. Research is also going on for the development of the full human eye from artificial means [2].

1.3 MONITORING, CONTROLS, AND HEALTH CARE

Monitoring and control of significant parameters associated with the human body include body temperature, blood pressure, body weight, blood sugar level, liver conditions, and cholesterol level. There are various instruments and sensors used to serve this purpose, and examples are a thermometer and various types of tests. While developing any socket or implant, the sensor and instrumentation employed for the measurement of pressure are expected to have a high degree of accuracy. Different types of pressure-sensing technology include flexible thin-film piezo-resistive sensors, fiber Bragg grating (FBG) sensors, and F-socket sensor mats. The strain gauge-based transducers are employed for the measurement of pressure and shear stress at different points in the prosthetic socket. The development of a prosthetic socket requires monitoring of pressure at different locations within the socket. The objective of monitoring these values is to eliminate harms like skin breakdown, painful sores, and soft tissue damage. This is performed by placing strain gauge at critical locations between the socket and the amputee. Conditions are then monitored for standing still as well as while walking. In a study conducted at MNIT Jaipur, it was reported that parameters like stamp length, height of a person, and body weight are significantly influential. The measured pressure values were used to develop an artificial neural network (ANN)-based model through which these findings were observed [10]. Figure 1.8 shows the different views of a prosthesis mounted with strain gauges.

1.4   BIO-MECHANICS

The development of implants and artificial organs requires thorough understanding of the mechanics and mechanism of stress and strain associated with these organs. Some examples are the magnitude of pressure produced in the human heart and the

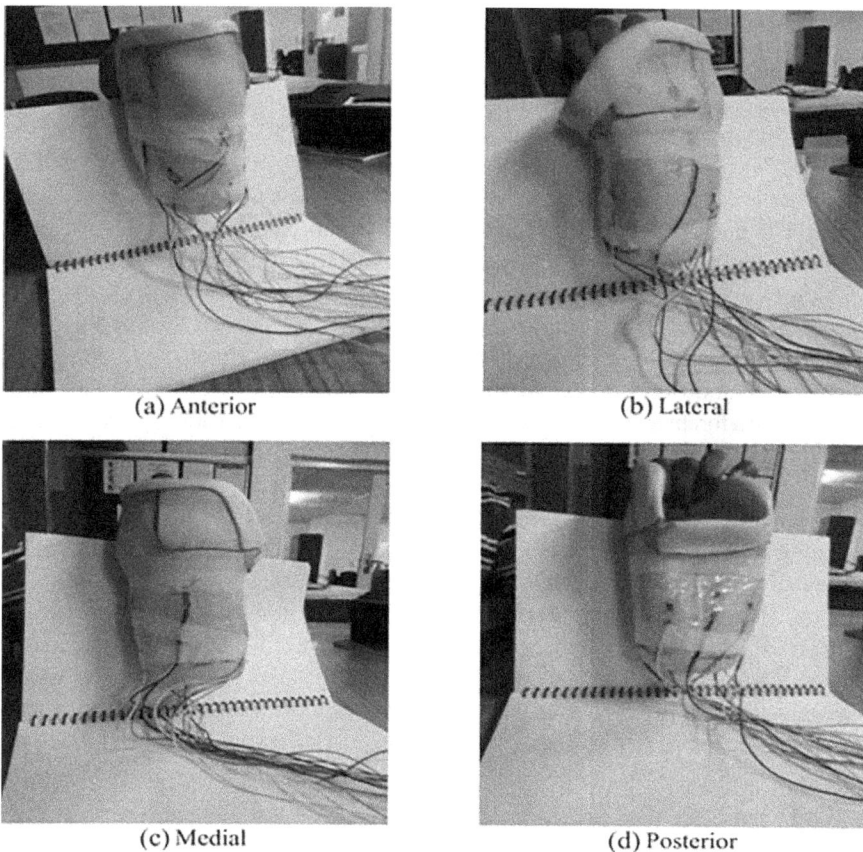

(a) Anterior   (b) Lateral

(c) Medial   (d) Posterior

FIGURE 1.8   Different views of a prosthesis mounted with strain gauges [10].

magnitude of stress experienced by prosthetic implants and amputees. The behavior of fluids present in the human body is a vital area to be studied before any implementation of artificial implants or use of instruments frequently used in diagnoses and treatments in the public health sector. The fluid flow and exchange in the human body have been understood for the development of artificial arteries and veins. Veins, for example, are channels through which blood flow takes place. The physical properties of veins like rigidity and elasticity are of extreme importance. To characterize the blood cells, it is essential to understand the mechanism of various physical and chemical interactions between blood and different internal organs. Abhishek et al. detailed the micro-fluidic method for the biological cell mechanophenotyping. The motivation for the development of a new method was the shortcomings of the slow and sophisticated conventional methods for the mechanical characterization of a biological cell. Typical methods like using optical tweezers (OT), atomic force microscopy (AFM), and micropipette aspiration (MA) perform inefficiently for time-sensitive analysis. Micro-fluidic methods offer a unique approach by applying the concept of fluid mechanics at the micrometer scale for the mechanical characterization of a cell. There are three different micro-fluidic techniques to serve the purpose of mechanophenotyping termed as:

- Aspiration-induced technique,
- Fluid-induced technique, and
- Structure-induced technique.

To make the characterization more rapid, researchers have integrated a micro-fluidic device with an electrode and optical fiber [8]. In another work, bio-mechanical characterization of a cell was performed. It was intended to understand the effect of compression rate on the cell, the associated volume loss, and the effect of the compression on the integrity of the nuclear envelope. The viscous-elastic behavior of the cell is an influential factor. The cell deformation behavior was studied on the application of compression at different rates. Microvideography was employed coupled with AFM to study the aforementioned behaviors. Results revealed a transition in the behavior of cells under compression from elastic with conserved volume to viscous-elastic behavior associated with volume loss. The associated volume loss was governed by the mechanical properties of the cell and the time scale of compression. Volume exchange for convective transfer (VECT) is a phenomenon that says cells take up the surrounding molecules as a recovery from the volume loss. In this study, it was found that the VECT has a minimal effect on the nuclear integrity of the cell. Ericksen number, which is a dimensionless factor, has been reported to be used for parameterization of compression rate and cell viscous-elastic properties to predict the associated volume loss. These findings are vital for future clinical use. Figure 1.9 shows that micro-fluidic ridge-based cell compressions cause volume exchange [9].

1.5 MATERIALS

Materials used in bio-mechanical applications are of extreme importance. There are high expectations from these materials, failing which may have fatal consequences

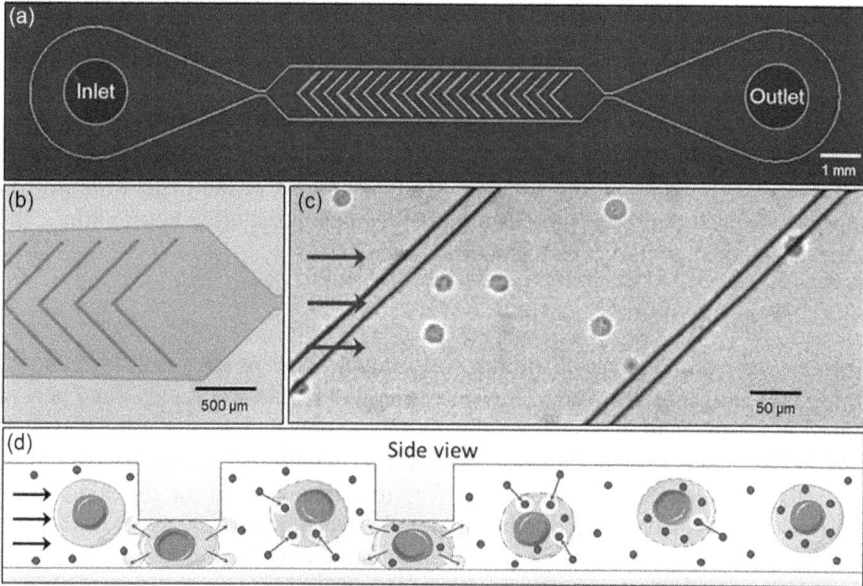

FIGURE 1.9 Micro-fluidic ridge-based cell compressions cause volume exchange. (a) Schematic of the device layout. See the Experimental Section for device design details. (b) Optical micrograph of a microchannel with chevron ridge geometry. (c) Still-frame image from a video of K562 cells flowing through the microchannel and ridges under a light microscope. (d) Schematic of cell permeabilization and volume loss, subsequent recovery, and repeated volume exchange with compressions [9].

for the patients. The challenges associated with these materials are not obvious; as such, it requires the keen attention of the researcher developing these materials for application in medical science. The body type, weight, height, and blood are the different variable factors associated with patients. Along with these factors, the blood pressure and the various contents of blood, i.e., hemoglobin, RBC, WBC, platelet, plasma, electrolytes, water percentage, etc. vary for a person over the course of time and the diet followed by the person.

Collectively these factors create a dynamic biological environment. When a foreign material is introduced into this environment, there are different kinds of possibilities associated. The response of the material against this biological environment depends on the physical as well chemical and mechanical properties of the material. Before moving further toward the type of materials, it is important to identify the associated challenges.

1.5.1 TOXIC AND ALLERGIC BEHAVIOR

While present in the body, the implant materials are always in contact with blood and the surrounding body, which might result in the formation of a blood clot, serious infections, and allergies. The compatibility of the material within the body must be considered.

1.5.2 Surface Roughness, Hardness, and Stiffness

Another important issue associated with the material is the tribological behavior of the material at the interface of the material and tissue.

The relative motion induced at the interface results in surface rubbing, which in turn produces pain and discomfort to the patient and damage to the associated bone or soft tissue. In addition, the strength and the stiffness of the material are again important aspects, and the materials used in the implant should be able to mimic the same mechanical properties as the natural organ.

1.5.3 Possibility of Corrosion

The exposure of the material to body fluid might result in chemical degradation, commonly termed as corrosion. This corrosion will reduce the strength and performance of the implant. Considering the above-mentioned challenges, the materials used in biomedical engineering must possess corrosion resistance, biocompatibility, and satisfactory mechanical properties. The materials used in the development of prosthetic sockets have a minor relaxation in the biocompatibility aspect because of the reason that they are exposed in contact with the outer skin of the amputee and as such the prosthetic material is expected to possess properties that are compatible with the outer skin and the accompanying soft tissue below it; since it is not in contact with the blood, the danger of corrosion and formation of the blood clot is ruled out; however, the weight and stiffness along with the tribological aspect at the interface of skin and socket must be considered at the time of development [10–12]. Figure 1.10 shows different types of materials used in bio-mechanical engineering.

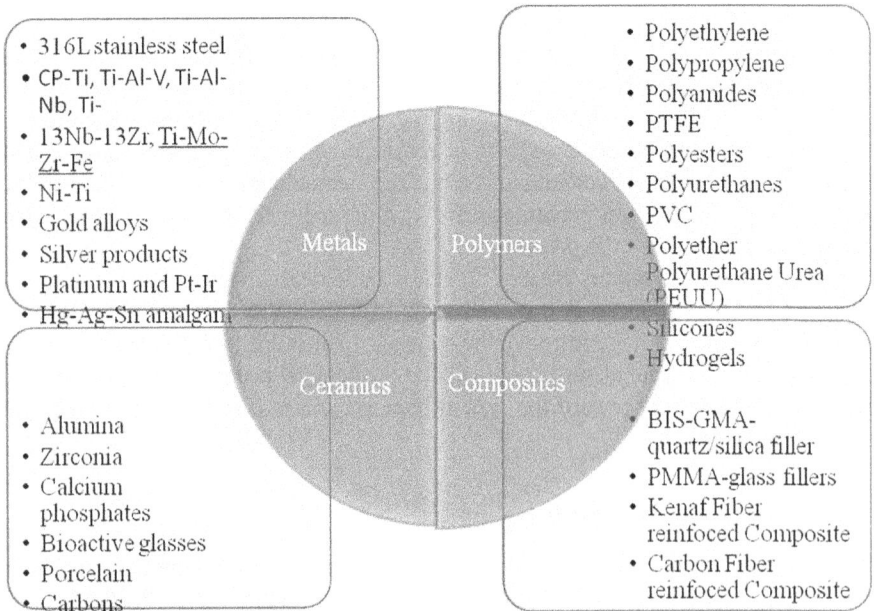

FIGURE 1.10   Different types of materials used in bio-mechanical engineering.

1.6 CONCLUSION

The available literature shown above proves that the field of bio-mechanical engineering is expanding with the advancements in technology. The collective efforts from the researchers belonging to different disciplines have contributed to the development of the associated parts of bio-mechanical engineering. However, the most influential factor is the development of suitable materials. With emerging changes in materials, dimensions are now opening up for progress in bio-mechanical engineering. Apart from this, advancements are also observed in the fabrication of artificial organs and prostheses. These researches are orientated to achieve a more user-friendly and durable substitute against the failed natural organ or the body part. Devices are now available to develop a thorough understanding of the behavior of the cell present in the human body as reported in recent studies. Together, considering all the aspects covered under bio-mechanical engineering, it can be concluded that the area is vast and has ample opportunity for future research and development.

REFERENCES

1. Brighton, J. A. (1977). *Why a Journal of Biomechanical Engineering?* DOI: 10.1115/1.3426262
2. Gebelein, C. G. (1984). *The Basics of Artificial Organs.* DOI:10.1021/bk-1984-0256. ch001
3. Quintero-Quiroz, C., & Pérez, V. Z. (2019). Materials for lower limb prosthetic and orthotic interfaces and sockets: Evolution and associated skin problems. *Revista de la Facultad de Medicina, 67*(1), 117–125.
4. Nayak, C., Singh, A., Chaudhary, H., & Tripathi, A. (2016). A novel approach for customized prosthetic socket design. *Biomedical Engineering: Applications, Basis and Communications, 28*(03), 1650022.
5. Nayak, C., Singh, A., & Chaudhary, H. (2017). Topology optimisation of transtibial prosthesis socket using finite element analysis. *International Journal of Biomedical Engineering and Technology, 24*(4), 323–337.
6. Versluys, R., Beyl, P., Van Damme, M., Desomer, A., Van Ham, R., & Lefeber, D. (2009). Prosthetic feet: State-of-the-art review and the importance of mimicking human ankle–foot biomechanics. *Disability and Rehabilitation: Assistive Technology, 4*(2), 65–75.
7. Cohn, W. E., Timms, D. L., & Frazier, O. H. (2015). Total artificial hearts: past, present, and future. *Nature Reviews Cardiology, 12*(10), 609–617.
8. Raj, A., & Sen, A. K. (2018). Microfluidic sensors for mechanophenotyping of biological cells. In Bhattacharya, S., Agarwal, A., Chanda, N., Pandey, A., & Sen, A. (eds), *Environmental, Chemical and Medical Sensors (Energy, Environment, and Sustainability)*, (pp. 389–408). Springer, Singapore. DOI:10.1007/978-981-10-7751-7_17
9. Liu, A., Yu, T., Young, K., Stone, N., Hanasoge, S., Kirby, T. J., ... Sulchek, T. (2020). Cell mechanical and physiological behavior in the regime of rapid mechanical compressions that lead to cell volume change. *Small, 16*(2), 1903857.
10. Nayak, C., Singh, A., & Chaudhary, H., (2017). *Customized Design and Development of Transtibial Prosthetic Socket for Improved Comfort Using Reverse Engineering & Additive Manufacturing.* Ph.D. Thesis, MNIT, Jaipur.
11. Hernandez, S. (2003). Overview of biomaterials and their use in medical devices. In ASM International *Handbook of Materials for Medical Devices (06974G)*, Edited by J.R. Davis, ASM International Ohio USA, 2003, pages 1-12, ISBN: 0-87170-790-X.

12. Jain, S., & Parashar, V. (2021). Critical review on the impact of EDM process on bio-medical materials. *Materials and Manufacturing Processes*, *36*(15), 1701–1724.

13. Ramadhani, G. A., Susmartini, S., Herdiman, L., & Priadythama, I. (2020). Advanced composite-based material selection for prosthetic socket application in developing countries. *Cogent Engineering*, *7*(1), 1745553.

2 Introduction to Cross Rolling of Biomedical Alloys

V. Murugabalaji and Matruprasad Rout
National Institute of Technology Tiruchirappalli

CONTENTS

2.1 INTRODUCTION

Biomedical alloys, as the name indicates, are extensively used in the medical field for various ailments. The performance of these alloys in the physiological environment is of major concern for their compatibility. Metallic alloys are remarkably employed in biomedical applications for the implantation of failed hard tissues and bones of the body [1]. The important characteristics required for the biomaterials to be used as implants include high strength, low modulus of elasticity, excellent resistance to wear and corrosion, and good biocompatibility in the physiological environment [2]. The biomaterials are mainly subjected to chemical and mechanical degradation, which leads to the toxicity and fracture of the material, respectively. These drastic effects can be overcome by several techniques, mainly selective alloying and thermomechanical processing [3]. The key challenges in processing these alloys to make them biocompatible are improving their properties like strength, ductility, corrosion resistance, formability, fatigue life cycle, etc. Thermomechanical processing can help in

DOI: 10.1201/9781003286806-2

bringing the microstructural alterations like fragmented precipitates, new phase formations, reduced anisotropy, etc., which can help in improving the biocompatibility of the alloys [4,5]. This chapter discusses the thermomechanical processing of biomedical alloys through the cross rolling (CR) process, a technique of rolling metallic sheets in which the strain path is altered by 90° in between consecutive passes [6]. The advantages of CR of biomedical alloys over unidirectional rolling (UR), where there is no change in the strain path, are also included. The various techniques used by the researchers to study the microstructural aspects, textural characteristics and various properties of the cross-rolled biomedical alloys are discussed.

2.2 CROSS ROLLING

The rolling process is defined as the process of plastically deforming a material between two rollers rotating in opposing directions, where the gap between the rollers determines the final thickness of the material [7]. The deformation in the rolling process is referred to as plane strain deformation since neither elongation nor shortening of the dimensions of the material occurs in the transverse direction (TD) of rolling [8]. CR can be defined as the rolling process with the change in RD by 90° about the normal direction (ND) [7]. The change in RD is obtained by the rotation of the material on the rolling plane and hence, the length and width of the material are constraints for the CR process. Depending upon the sequence of change in the RD, the CR process can be classified as follows [6]: two-step cross rolling (TSCR), which is also termed as pseudo-cross rolling, and multistep cross rolling (MSCR), also termed as true cross rolling. In the former, the RD is changed only after obtaining 50% of the total required thickness reduction, whereas in the latter case, the RD is changed after each pass. On the other hand, rolling with a change in RD by 180° is termed as reverse rolling (RR), and without change in RD, the rolling is termed as UR. A schematic of these processes, indicating the orientation of the material to be rolled, is shown in Figure 2.1.

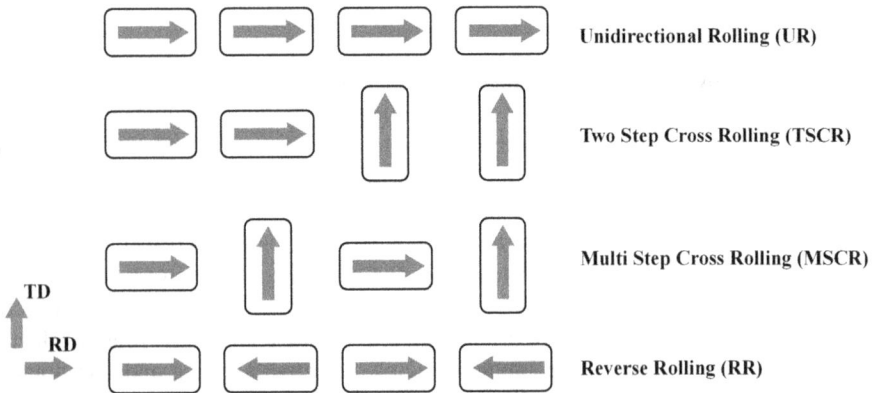

FIGURE 2.1   Representation of the change in rolling direction in different types of CR processes.

2.3 PROPERTY REQUISITES AND TESTING METHODS FOR BIOMEDICAL MATERIALS

2.3.1 PROPERTY REQUISITES FOR BIOMEDICAL MATERIALS

Biomedical implants are generally used in orthopaedics, cardiovascular stents, pacemakers, neural prosthetics, defibrillators and drug delivery systems [9,10]. The important properties required for biomedical applications as stents in interventional cardiology include the degradation rate, matching the tissue's healing time, adequate tensile properties, good biocompatibility and least cytotoxicity. In addition, homogeneous and isotropic materials must be used for cardiovascular applications to avoid catastrophic failures in the deployment sites [11]. The biomaterials used to replace hard tissues and bones as implants must have high fatigue and fretting fatigue life, good wear properties and functionalities in addition to the above-said requisites for a stent material [12]. Researchers followed different metal processing techniques like selective alloying of metal sheets [13,14], electrodeposition/electroforming of the material [15] and thermomechanical processing of the material [16] to achieve these properties. However, the present chapter focuses on the CR process only and the properties for cross-rolled biomedical alloys, studied by different researchers, are discussed here. These include microstructure, texture, mechanical and corrosion properties.

2.3.2 TESTING METHODS TO STUDY THE PROPERTIES OF BIOMEDICAL MATERIALS

2.3.2.1 Microstructural and Textural Characterisation

The microstructural investigations of the material are performed to understand the changes that could have occurred during the processing of the metal alloys. Usually, the microstructural characterisation studies are carried out using an optical microscope, a scanning electron microscope (SEM – analysing signals from electrons interacting with the atoms of the target specimen), a transmission electron microscope (TEM – analysing image from electrons transmitted through the target specimen) and X-ray diffraction (XRD – analysing the data from the diffraction of X-rays on the target specimen) to understand the underlying principles of mechanical deformation that could have occurred during the rolling process [17,18]. The evolution of the deformed microstructure is found to occur in three stages, *viz.* recovery, recrystallisation and grain growth [19]. Stacking fault energy (SFE) plays a vital role in the evolution of the deformed microstructure. The materials with low SFE show less tendency of recovery and recrystallisation is considered the major mechanism for microstructure evolution [20]. Dynamic recrystallisation (DRX) is the crucial phenomenon in enhancing the ductility of the specimen by the generation of strain-free grains during deformation. The DRX behaviour of the material significantly affects the microstructure and load requirement for processing the material [21]. The microstructure of the rolled specimen is generally viewed longitudinally to address the features of the deformation [22]. The characteristics of the microstructure evolved by the CR of the material are entirely different from those of the conventional rolling process, i.e. UR [23].

Texture refers to the measure of similarity in the orientation of the crystal network in the constitutive grains of a polycrystalline material [24]. The texture or preferred orientation is a major factor that influences the anisotropy and material properties required for specific applications. Thus, the texture analysis is of major research interest for metal-forming applications [25]. The texture components are studied by the interpretation of pole figures and inverse pole figures. The orientation distribution functions (ODFs) are also used to study the texture components efficiently. Techniques like electron backscattered diffraction (EBSD – analysing the diffraction pattern of backscattered electrons) and XRD are generally used to study texture. Interested readers may refer to other available books on texture to have a better understanding [8,26].

2.3.2.2 Mechanical Characterisation

The mechanical properties like elongation percentage, yield strength, ultimate strength, etc. are usually measured by the tensile test, whereas the microhardness is measured by the Vickers hardness test, Knoop hardness test, etc. [27,28]. The conventional strategy followed by the researchers to measure the anisotropy in mechanical properties of the sheets is to conduct the tensile tests along three different directions of the sheet *viz.* RD, TD and 45° to the RD, as shown in Figure 2.2. The anisotropy is characterised by the Lankford parameter R, which is the ratio of the strain measured in the width direction (ε_w) to the strain measured in the thickness direction (ε_t) [29].

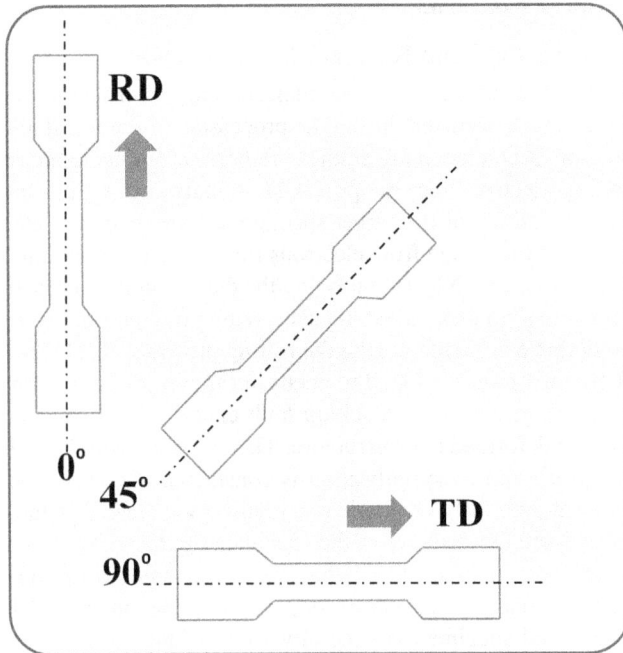

FIGURE 2.2   Schematic representation of tensile specimen samples to measure tensile properties along different directions.

The average R value ($\bar{R}$) and the planar anisotropy ($|\Delta R|$) are determined using equations (2.1) and (2.2), respectively [30]:

$$\bar{R} = \frac{R_{0°} + 2R_{45°} + R_{90°}}{4} \tag{2.1}$$

$$|\Delta R| = \frac{|R_{0°} - 2R_{45°} + R_{90°}|}{2} \tag{2.2}$$

where the subscripts 0°, 45° and 90° represent the tensile specimen direction with respect to RD.

Formability is an important factor in fabricating biomedical stents of extremely small thickness [4]. So, this should also be assessed for the biomedical alloy for its effective use as a biomaterial. The formability of sheets depends upon various factors *viz.* crystal structure of the material, type of rolling employed, annealing temperature, microstructure, texture, etc. [31]. A sheet metal is assessed with its ability to distribute strain uniformly and withstand in-plane compressive and shear stresses without wrinkling and fracturing [32]. It should also attain high strain ranges without being necked or fractured, retaining its shape and surface quality [32]. Various techniques like the Erichsen test, conical cup test and limit dome height (LDH) test are applied by the researchers to evaluate the formability of sheet metals [33–35]. In the Erichsen test, a sheet specimen is stretched with a hemispherical punch until being fractured. The depth of indentation of the punch marked in the specimen is expressed in millimetres and is called the Erichsen index, which is considered as the measure of formability [36]. The other available formability measures are not discussed in this section as they are not used to date for biomedical alloys.

2.3.2.3 Corrosion Characteristics

The biodegradation of a metal is an intricate phenomenon that depends on many metallurgical parameters such as crystallographic texture, average grain size and distribution, precipitation of impurities during processing, amount of cold working and procedure involved, characteristics of thermal processing and working environment [16]. The biodegradation of metal alloys is commonly studied using an immersion-based test called a static immersion test and an electrochemical test called a potentiodynamic polarisation test. In the static immersion test, the samples are prepared by wet grinding (generally, with SiC papers between 120 and 4000 grit.) after which it is cleansed with C_2H_5OH (ethanol), dried to get rid of the moisture and then weighted. The corrosion test specimen is immersed in Hanks' solution in the beaker, separately, for 336 hours (14 days) maintained at a temperature of 37°C. After 336 hours (14 days) of immersion, the samples were taken out from the Hanks solution, rinsed with distilled water, cleansed with C_2H_5OH, dried to get rid of moisture and then weighted. The ACR (average corrosion rate) is calculated based on the mass loss using equation (2.3) from [4].

$$ACR = 8.76 \times 10^4 \times \frac{W}{A \times t \times \rho} \tag{2.3}$$

where 'ACR' is in mm/year, 'W' represents the loss of mass after 336 hours, 'A' is the surface area of the sample exposed in solution (cm^2), 't' is the exposure time (hours) and 'ρ' is the material density [4]. An electrode cell system is used to perform the potentiodynamic polarisation test in which the sample (prepared by wet grinding using SiC papers with a grit size between 120 and 4000 and then cleansed with C_2H_5OH and dried) is made as the working electrode. The test is carried out at a standard scanning rate and potential range and the open circuit potential (OCP) measurement is done. The corrosion rate is determined by measuring the corrosion current density from the Tafel curve (a curve plotted against potential and current density) [4].

2.4 CROSS ROLLING OF BIOMEDICAL ALLOYS

2.4.1 MICROSTRUCTURAL AND TEXTURAL CHARACTERISATION

Polycrystalline pure iron attracted the interest of researchers after its first experimentation as a biodegradable material for cardiovascular applications in 2001 [37]. Obayi et al. [4] performed UR and CR in high-purity ARMCO iron sheets of 2 mm thickness with a thickness reduction of 75%. They made samples of $10 \times 10 \, mm^2$ from both unidirectional and cross-rolled sheets, which were subjected to annealing at 550°C and 900°C for 2 hours and then air-cooled to room temperature. The texture studies indicate the formation of a higher fraction of {111} basal texture in CR samples, which leads to more expansion during annealing of CR samples than UR samples, thereby leading to higher plastic strain ratios. At the same annealing temperatures, EBSD experiments show that the grain size of CR samples is larger than UR samples. They attributed this effect to the lower density of dislocations in the CR samples than in the UR samples and the higher recrystallisation rate in the UR samples with strong texture.

Recently, Ni-free titanium alloys were developed to avoid hypersensitivity and cytotoxicity effects of Ni. Wang et al. [38] developed a Ti–35Nb–2Ta–3Zr alloy and studied the changes in the microstructure and mechanical properties after CR at different final reduction ratios (40%, 60% and 99%). When the reduction ratio was 40%, microstructural examination confirmed the presence of stress-induced α'' martensite. The number of α phases was increased at 60% reduction and at 99% reduction, the matrix and plate-shaped α phases are purified into balanced granules with diameters ranging from 20 to 100 nm (observed through TEM images). The cold MSCR of β-titanium alloy for 80% thickness reduction by Gurao et al. [39] showed the presence of strong (556) $\left[5\bar{1} \ \bar{1}5 \right]$ components in UR samples and (111) $\left[11\bar{2} \right]$ components in MSCR samples after recrystallisation. They attributed this to the fact that the accumulation of defects in UR samples is more thereby forming a strong texture in UR samples compared to MSCR samples [39]. The effects of CR on the microstructural and tensile characteristics of zinc-based bio-absorbable alloys were studied by Ramirez–Ledesma et al. [40]. They found that the CR samples developed improved ductility as the CR process facilitates enormous grain growth. In contrast, the UR provides higher grain refinement and strength, resulting in less isotropic microstructural characteristics than CR samples. The literature shows that CR is commonly applied for the symmetrisation of rolling textures that yield comparatively homogeneous mechanical properties of metals and alloys.

Magnesium alloys are of lightweight and possess good biocompatibility, which make them suitable for their usage as orthopaedic implants in medical applications [41]. Chen et al. [42] investigated the effective ways to improve the microstructure and anisotropy in mechanical properties of an AZ31 magnesium alloy sheet with a strong initial basal texture. They found that MSCR yields weak and symmetric texture and the mechanical properties are improved compared to UR. They also observed that the microstructure produced by CR is finer and more homogeneous compared to UR. On the other hand, weaker basal texture and formation of rotated grains, more scattered in sheet plane, lead to reduced anisotropy in the mechanical properties for CR than UR samples of Mg–0.6%Zr–1.0%Cd sheets [5]. Catorceno et al. [43] studied the effect of CR on the evolution of microstructures in an AZ31B magnesium alloy sheet for different reductions at different temperatures (25°C, 100°C, 200°C, 250°C and 300°C). They found that CR of the AZ31B magnesium alloy produced microstructures depending on the degree of deformation and rolling temperature. The heterogeneous microstructure is formed with small, unbranched grains surrounded by coarse twining grains and shear bands at reduced strain rates, while twinning and shear band formation are predominant at increased strain rates. They observed that during cold CR, catastrophic failure of a workpiece material occurred due to the huge production of mechanical twins and shear bands. On the other hand, for hot CR, the ductility was enhanced due to the DRX. The evolution of different textures and important applications of some of the cross-rolled alloys are summarised in Table 2.1.

TABLE 2.1
Texture Evolution and Applications of Some Cross-Rolled Biomedical Alloys

Alloy Material	Texture	Applications	Reference
Pure iron	{111} basal texture – CR and annealing at 550°C and 900°C	Used as a stent material in cardiovascular applications	Obayi et al. [4]
Ti–35Nb–2Ta–3Zr alloy	Texture not analysed	Bone fixation and spinal fixation applications	Wang et al. [38]
Zn–5.0 Ag–0.5 Mg and Zn–10.0 Ag–1.0 Mg	Texture not analysed	Used as a stent material in cardiovascular applications	Ramirez–Ledesma et al. [27]
AZ31 Mg alloy	Weak {0001} basal textures	Implants in orthopaedic applications	Chen et al. [42]
	Cold CR produced strong basal texture and with an increase in temperature and reductions, weal basal texture is formed		Catorceno et al. [43]
	Low intensity (0002) texture		Chino et al. [33]
Pure titanium sheet	Weak texture with an intensity of 1.8	In dental and orthopaedic reconstructive surgery	Liu et al. [44]
β-Titanium alloy	(111) [11$\bar{2}$] component after MSCR and recrystallisation	Used as implants in orthopaedic and dental applications	Gurao et al. [39]

2.4.2 Mechanical Characterisation Investigations

Works of Obayi et al. [4] on pure ARMCO iron sheets indicated that cross-rolled sheets possess more ductility than unidirectionally rolled samples and the cross-rolled samples, annealed at 550°C, showed better ductility and isotropic properties than other samples. Due to their high elastic limit-to-density ratio, strong corrosion resistance and outstanding biocompatibility, titanium and titanium-based alloys have been widely used in medical sectors [45]. Ma et al. [46] conducted cold UR and TSCR on β-titanium alloy produced by forging at 950°C followed by hot rolling at 850°C to produce sheets of 2 mm thickness. They performed solution treatment of sheets at 800°C (below a β-transition temperature of 815 ± 10°C) for 30 minutes. The tensile test result of TSCR sheets reveals similar elongation and tensile properties in different directions, whereas a decrease in plasticity with the increase in the angle between the tensile direction and RD was observed for the UR samples. The tensile tests carried out by Wang et al. [38] for cross-rolled Ni-free titanium alloy (Ti–35Nb–2Ta–3Zr) along RD, TD and 45° to RD indicate that CR has induced isotropy in the samples, and the shape of the stress–strain curve along these three directions also looked similar.

Commercially pure titanium (CP-Ti), being an HCP material, exhibits poor ductility and anisotropic behaviour at room temperature [47]. Therefore, research works are focused on improving the above properties. Liu et al. [44] carried out their research on pure titanium sheets by performing rolling in three different routes, *viz.* two UR along RD and TD directions and one CR. They found that CR samples exhibited isotropic properties (tensile test) when loaded along three different directions (RD, 45° and TD). The deep drawing test and Erichsen tests also showed better results for the CR samples when compared to the UR samples. The improvement in properties of CR samples is due to the weakened texture developed during CR. Stretch formability is one of the desirable properties for the use of Mg alloys in a variety of applications. However, their poor formability at room temperature led to many research works on these alloys to improve their formability [48]. The limitation in the number of active slip systems for the HCP structure is found to be the reason for the formability limitations at room temperatures [49]. Kaya et al. [50] observed significant improvement in the formability of Mg alloys at high temperatures when compared to room temperature. Similarly, as reported by Chen et al. [35], good stretchability and drawability for AZ31 Mg alloys can be observed in the range of temperatures between 150°C and 300°C. Zhang et al. [51] performed deep drawing tests on AZ31 Mg alloy sheets and found that the extruded sheets exhibited good formability in the range of temperatures between 250°C and 350°C, whereas extruded and cross-rolled sheets showed good formability from 105°C to 170°C. Formability improvements at low temperatures by the CR of AZ31 Mg alloy sheets have also been reported by Xu et al. [52]. The improvement in formability is attributed to the grain refinement induced by the CR process.

Chino et al. [33] performed UR and CR experiments to study the press formability of the AZ31 Mg alloy sheets. Prior to the rolling operation, the material was heat-treated for 24 hours at 400°C and then annealed for 30 minutes at 400°C. Erichsen tests carried out at 220°C, 240°C and 260°C revealed higher Erichsen values for CR samples at 220°C and 240°C. They conclude that the higher Erichsen values for the CR samples were due to the reduction of (0002) texture intensity by the change in RD. At 260°C, the values are almost identical, indicating that texture control affects formability at lower temperatures around 220°C. Their results are in good agreement with the relationship between Erichsen values and texture of AZ31 Mg alloy sheets, developed by Iwanaga et al. [34]. In another work, Chino et al. [53] conducted the RR along with the UR and CR for the same material and found that the RR and CR exhibited more press formability. They found that the press formability of the sheets does not depend upon the elongation for failure, exponent of strain hardening, average R value $\left(\bar{R}\right)$ and planar anisotropy value ΔR. They claimed that the formation of minor texture during the RR and CR processes resulted in reduced strain anisotropy, resulting in enhanced press formability [53]. In addition to the routes like UR and CR, Zhang et al. [54] also examined the effect of change in RD by 45° after each CR path (i.e. RD → TD → 45° to TD). They found that for the AZ31 Mg alloy, CR and CR with change in RD by 45° are very effective in yielding weakened basal texture and grain refinement. Moreover, the Erichsen test results indicated an increase in the Erichsen value by 28% and 31% for CR and CR with a change in RD by 45°, respectively.

2.4.3 CORROSION CHARACTERISATION INVESTIGATIONS

The rate of corrosion decreases as the grain size of pure iron decreases due to the surface passivation of the grain boundary [55]. The work of Obayi et al. [4] to find the ACR of pure ARMCO iron samples through the static immersion test and potentiodynamic polarisation test indicates that the samples are cross-rolled and annealed at 900°C corroded less than the non-annealed and unidirectionally rolled samples. They also found that the grain boundary corrosion was reduced in cross-rolled samples. Annealing reduces the imperfection density and thereby, corrosion rates are reduced in annealed samples, as reported by Obayi et al. [4]. This was in good agreement with the earlier works reported while studying the effects of annealing on corrosion of biomaterials by other researchers [56,57]. They also found, through the SEM images, that grain boundary corrosion was predominant in UR than in CR as a result of higher dislocation density.

2.5 SUMMARY

From the literature, it is clear that CR of biomedical alloys enhances the biomedical requirements of the alloy. The key aspects can be summarised as follows:

- The CR of pure iron yields {111} basal texture after annealing and it is very helpful in achieving good tensile characteristics. The corrosion rate also tends to be lower in these samples due to reduced imperfection density.
- The textures of pure titanium and β-titanium alloys are also weakened by the CR process, and they can then be effectively used in dental and orthopaedic applications by enhancing their mechanical properties. In Ni-free titanium alloy (Ti–35Nb–2Ta–3Zr), the CR induces severe plastic deformation and

results in a grain size of few nanometres. It also improves the isotropic properties and tensile strength of the alloy, which enhance its use as a bio-material in bone and spine fixation applications.

- Zinc-based bio-absorbable alloys, *viz.* Zn–5.0Ag–0.5Mg and Zn–10.0Ag–1.0 Mg, after CR resulted in improvement in ductility and enormous grain growth. This makes them favourable for their use as stents for cardiovascular applications.
- Mg alloys are also the beneficiaries of CR as they attain a weak basal texture after CR, making them more formable. This makes them effective in their use as biomaterials for cardiovascular applications.

2.6 CONCLUDING REMARKS

This chapter, based on the past research work, gives an overall knowledge on the role of the CR process on microstructure and texture development and hence on altering the properties, especially the mechanical and corrosion properties, of biomedical alloys. The CR of biomedical alloys is not explored much and only the microstructure, texture, tensile properties and few corrosion studies have been done. The change in RD affects the grain orientation and thereby affects the texture of the material. This will further change the microstructural aspects and mechanical properties of the material when accompanied by subsequent annealing. So, a detailed study on the CR of various biomaterials will explore the scope for its application in various fields of biomedical applications.

REFERENCES

1. Li, Y., Yang, C., Zhao, H., Qu, S., Li, X., Li, Y. (2014), New developments of ti-based alloys for biomedical applications. *Materials*, 7, 1709–1800. doi: 10.3390/ma7031709.
2. Temenoff, J.S. Mikos, A. (2008), *Biomaterials: The Intersection of Biology and Materials Science* (Volume 1). Pearson/Prentice Hall, Upper Saddle River, NJ.
3. Hanawa, T. (2006), Recent development of new alloys for biomedical use. *Materials Science Forum*, 512, 243–248. doi: 10.4028/www.scientific.net/msf.512.243.
4. Obayi, C. S., Tolouei, R., Paternoster, C., Turgeon, S., Okorie, B. A., Obikwelu, D. O., Cassar, G., Buhagiar, J., Mantovani, D. (2015), Influence of cross-rolling on the micro-texture and biodegradation of pure iron as biodegradable material for medical implants. *Acta Biomaterialia*, 17, 68–77. doi: 10.1016/j.actbio.2015.01.024.
5. Chen, Chen, Z., Yi, L., Xiong, J., Liu, C. (2014), Effects of texture on anisotropy of mechanical properties in annealed Mg-0.6%Zr-1.0%Cd sheets by unidirectional and cross rolling. *Materials Science and Engineering A*, 615, 324–330. doi: 10.1016/j.msea.2014.07.089.
6. Suwas, S., Gurao, N. P. (2014), Development of microstructures and textures by cross rolling. *Comprehensive Materials Processing*, 81–106. doi: 10.1016/B978-0-08-096532-1.00308-3. Elsevier.
7. Rout, M., Pal, S. K., Singh, S. B. (2015), Cross rolling: A metal forming process, 41–64. doi: 10.1007/978-3-319-20152-8_2.
8. Bocker, A., Klein, H., Bunge, H. J. (1990), Development of cross-rolling textures in ARMCO - iron. *Textures and Microstructures*, 12, 155–174.
9. Regar, E., Sianos, G., Serruys, P. W. (2001), Stent development and local drug delivery. *British Medical Bulletin*, 59, 227–248. doi: 10.1093/bmb/59.1.227.

10. Greatbatch, W., Holmes, C. F. (2002), History of implantable devices. *IEEE Engineering in Medicine and Biology Magazine*, 10, 38–41. doi: 10.1109/51.84185.
11. Hermawan, H., Mantovani, D. (2013), Process of prototyping coronary stents from biodegradable Fe-Mn alloys. *Acta Biomaterialia*, 9, 8585–8592. doi: 10.1016/j. actbio.2013.04.027.
12. Niinomi, M. (2008), Mechanical biocompatibilities of titanium alloys for biomedical applications. *Journal of the Mechanical Behavior of Biomedical Materials*, 1, 30–42. doi: 10.1016/j.jmbbm.2007.07.001.
13. Liu, B., Zheng, Y. F. (2011), Effects of alloying elements (Mn, Co, Al, W, Sn, B, C and S) on biodegradability and in vitro biocompatibility of pure iron. *Acta Biomaterialia*, 7, 1407–1420. doi: 10.1016/j.actbio.2010.11.001.
14. Schinhammer, M., Hänzi, A. C., Löffler, J. F., Uggowitzer, P. J. (2010), Design strategy for biodegradable Fe-based alloys for medical applications. *Acta Biomaterialia*, 6, 1705–1713. doi: 10.1016/j.actbio.2009.07.039.
15. Moravej, M., Purnama, A., Fiset, M., Couet, J., Mantovani, D. (2010), Electroformed pure iron as a new biomaterial for degradable stents: In vitro degradation and preliminary cell viability studies. *Acta Biomaterialia*, 6, 1843–1851. doi: 10.1016/j.actbio.2010.01.008.
16. Nie, F. L., Zheng, Y. F., Wei, S. C., Hu, C., Yang, G. (2010), In vitro corrosion, cytotoxicity and hemocompatibility of bulk nanocrystalline pure iron. *Biomedical Materials*, 5. doi: 10.1088/1748-6041/5/6/065015.
17. Fu, X., Ji, Y., Cheng, X., Dong, C., Fan, Y., Li, X. (2020), Effect of grain size and its uniformity on corrosion resistance of rolled 316L stainless steel by EBSD and TEM. *Materials Today Communications*, 25, 101429. doi: 10.1016/j.mtcomm.2020.101429.
18. Zhang, B. P., Tu, Y. F., Chen, J. Y., Zhang, H. L., Kang, Y. L., Suzuki, H. G. (2007), Preparation and characterization of as-rolled AZ31 magnesium alloy sheets. *Journal of Materials Processing Technology*, 184, 102–107. doi: 10.1016/j.jmatprotec.2006.11.009.
19. Rout, M., Ranjan, R., Pal, S. K., Singh, S. B. (2018), EBSD study of microstructure evolution during axisymmetric hot compression of 304LN stainless steel. *Materials Science and Engineering A*, 711, 378–388. doi: 10.1016/j.msea.2017.11.059.
20. Rollett, A., Humphreys, F., Rohrer, G. S., Hatherly, M. (2004), *Recrystallization and Related Annealing Phenomena*: 2nd ed., 1–628. doi: 10.1016/B978-0-08-044164-1.X5000-2.
21. El Wahabi, M., Cabrera, J. M., Prado, J. M. (2003), Hot working of two AISI 304 steels: A comparative study. *Materials Science and Engineering A*, 343, 116–125. doi: 10.1016/S0921-5093(02)00357-X.
22. Liu Q., Juul Jensen, D., Hansen, N. (1998), Effect of grain orientation on deformation structure in cold-rolled polycrystalline aluminium. *Acta Materialia*, 46, 5819–5838. doi: 10.1016/S1359-6454(98)00229-8.
23. Nayan, N., Mishra, S., Prakash, A., Murty, S. V. S. N., Prasad, M. J. N. V., Samajdar, I. (2019), Effect of cross-rolling on microstructure and texture evolution and tensile behavior of aluminium-copper-lithium (AA2195) alloy. *Materials Science and Engineering A*, 740–741, 252–261. doi: 10.1016/j.msea.2018.10.089.
24. Suwas, S., Gurao, N. P. (2008), Crystallographic texture in materials. *Journal of the Indian Institute of Science*, 88, 151–177.
25. Engler, O. (2012), Control of texture and earing in aluminium alloy AA 3105 sheet for packaging applications. *Materials Science and Engineering A*, 538, 69–80. doi: 10.1016/j.msea.2012.01.015.
26. Engler and Randle, V. (2008), *Introduction to Texture Analysis: Macrotexture, Microtexture, and Orientation Mapping*: 2nd ed. CRC Press, doi: 10.1142/9781848161160_0001.
27. Ramirez-Ledesma, A. L., Roncagliolo-Barrera, P., Paternoster, C., Casati, R., Lopez, H., Vedani, M., Mantovani, D. (2020), Microstructural precipitation evolution and in vitro degradation behavior of a novel chill-cast Zn-based absorbable alloy for medical applications. *Metals*, 10, 1–20. doi: 10.3390/met10050586.

28. Blau, P. J. (1980), Use of a two-diagonal Measurement method for reducing scatter in Knoop microhardness testing. *Scripta Metallurgica*, 14, 719–724.

29. Oertel, C. G., Hünsche, I., Skrotzki, W., Lorich, A., Knabl, W., Resch, J., Trenkwalder, T. (2010), Influence of cross rolling and heat treatment on texture and forming properties of molybdenum sheets. *International Journal of Refractory Metals and Hard Materials*, 28, 722–727. doi: 10.1016/j.ijrmhm.2010.07.003.

30. Narayanasamy, R., Narayanan, C. S. (2008), Forming, fracture and wrinkling limit diagram for if steel sheets of different thickness. *Materials and Design*, 29, 1467–1475. doi: 10.1016/j.matdes.2006.09.017.

31. Ghosh, A., Roy, A., Ghosh, A., Ghosh, M. (2021), Influence of temperature on microstructure, crystallographic texture and mechanical properties of EN AW 6016 alloy during plane strain compression. *Materials Today Communications*, 26, 101808. doi: 10.1016/j.mtcomm.2020.101808.

32. Semiatin, S. L. (2018), *Metalworking: Sheet Forming*. ASM International, Materials Park, OH.

33. Chino, Y., Lee, J. S., Sassa, K., Kamiya, A., Mabuchi, M. (2006), Press formability of a rolled AZ31 Mg alloy sheet with controlled texture. *Materials Letters*, 60, 173–176. doi: 10.1016/j.matlet.2005.08.012.

34. Iwanaga, K., Tashiro, H., Okamoto, H., Shimizu, K. (2004), Improvement of formability from room temperature to warm temperature in AZ-31 magnesium alloy. *Journal of Materials Processing Technology*, 155–156, 1313–1316. doi: 10.1016/j.jmatprotec.2004.04.181.

35. Chen, F. K., Huang, T. B. (2003), Formability of stamping magnesium-alloy AZ31 sheets. *Journal of Materials Processing Technology*, 142, 643–647. doi: 10.1016/S0924-0136(03)00684-8.

36. Banabic, D., Bunge, H. J., Pohlandt, K., Tekkaya, A. E. (2000), *Formability of Metallic Materials : Plastic Anisotropy, Formability Testing, Forming Limits*. Eng. Mater, Springer Verlag. doi: 10.1007/978-3-662-04013-3.

37. Peuster, M., Wohlsein, P., Brügmann, M., Ehlerding, M., Seidler, K., Fink, C., Brauer, H., Fischer, A., Hausdorf, G. (2001), A novel approach to temporary stenting: Degradable cardiovascular stents produced from corrodible metal - Results 6–18 months after implantation into New Zealand white rabbits. *Heart*, 86, 563–569. doi: 10.1136/heart.86.5.563.

38. Wang, L., Lu, W., Qin, J., Zhang, F., Zhang, D. (2008), Change in microstructures and mechanical properties of biomedical Ti-Nb-Ta-Zr system alloy through cross-rolling. *Materials Transactions*, 49, 1791–1795. doi: 10.2320/matertrans.MRA2008040.

39. Gurao, N. P., Ali A, A., Suwas, S. (2009), Study of texture evolution in metastable β-Ti alloy as a function of strain path and its effect on α transformation texture. *Materials Science and Engineering A*, 504, 24–35. doi: 10.1016/j.msea.2008.11.053.

40. Ramirez–Ledesma, A. L., Domínguez–Contreras, L. A., Juarez–Islas, J. A., Paternoster, C., Mantovani, D. (2020), Influence of cross – Rolling on the microstructure and mechanical properties of Zn bioabsorbable alloys. *Materials Letters*, 279. doi: 10.1016/j.matlet.2020.128504.

41. Eddy Jai Poinern, G., Brundavanam, S., Fawcett, D. (2013), Biomedical magnesium alloys: A review of material properties, surface modifications and potential as a biodegradable orthopaedic implant. *American Journal of Biomedical Engineering*, 2, 218–240. doi: 10.5923/j.ajbe.20120206.02.

42. Chen, P., Xing, S., D., Xiao, R., Huang, G. J., Liu, Q. (2010), Influence of rolling ways on microstructure and anisotropy of AZ31 alloy sheet. *Transactions of Nonferrous Metals Society of China (English Edition)*, 20, s589–s593. doi: 10.1016/S1003-6326(10)60544-4.

43. Catorceno, L. L. C., de Abreu, H. F. G., Padilha, A. F. (2018), Effects of cold and warm cross-rolling on microstructure and texture evolution of AZ31B magnesium alloy sheet. *Journal of Magnesium and Alloys*, 6, 121–133. doi: 10.1016/j.jma.2018.04.004.

44. Liu, D.-k., Huang, G., Gong, G., Wang, G., Pan, F. (2017), Influence of different rolling routes on mechanical anisotropy and formability of commercially pure titanium sheet. *Transactions of Nonferrous Metals Society of China*, 27, 1306–1312. doi: 10.1016/S1003-6326(17)60151-1.

45. Kim, W. J., Yoo, S. J., Lee, J. B. (2010), Microstructure and mechanical properties of pure Ti processed by high-ratio differential speed rolling at room temperature. *Scripta Materialia*, 62, 451–454. doi: 10.1016/j.scriptamat.2009.12.008.

46. Ma, Y., Du, Z., Cui, X., Cheng, J., Liu, G., Gong, T., Liu, H., Wang, X., Chen, Y. (2018), Effect of cold rolling process on microstructure and mechanical properties of high strength β titanium alloy thin sheets. *Progress in Natural Science: Materials International*, 28, 711–717. doi: 10.1016/j.pnsc.2018.10.004.

47. Zhang, X. H., Tang, B., Zhang, X. L., Kou, H. C., Li, J. S., Zhou, L. (2012), Microstructure and texture of commercially pure titanium in cold deep drawing. *Transactions of Nonferrous Metals Society of China (English Edition)*, 22, 496–502. doi: 10.1016/S1003-6326(11)61204-1.

48. Altan, T., ErmanTekkaya, A. (1992), *Sheet Metal Forming : Processes and Applications.* ASM International, Materials Park, OH.

49. Liu, Q., Roy, A., Silberschmidt, V. V. (2017), Temperature-dependent crystal-plasticity model for magnesium: A bottom-up approach. *Mechanics of Materials*, 113, 44–56. doi: 10.1016/j.mechmat.2017.07.008.

50. Kaya, S., Altan, T., Groche, P., Klöpsch, C. (2008), Determination of the flow stress of magnesium AZ31-O sheet at elevated temperatures using the hydraulic bulge test. *International Journal of Machine Tools and Manufacture*, 48, 550–557. doi: 10.1016/j.ijmachtools.2007.06.011.

51. Zhang, S.H., Xu, Y. C., Palumbo, G., Pinto, S., Tricarico, L., Wang, Z. T., Zhang, Q. L. (2005), Formability and process conditions of magnesium alloy sheets. *Materials Science Forum*, 488–489, 453–456. doi: 10.4028/www.scientific.net/msf.488-489.453.

52. Xu, Y. C., Zhang, S. H., Liu, H. M., Wang, Z. T., Zheng, W. T., Zhang, Q. L., Xu, Y. (2005), Improved formability and deep drawing of cross-rolled magnesium alloy sheets at elevated temperatures. 489, 461–464. doi: 10.4028/www.scientific.net/MSF.488-489.461.

53. Chino, Y., Sassa, K., Kamiya, A., Mabuchi, M. (2006), Influence of rolling routes on press formability of a rolled AZ31 Mg alloy sheet. *Materials Transactions*, 47, 2555–2560. doi: 10.2320/matertrans.47.2555.

54. Zhang, H., Huang, G., Jørgen, H., Wang, L., Pan, F. (2013), Influence of different rolling routes on the microstructure evolution and properties of AZ31 magnesium alloy sheets. *Materials and Design*, 50, 667–673. doi: 10.1016/j.matdes.2013.03.053.

55. Ralston, K. D., Birbilis, N., Davies, C. H. J. (2010), Revealing the relationship between grain size and corrosion rate of metals. *Scripta Materialia*, 63, 1201–1204. doi: 10.1016/j.scriptamat.2010.08.035.

56. Hermawan, H., Alamdari, H., Mantovani, D., Dubé, D. (2008), Iron-manganese: New class of metallic degradable biomaterials prepared by powder metallurgy. *Powder Metallurgy*, 51, 38–45. doi: 10.1179/174329008X284868.

57. Moravej, M., Amira, S., Prima, F., Rahem, A., Fiset, M., Mantovani, D. (2011), Effect of electrodeposition current density on the microstructure and the degradation of electroformed iron for degradable stents. *Materials Science and Engineering B: Solid-State Materials for Advanced Technology*, 176, 1812–1822. doi: 10.1016/j.mseb.2011.02.031.

3 Additive Manufacturing and Characterisation of Biomedical Materials

Mainak Saha
Indian Institute of Technology Madras

Manab Mallik
National Institute of Technology Durgapur

CONTENTS

DOI: 10.1201/9781003286806-3

3.1   INTRODUCTION

In terms of addressing design complexities and versatility in material selection, additive manufacturing (AM) turns out to be highly advantageous over traditional manufacturing techniques, particularly, in terms of following the 'bottom up' approach where a structure can be fabricated into a pre-designed shape using a 'layer-by-layer' deposition [1–4]. These make AM techniques suitable for most of the industrial sectors, especially the medical sector, where AM-based biomedical materials, presently find a number of applications in orthopaedics [5–8], cardiology [5,9,10], respirology [7,11] and urology [5,12]. In spite of the tremendous advantage offered by AM techniques in addressing design complexities in a wide range of materials ranging from metallic materials to Functionally Graded Materials (FGM) [2,12], the primary challenge still remains in obtaining 'real, robust and functional' objects of engineering interest [3,13,14]. Moreover, the other challenges include: (i) size limitations [1,15], (ii) quality consistency [16], (iii) scaling issues [17,18] and (iv) high material cost [16,18,19]. In this context, there are mainly two parameters: (i) process parameters, which primarily influence material processing during AM, and (ii) structural parameters, which provide a 'post-mortem analysis' in terms of microstructural features of AM products and hence are very essential for selection of materials for AM [20]. Optimisation of these two parameters is extremely necessary for overcoming the aforementioned challenges associated with AM [21–23]. At present, there are a number of reports on understanding the process parameters in AM techniques for a wide range of materials [24–27]. However, there are very few reports on understanding structural parameters especially in the context of AM biomedical materials [18].

On the other hand, the common characterisation techniques used for determining the influence of surface modification techniques on the biocompatibility of biomedical materials are time-of-flight secondary ion mass spectrometry (ToF-SIMS), infrared (IR) spectroscopy, X-ray photoelectron spectroscopy (XPS) techniques and atomic force microscopy (AFM) [28,29]. However, AFM provides information on only the surface topography with no information on the surface chemical composition, whereas IR spectroscopy, ToF-SIMS and XPS techniques provide information on only the surface chemistry of these materials. In the recent decade, the emergence of a novel 'correlative microscopy' methodology involving the use of a number of different characterisation techniques for correlation of structural information with chemical evidence from the same section in a particular microstructure has proven to be an extremely powerful tool for addressing AM-based selection and processing challenges in AM-based metallic materials [24–26]. However, owing primarily to challenges in sample preparation, there is hardly any report on employing the novel aforementioned methodology for structure–property correlation in biomedical materials. The present chapter is aimed at highlighting the importance of parametric optimisation along with the need to employ the novel 'correlative microscopy' methodology as a tool to address the challenges involved in material selection and processing in AM through a discussion on the recent developments on AM-based biomedical materials based on a number of interesting case studies. Moreover, the present chapter intends to provide a future outlook in the direction of AM of biomedical materials from the authors' viewpoint.

3.2   CLASSIFICATION OF BIOMATERIALS

Biomaterials interact with biological systems and they may be either natural or synthetic [30]. Moreover, in medical applications, they are primarily meant for replacing a natural function. Biomaterials may be categorised on the basis of their biocompatibility levels as being bioactive, biodegradable, bioinert and/or biotolerant. A bioactive material in the environment of bone tissue may create an environment, which is compatible with osteogenesis through the formation of chemical bonds with bone tissues [31]. Bioactive materials may be categorised into two different classes: osteoconductive and osteoinductive materials [32].

Osteoconductive materials (such as hydroxyapatite and $Ca_3(PO_4)_2$) allow the growth of bone tissues along the bioactive material surface [32]. Osteoinductive materials stimulate the growth of new bones. Some osteoinductive materials (such as bioactive glasses) are also known as osteoproductive materials by which bone growth can be stimulated away from the site of the implant [33,34]. When a bioactive material is implanted into the human body, it stimulates a biological response from the body, which leads to a series of biophysical and biochemical reactions between the implant and tissue leading to a strong chemical bonding between the implant and the tissue [35,36]. Although biotolerant materials are accepted by the host, they are detached from the host tissue by the construction of a fibrous (scar) tissue. The layer of the scar tissue is stimulated by the discharge of ions and chemical compounds (including corrosion products) from the implant [33,37,38]. Most metals and artificial (or, synthetic) polymers fall into this category. Bioinert materials (such as Ti and its alloys) are stable and do not react with body fluids or tissues [39]. Fibrous tissues encapsulate these materials to isolate them from the neighbouring bone [39]. This is similar to the tendency of biotolerant materials [35]. Biodegradable materials (such as polyglycolic and polylactic acids, calcium phosphates and Mg) dissolve upon coming in contact with the body fluids [36]. The products (formed after dissolution) are secreted via the kidneys [35]. These materials find applications in medical goods such as surgical sutures and controlled drug release [36,38].

3.3   CLASSIFICATION OF ADDITIVE MANUFACTURING TECHNIQUES FOR BIOMATERIAL FABRICATION

Figure 3.1 shows the common classification scheme followed for biomaterials. Besides, a number of AM techniques are available for medical and tissue engineering applications, which are:

- **Powder bed fusion (PBF)**: PBF techniques utilise either laser or electron beam to selectively consolidate powder particles. These methods include selective laser melting (SLM), electron beam melting (EBM) and selective

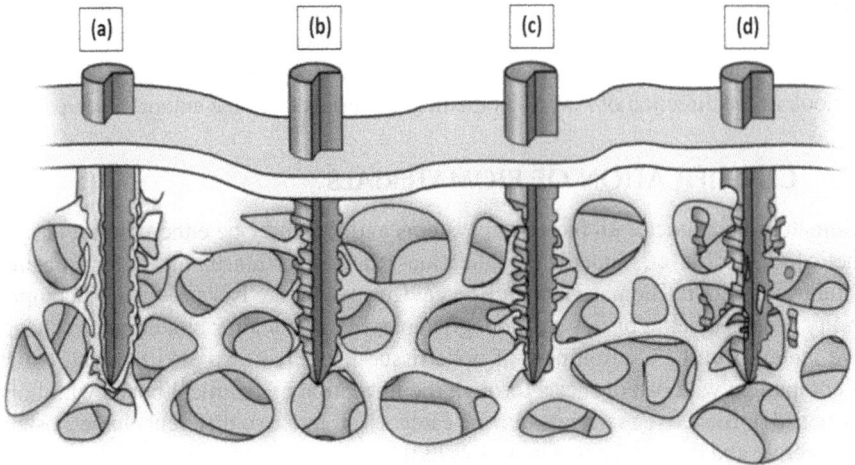

FIGURE 3.1 Biomaterial classifications illustrated using a bone screw: (a) biotolerant, (b) bioinert, (c) bioactive and (d) biodegradable [38].

laser sintering (SLS). Among these, SLM and EBM both melt completely and undergo fusion with the powder, whereas in the SLS technique, the powder is heated to the point where it can undergo fusion at a molecular level. In all PBF techniques, there is a layerwise spreading of material powder.

- **Binder jet 3D printing (BJ3DP)**: This technique is similar to the PBF technique in terms of utilisation of material powders, which are spread one on top of the other layer. However, unlike PBF, which involves melting and fusion of the powder particles, in this method, the binder is used for consolidation across different layers.
- **Material extrusion (or fused deposition modelling (FDM))**: This technique involves pushing of raw materials in the form of polymer wires through a heated nozzle. The material is deposited in the form of polymer roads, which are arranged to define the cross-section of a component and are consequently stacked in a layerwise manner.
- **Material jetting**: A liquid photopolymer resin cured with ultraviolet (UV) or near-UV radiation is used in this method. Similar to the FDM technique, a nozzle moving horizontally across the building platform is used to deposit the material. The material is subsequently cured followed by the consolidation of the resulting cross-section in a layer-by-layer manner as the building platform undergoes a vertical motion.
- **Vat polymerisation**: This method employs photopolymer resins cured with UV radiation in a layerwise manner. In contrast to material jetting, the resin remains in a material vat, where the building platform is submerged. This is followed by the downward (or upward) motion of the building platform depending on the location of the source of radiation to create added layers one on top of the other.

3.4 METALLIC BIOMATERIALS

Owing to an excellent combination of high stiffness coupled with wear resistance, ductility and electrical and thermal conductivities, metallic materials commonly find applications in orthopaedic and orthodontic implants, artificial joints, bone and external fixators [40,41]. It is due to a unique combination of strength and ductility that even today, metallic implants cannot be completely replaced by the more bio-compatible ceramics and polymers [42]. Biocompatible metals are mainly classified as being biotolerant except for Ti and its alloys, which are bioinert. In addition, Ti and its alloys, Co–Cr alloys and stainless steel have been reported as the most commonly used biocompatible metals [43,44]. To date, only PBF techniques have been able to successfully process biocompatible metallic materials (for medical grade) [45,46]. Ti6Al4V is a common material for orthopaedic implants owing to its unique biocompatibility, exceptional corrosion resistance and high specific strength [47,48]. Ti6Al4V (α-β Ti alloy) is inert meaning that the material may undergo direct interaction with the neighbouring bone tissue without introducing any chemical reaction between the implant and the host tissue [49,50]. Once a bioinert material is implanted into the human body, it undergoes self-passivation by forming an adhesive oxide layer, which prevents both electronic and ionic flow in the body fluid or adjoining tissue [48,51]. V in Ti-6Al-4V acts as a β stabiliser, whereas Al acts as an α stabiliser, which simultaneously contributes to strengthening and a decrease in density of the alloy [52–54].

Stainless steel (SS), on the other hand, is a common material for biomedical implants [55,56]. In addition, it is a low-cost material. The AISI3xx series (mainly 304 and 316L grades) with a fully austenitic microstructure is utilised in medical applications [57–59]. Although the aforementioned SS grades do not offer the same level of biocompatibility as in Ti6Al4V, they are biotolerant. Figure 3.2 shows the SEM images (at two different magnifications: 100× and 500×) of the Ti–6Al–4V alloy fabricated using the EBM technique. With surface treatments, it is possible to increase both the biocompatibility and corrosion resistance of the aforementioned SS grades [60,61]. Owing to the excellent combination of high strength coupled with

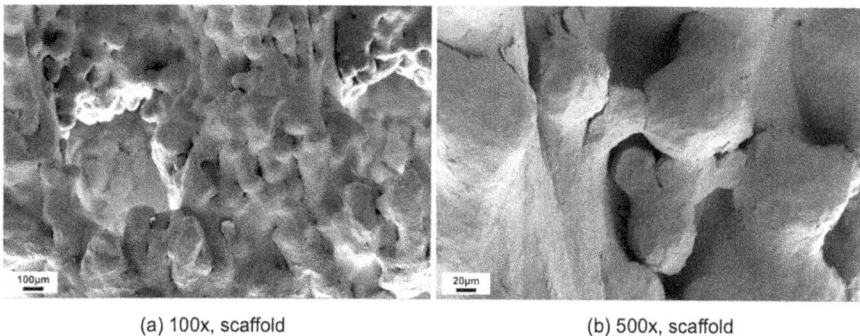

(a) 100x, scaffold   (b) 500x, scaffold

FIGURE 3.2 SEM images at different magnifications: (a) 100× and (b) 500× of Ti–6Al–4V scaffolds (mean pore size ≈ 800 μm) fabricated using the EBM technique [38].

corrosion resistance, SS is often used in bone plates, spinal fixation, knee and hip components [51,62]. Co–Cr alloys are another class of biotolerant materials. These alloys possess high wear resistance [63]. Cr forms an oxide layer on the surface of the alloy making it corrosion resistant in a biological environment whereas Co ensures a continuous phase resulting in homogeneous properties [64]. This makes Co–Cr alloys suitable candidates for bone implant applications [65–67]. Xie [68] has reported that even though the metals do not express bioactive properties, the biocompatibility of most metals may be enhanced by creating bio-inspired surfaces. Although AM-based metals have been widely used in the dental industry, AM has the potential to set up new possibilities for long-lasting orthopaedic implants for load-bearing applications. Table 3.1 summarises the classification, fabrication technique and application of some of the commonly used metallic biomaterials. Table 3.2 shows different AM-based techniques for the production of metallic biomaterials and Table 3.3 shows a summary of some of the most commonly used AM-based methods for the production of metallic biomaterials.

3.5 BIOCERAMICS

Owing to their excellent biocompatibility, these materials find applications as implants for bones, joints and teeth. These may be either bioinert or bioactive [77]. Bioactive ceramics may further be classified as either degradable or non-degradable [78]. These ceramics are commonly integrated with bone tissues via chemical reactions, which lead to the formation of hydroxycarbonate apatite without any inflammation.

TABLE 3.1

Classification, AM-Based Fabrication Techniques and Application of Some Commonly Used Metallic Biomaterials [38]

Biomaterial	Classification	Fabrication Technique	Application	Reference
Gold	Biotolerant	PBF (SLM) and binder jetting	Dental restorations	[69]
Co–Cr–Mo alloys		PBF (EBM and SLM)	Orthopaedic and dental implants	[70]
Stainless steel		PBF (EBM and SLM) and material extrusion	Cardiovascular stents and orthopaedic implants	[70], [71]
Niobium		PBF (EBM)	Vascular stents and coating for orthopaedic implants	[72]
Tantalum		PBF (EBM and SLM)	Orthopaedic implants	[73]
Commercially pure Ti	Bioinert	PBF (EBM and SLM)	Orthopaedic and dental implants	[74]
α-β Ti alloy (Ti–6Al–4V)		PBF (EBM and SLM)	Orthopaedic and dental implants	[75]

EBM, Electron Beam Melting; SLM, Selective Laser Melting.

TABLE 3.2

Comparison of Different AM-Based Methods for the Fabrication of Metallic Biomaterials [76]

AM-Based Technique	Resolution	Build Speed	Surface Roughness	Power Efficiency	Build Volume	Residual Stress	Cost
3DP	P	F	P		B	L	L
SLS	G	Sl	E	P	S	H	H
SLM	G	Sl	E	P	S	H	H
EBM	M	F	G	G	S	M	H
DMLS	G	Sl	E	P	S	L	H
DMD	P	F	P	P	B	H	M
EBAM	M	M	G	G	S	M	H

B, Big; DMD, Direct Metal Deposition; DMLS, Direct Metal Laser Sintering; E, Excellent; EBAM, Electron Beam Additive Manufacturing; EBM, Electron Beam Melting; F, Fast; G, Good; H, High; L, Low; M, Moderate; P, Poor; S, Small; Sl, Slow; SLM, Selective Laser Melting; SLS, Selective Laser Sintering; 3DP, 3D Printing.

The bond (formed between the bone tissues and bioactive ceramics) is stronger than the bone itself [79]. Common examples of these ceramics are bioglass and calcium phosphates [80,81]. Some calcium phosphates are based on hydroxyapatite (HA) and tricalcium phosphate (TCP) and have been considered for bone replacement applications [81]. $HA(Ca_{10}(PO_4)_6(OH)_2)$ is a bioactive ceramic with structure and chemistry in close resemblance with those of bone minerals and finds applications in scaffolds [79]. These ceramics are designed to undergo gradual degradation in a predetermined time frame. TCP $(Ca_3(PO_4)_2)$ is another common bioactive ceramic with a chemical composition similar to that of bone tissue minerals [77]. It has good resorbability and bioactivity with higher rates of biodegradation as compared to that of HA under in-vivo conditions [78].

Considering the brittle nature and poor fatigue properties of ceramics, they are less suitable for load-bearing applications unlike most metallic materials [68]. However, bioactive materials, (such as HA and bioglass) are used as bioactive coatings on metallic implants for load-bearing applications [82]. Ceramic coatings on metal implants offer three major advantages, viz. (i) enhancement of bone formation, (ii) direct bonding of the costing with the adjoining bone and (iii) reduction of metal corrosion as well as the release of corrosion products. Electrophoretic deposition [83], plasma spraying [84] and dip coating [78,85] have been reported as common fabrication techniques for bioceramics.

Bioinert ceramics, on the other hand, possess excellent chemical stability and high mechanical strength in vivo. In addition, these are chemically inert and have a lower coefficient of friction and wear rate as compared to those of most metallic materials [43]. Hence, these ceramics often find applications as femoral heads of hip implants [81]. Common examples of bioinert ceramics are Al_2O_3 and ZrO_2 [82,83]. Al_2O_3 (or alumina) has a low coefficient of friction, high hardness combined with excellent wear and corrosion resistance [77]. Owing to these properties, Al_2O_3 has been developed

TABLE 3.3

Summary of Some Common AM-Based Techniques Used for the Fabrication of Metallic Biomaterials [76]

AM-Based Technique	Characteristics	Applicable for Metallic Materials in Biomedical Applications	Advantages and Disadvantages	Classification
DMLS	• A thin layer of metal powder is printed. • Laser moves slowly across the surface to sinter metal powder. • Sintering of additional powder layers.	Stainless steel, Ti	Advantage(s): • Fabrication of parts free from internal stresses. Disadvantage(s): • Expensive; limited use of high-end applications. • Not suitable for low-ductility materials that require a heating stage.	PBF
DMD	• Melting of powder particles using laser or other energy sources followed by layerwise deposition.	Fe, Ti	Advantage(s): • No limitation of parts. Large metal parts may be fabricated. • Versatile. Disadvantage(s): • Poor surface finish.	DED
EBAM	• Conversion of the CAD model to CNC code. • Deposition of metal using an electron beam gun, via layerwise deposition of powder or wire feedstock until the near-net-shape is attained. • Heat treatment and machining as finishing treatments.	Ti, stainless steel, Zn alloy, Ta, W	Advantage(s): • No limitation of parts. Large metal parts may be fabricated. • Excellent material utilisation. • Utilisation of multiple wire feed with a single EB gun. Disadvantage(s): • Low processing accuracy and poor surface finish.	DED

(Continued)

TABLE 3.3 (Continued)
Summary of Some Common AM-Based Techniques Used for the Fabrication of Metallic Biomaterials [76]

AM-Based Technique	Characteristics	Applicable for Metallic Materials in Biomedical Applications	Advantages and Disadvantages	Classification
3DP	• Adding binder on metal powder. • Curing the binder. • Sintering the powder. • Infiltrating with a second metal (optionally).	Stainless steel, Co–Cr alloys, Fe, Zr, W	Advantage(s): • Ability to create shapes with high design complexity. • Extensive laser optimisation is not required. • Heat source during processing is not needed. • Build plate is not required. Disadvantage(s): • Fabricated parts need extensive post-processing. • Porosity in final parts. • Part reparation is not available.	Binder jetting
SLS	• Preparation of powder bed followed by layerwise deposition of powder. • Sintering each layer according to the CAD file, using a laser source.	Stainless steel, Co–Cr alloys, Ti	Advantage(s): • No requirement of support and post-processing. Disadvantage(s): • Heat treatment and material infiltration are necessary. • Porous part and rough surface in final parts. • Thermal distortion in the finished parts. • No option for part reparation.	PBF

(Continued)

TABLE 3.3 (Continued)
Summary of Some Common AM-Based Techniques Used for the Fabrication of Metallic Biomaterials [76]

AM-Based Technique	Characteristics	Applicable for Metallic Materials in Biomedical Applications	Advantages and Disadvantages	Classification
SLM	• Distribution of atomised fine metal powder onto a substrate plate as thin layers (20–100 μm) using a coating mechanism. • Each slice (2D) of the part undergoes fusion by selective melting of the powder particles. • Repetition of the process in a layer-by-layer fashion until fabrication is completed.	Stainless steel, Fe-based alloys, Ti, Au, Ag	Advantage(s): • Fabrication of a near-net-shape component with full density by thorough melting of the powder particles and without post-processing. • High precision is attained (~10 μm). Disadvantage(s): • High-quality requirements for metal powders coupled with limited part size. • High residual thermal stress leads to distortion.	PBF
EBM	• Reading of the data from a 3D CAD model and subsequent layerwise deposition of powder particles. • These layers are melted, using an electron beam under high-vacuum conditions.	Ti alloys, Co–Cr alloy	Advantage(s): • Preheating of the powder helps in the lowering of thermal stresses. • Vacuum is maintained to avoid oxidation. Disadvantage(s): • Complex internal cavities in the fabricated part. • Rougher texture and lower precision when compared to the laser beam manufacturing technique.	PBF

DED, Direct Energy Deposition; DMD, Direct Metal Deposition; DMLS, Direct Metal Laser Sintering; EBAM, Electron Beam Additive Manufacturing; EBM, Electron Beam Melting; PBF, Powder Bed Fusion; SLM, Selective Laser Melting; SLS, Selective Laser Sintering; 3DP, 3D Printing.

as an alternative to surgical metal alloys for orthopaedic and dental applications [86]. ZrO_2 (or zirconia) derived from Zr is commonly used in a number of prosthetic devices owing to its high strength and wear resistance [44]. ZrO_2 is also used as a coating on Ti in dental implants [85]. In addition, it has been shown that ZrO_2 implants accumulate fewer bacteria as compared to commercially pure Ti implants in vivo [48].

AM can be a powerful tool to fabricate dental implants. Not only does the layer-by-layer approach (followed in AM-based techniques) reduce material consumption, but it also allows the fabrication of complex-shaped components. Recently, lithium disilicate glass-ceramic dental restorations have been manufactured using a stereolithography-based AM technique, with a high flexural strength (>400 MPa) [87]. Mitteramskogler et al. [87] have utilised the vat polymerisation technique and utilised a modified digital light processing system to improve the geometrical accuracy of 45 vol% ZrO_2 green parts [87]. ZrO_2-toughened Al_2O_3 ceramics have also been fabricated using the vat polymerisation technique [77]. Liu et al. [88] have manufactured HA porous scaffolds using the vat polymerisation technique. Moreover, the aforementioned scaffolds have been reported to demonstrate good in-vitro biocompatibility for orthopaedic applications. Schmidleithner et al. [71] have also used the vat polymerisation technique to manufacture TCP scaffolds (with <2 vol.% error in porosity and <6% deviation from the mean pore size) for the regeneration of bone tissues. Table 3.4 summarises the classification, fabrication technique and application of some of the commonly used bioceramics.

3.6   BIOPOLYMERS AND CO-POLYMERS

From the viewpoint of biomaterials, polymers and co-polymers may be categorised into two different classes namely biodegradable and biotolerant [95]. Among metallic biomaterials and bioceramics, polymers exhibit minimum toughness (including both

TABLE 3.4
Classification, AM-Based Fabrication Techniques and Application of Some Commonly Used Bioceramics [38]

Bioceramic	Classification	Fabrication Technique	Application	Reference
Al oxide	Bioinert	Binder jetting, vat polymerisation	Osteosynthetic devices, bearing surfaces	[89]
Zirconium oxide		PBF (SLS)	Fixed partial dentures	[90]
Hydroxyapatite	Bioactive	Vat polymerisation, PBF (SLS), material extrusion and binder jetting	BTE	[91]
Bioglass		Vat photopolymerisation	BTE	[92]
Calcium silicate		PBF (SLS)	Tissue engineering	[93]
Tricalcium phosphate	Bioactive/ biodegradable	Binder jetting, vat polymerisation, material extrusion	BTE	[94]

BTE, Bone Tissue Engineering; PBF, Powder Bed Fusion; SLS, Selective Laser Sintering.

strength and ductility) [95]. As a result, biocompatible polymers and co-polymers (also known as biopolymers and co-polymers) are not used in load-bearing biomedical applications. However, owing to a high level of tunability in terms of interaction with the biological system, biodegradable polymers are widely investigated for applications in temporal devices [95]. AM-based biodegradable polymers, both natural and synthetic, are used for the fabrication of drug delivery vehicles (for controlled drug release), temporary 3D porous structures such as tissue engineering scaffolds and temporary prostheses [96]. The degradation of polymers may be further classified into hydrolytic and enzymatic polymeric degradation [96]. Enzymatic degradation refers to a state of degradation wherein the polymeric material undergoes degradation by the enzymes, which are secreted by the immune system, tissues or microbes present in a biological environment [97]. This kind of degradation is common in most natural polymers [97]. In addition, the rate of enzymatical degradation largely depends on the implantation site (especially on the availability of different enzymes at an implantation site) [96].

On the other hand, hydrolytically degradable polymers undergo degradation by the cleavage of hydrolytically sensitive bonds in the polymer, which consequently leads to polymer erosion [96]. Polymer erosion may be divided into bulk or surface erosion, or a combination of both. In surface erosion, erosion starts from the exterior of the material and the interior of the material does not degrade until all the surrounding material has been degraded [95]. On the contrary, bulk erosion is characterised by an equal amount of erosion occurring throughout the entire material [97]. Interplay of these erosion mechanisms determines the suitability of different biomaterials for biomedical applications. For instance, in the context of sustained drug delivery, surface erosion is preferred over bulk erosion [97]. This is advantageous for bone tissue engineering (BTE) applications meant for ensuring a gradual replacement of the scaffold implant with the adjoining bone tissues [97]. Figure 3.3 shows a flowchart of the design, fabrication and evaluation of BTE scaffolds.

The present research is mainly focussed on implementing AM-based techniques for fabricating customised implants. Guerra et al. have employed material extrusion techniques to fabricate stents using polycaprolactone (PCL)/polylactic acid (PLA) composites [96]. Moreover, the aforementioned printing technique was reported to be suitable for fabricating composite stents with an accuracy of ~85% to 95% combined with medium degradation rates and enhanced biocompatibility [97]. Jia et al. [98] have designed and fabricated self-expandable biodegradable vascular stents from PLA using the material extrusion technique. However, there are a number of limitations with biodegradable polymers when compared to conventional metallic bone fixators. There is a need to pre-drill holes for the biodegradable screws. Yeon et al. [99] have reported the manufacturing of a PLA/HA/Silk composite bone clip (using the material extrusion technique) implanted in the rat femur bone. Moreover, the bone clip was reported to show the excellent alignment of the bone segments [99]. Zhang et al. [100] have utilised the material extrusion technique to fabricate PCL scaffolds with three distinct mean pore sizes (215, 320 and 515 μm) [100]. In addition, the PCL scaffold with a mean pore size of ~215 μm showed fibrocartilaginous tissue formation and enhanced mechanical properties as compared to the other pore sizes [100]. Table. 3.5 shows the classification, fabrication techniques and applications of some commonly used biopolymers and co-polymers.

TABLE 3.5
Biopolymers and Co-polymers [38]

Biopolymer/Co-polymer	Classification	Fabrication Technique	Application	Reference
Polyethylene (PE)	Biotolerant	PBF (SLS)	Vascular prostheses, cardiac valves and hip joints	[101]
Poly(hexano-6-lactam) (PA6)		PBF (SLS)	Intravascular balloon catheters	[102]
Poly(methyl methacrylate) (PMMA)		PBF (SLS) and vat photopolymerisation	Anchoring of hip prostheses, vertebroplasties and eyeglass lenses	[103]
Poly(tetrafluorethylene) (PTFE)		Vat photopolymerisation	Orthopaedy and vascular clips	[104]
Poly(aryletherketone) (PAEK)	Bioactive	PBF (SLS)	Orthopaedic and spinal implants	[105]
Polyurethane (PUR)	Biostable and biodegradable	Vat photopolymerisation	Cardiovascular devices	[106]
Polycaprolactone (PCL)	Biodegradable	PBF (SLS) and material extrusion	Tissue engineering and controlled drug release	[104]
Poly(lactic acid) (PLA)		Material extrusion	Bioabsorbable fixation, bone regeneration and fixation and drug delivery	[103]
Poly(lactic acid-*co*-glycolic acid) (PLGA)		Material jetting and material extrusion	Therapeutic devices, drug delivery and tissue engineering	[102]

3.7 CHARACTERISATION OF BIOMATERIALS

3.7.1 STRUCTURAL AND CHEMICAL CHARACTERISATION

3.7.1.1 X-Ray Diffraction (XRD)

X-ray diffraction (XRD) is primarily used to determine the structure of materials [107]. A typical powder X-ray diffractometer consists of an X-ray generation source (Co, Cr, Cu and Mo are typically used as the source), a diffractometer, a monochromator and a detector. In addition, Bragg-Brentano geometry is followed in a typical powder XRD instrument [107].

In the powder XRD technique, a monochromatic X-ray beam is focussed on the material with an interplanar spacing d and the diffracted beam intensity is measured as a function of the angle between the incident and the diffracted beam (2θ, where θ is the angle between the incident X-ray beam and the Bragg plane). Bragg's law is used to determine d from 2θ [107]:

$$\lambda = 2d \sin\theta \tag{3.1}$$

where λ is the wavelength of the monochromatic X-ray beam. 2θ and d provide information such as the crystal structure, lattice parameter, unit cell dimension, crystallite size, residual stress, etc.

3.7.1.2 Infrared (IR) Spectroscopy

This is an optical technique for identifying the structure and chemical composition of complex compounds [106]. IR radiation (at various frequencies) is absorbed by different functional groups [76,108]. This enables IR spectroscopy to detect the different chemical functional groups in a molecule [108,109]. Similar to XRD (discussed in Section 3.7.1.1), this technique is non-destructive and can be used to analyse biomaterials irrespective of their state of matter (solid, liquid or gas) [110]. IR photons do not possess a sufficient amount of energy to cause electronic transitions in the valence shells of atoms, but the rotational and vibrational motion is excited by IR radiation [110]. The IR spectrum depicts the variation of absorption, reflection or transmission intensity with frequency or wavelength and may be further categorised into different sub-regions, namely, (i) near-IR (NIR) that ranges from ~800 to ~2500 nm, (ii) mid-IR (MIR) that extends from ~2500 to ~15000 nm and (iii) far-IR (FIR) that extends from ~15,000 to ~1,00,000 nm (FIR) [109]. The Fourier transform infrared (FTIR) spectrometer is easily accessible and usable due to its high signal-to-noise ratio [111]. In addition, it is capable of measuring all wavelengths. Thus, the whole spectral information is obtained in one go.

In the context of biomedical materials, the degree of conversion in dental composites and the polymerisation process have been examined by FTIR spectroscopy [112,113]. Moreover, attenuated total reflection FTIR (ATR-FTIR) spectroscopy is being recently used to characterise biomaterials. Non-compulsory pretreatment during sample preparation is the key advantage of the ATR-FTIR technique [114].

3.7.1.3 Raman Spectroscopy

Similar to XRD (discussed in Section 3.7.1.1) and IR spectroscopy (discussed in Section 3.7.1.2), this is another non-destructive characterisation technique. However, unlike XRD which is meant for structural characterisation of materials, this is a spectroscopy technique based on the molecular vibrations of materials and has shown promising potential as a spectroscopic technique in the field of biomaterials irrespective of their state of matter (solid, liquid or gas). This is unlike the existence of selection rules based on the structure factor calculations (for different crystal structures) in XRD, due to available excitations in vibrational mode, which are permitted in IR spectroscopy [115]. Optical fibres are utilised to collect the Raman spectra where there are interactions of photons with the specimen molecules. The chemical composition, molecular structure and identification of unknown materials have been examined by Raman spectroscopy. In this technique, the Raman intensity is plotted as a function of the Raman shift [116]. The distinction of frequencies among the incident and scattered Raman light beam is defined as the Raman shift.

3.7.1.4   X-Ray Photoelectron Spectroscopy (XPS)

The chemical composition of the external top surface (~1 to 10 nm) of any solid is characterised based on the photoelectric effect during the bombardment of the surface with X-ray photons. The expulsion of electrons appears operating monochromatic X-rays in an ultrahigh vacuum (UHV) [111], which is followed by the emission of electrons from the different shells of atoms. Detectors are utilised to measure their kinetic energy and frequency. The binding energy of electrons is a representative of the elements, which is influenced by the oxidation state, and the local bonding environment between atoms (especially the state of hybridisation). Therefore, XPS is capable of determining the chemical nature of the materials [111]. The application of XPS is limited in the context of biomaterials as they have a high chance of radiation damage caused by X-ray photons. Besides, XPS also enables the determination of the extent of the functionality and binding of biomolecules onto a number of surfaces. In the context of dental applications [111], XPS has been used to analyse tooth tissues in restorative dentistry for understanding the mechanisms of interaction among the hard tissue and the biomaterial [111,117].

3.7.1.5   Ultraviolet (UV)-Vis Spectroscopy

This technique is based on the variation of wavelength with the absorbance of UV radiation ($\lambda \approx 190\text{--}350$ nm) to visible light ($\lambda \approx 350\text{--}800$ nm) (in a material) [111,118]. The absorption (of UV radiation) occurs due to the transition (of electrons) from the ground state to the excited state with the magnitude depending on the Beer–Lambert relationship [109,111]:

$$A = abc \tag{3.2}$$

where A, a, b and c are the absorbance, the absorption coefficient (wavelength-dependent), the path length through the solution and the molar concentration, respectively. This technique is especially useful for providing both qualitative and quantitative information on dental biomaterials and composites.

3.7.1.6   Nuclear Magnetic Resonance (NMR) Spectroscopy

NMR follows the non-destructive principle and is utilised for determining the chemical composition and conformations of biomolecules [111]. In NMR spectroscopy, the nuclei of atoms are investigated and the behaviour of specific atoms (1H, 13C, 15N, 31P and 19F) is analysed on being exposed to an external magnetic field, which leads to a spin-nuclei mechanism [112]. The mechanisms of biomineralisation (the ones used for bone repair and hard tissue regeneration of the teeth) can be understood utilising NMR applied at the molecular level [116].

3.7.1.7 Mercury Intrusion Porosimetry (MIP)

Recently, porous biomaterials have gained attention for applications in scaffolds for tissue engineering and drug delivery system. The in-growth of mineralised tissue requires a minimum pore size of ~50 μm [109]. In this context, it is worth mentioning that larger pore sizes degrade the mechanical properties and also lead to an increase in the depth of infiltration of these tissues into the biomaterial [111]. Smaller pore sizes, on the other hand, lead to large surface areas, resulting in a higher adsorption of cell-inducing proteins. MIP is used to determine the pore sizes and porosity in a number of biomaterials (especially bioceramics) [111].

3.7.1.8 Scanning Electron Microscopy (SEM)

SEM is the most widely used microscopy tool utilised for analysing the microstructure of the materials [111]. In SEM, a low-energy electron beam scans the sample surface [109]. As the beam reaches the material, a number of different interactions occur, which lead to the emission of electrons and characteristic X-rays from the vicinity of the sample surface [109,119]. To form an image, special types of detectors are utilised for receiving signals emitted from the sample [111]. For instance, secondary electrons (SEs) generated from near the sample surface provide information about the surface topography whereas backscattered electrons (BSE) generated from a greater depth in the sample show the atomic number (Z) contrast between the different phases in a given microstructure and can also be used to generate information about the orientation of different grains in a polycrystalline material (through tilting the specimen to ~70° with respect to the horizontal level) by tilting the specimen and allowing the BSEs to undergo diffraction and finally detecting the Kikuchi bands (formed due to the diffraction of BSEs) through special detectors. This SEM-based technique is also known as electron backscatter diffraction (EBSD) [120]. On the other hand, energy dispersive spectroscopy (EDS) detectors, providing information on the chemical composition of different phases in a multiphase microstructure, detect the characteristic X-rays generated from within the specimen (at a much higher depth when compared with those of SE and BSE). Different modes of SEM are used for the characterisation of biomaterials such as EDS mapping, secondary electron (SE) imaging and backscattered electrons (BSE) imaging. The main components of a typical SEM are:

- **The electron gun**: for the emission of electrons which are then accelerated from ~0.1 to 30 keV.
- **Hairpin tungsten gun**: to form high-resolution images from a high-diameter electron beam.
- **Electromagnetic lenses and apertures**: meant to focus electron beam to form a small high-intensity spot on the specimen.
- **High-vacuum environment**: for preventing electron scattering.

3.7.1.9   Transmission Electron Microscopy (TEM)

This technique is used to fetch information about the crystal structure, chemical composition and morphology of biomaterials with a higher resolution than that may be achieved with a typical SEM. Here, electrons (with energy $\approx 120–300\,kV$) emitted from an electron gun (mainly of two types: thermionic and field emission) are directed by the electrostatic lenses onto an electro transparent specimen (thickness $< 50\,nm$) and undergo dynamic scattering in the specimen [109,111]. Owing to the dynamic scattering events undergone by the electrons with the electron transparent sample, a fraction of the electrons undergo scattering (or absorption) while another fraction passes through the sample depending on the sample density. These electrons, which pass through the thin sample and hit the detector, form an image on the fluorescent screen placed at the bottom of the TEM. The denser the sample, the lesser the probability of electrons to pass through it, and consequently, the image formed (in bright field (BF) mode) is darker [121,122]. The main limitations include the smaller field of view of TEM compared to SEM, chances of sample damage if the beam energy is excessively high (very common for sensitive biological materials), poor contrast in low atomic number (Z) materials, sample preparation (both conventional and focussed ion beam (FIB)-based) requiring huge effort and skills, expertise in equipment handling and data interpretation and low depth of resolution [123,124]. Figure 3.3 shows the TEM-BF image of human chondrocytes grown at the surface and within the bulk.

3.7.1.10   Atomic Force Microscopy (AFM)

AFM is utilised to track the contour of a wide variety of surfaces (hard or soft, insulator or conductor).

The topography formed by AFM reveals the 3D surface features with a spatial resolution of the order of a few nm [126]. Here, a sharp tip (nearly one atom thick and made of Si or Si nitride) is used to record the topography of the sample [126]. The force acting between the probe tip and the surface of the sample leads to an elastic deflection of the beam (which is directly proportional to the magnitude of the inter-atomic forces) to which the tip is attached. The deflection of the beam is analysed utilising an optical system [126]. Based on the nature of tip–surface interactions, different modes of AFM are as follows:

- **Dynamic force (or tapping mode)**: It involves oscillation and movement of the tip in the vicinity of the surface of the sample, leading to an intermittent contact between the probe and the sample surface.
- **Contact mode**: It involves movement of the probe over the sample surface that experiences a strong repulsion from the sample surface leading to the bending of the beam.
- **Non-contact mode**: It involves movement of the tip adjacent to the surface (at a distance further than that for the dynamic mode), and hence, it does not come in contact with the sample surface. The interaction forces (between the sample surface and the tip) in this mode are very low (of the order of a few pN). This mode is especially useful for soft biomaterials since this does not damage their surfaces.

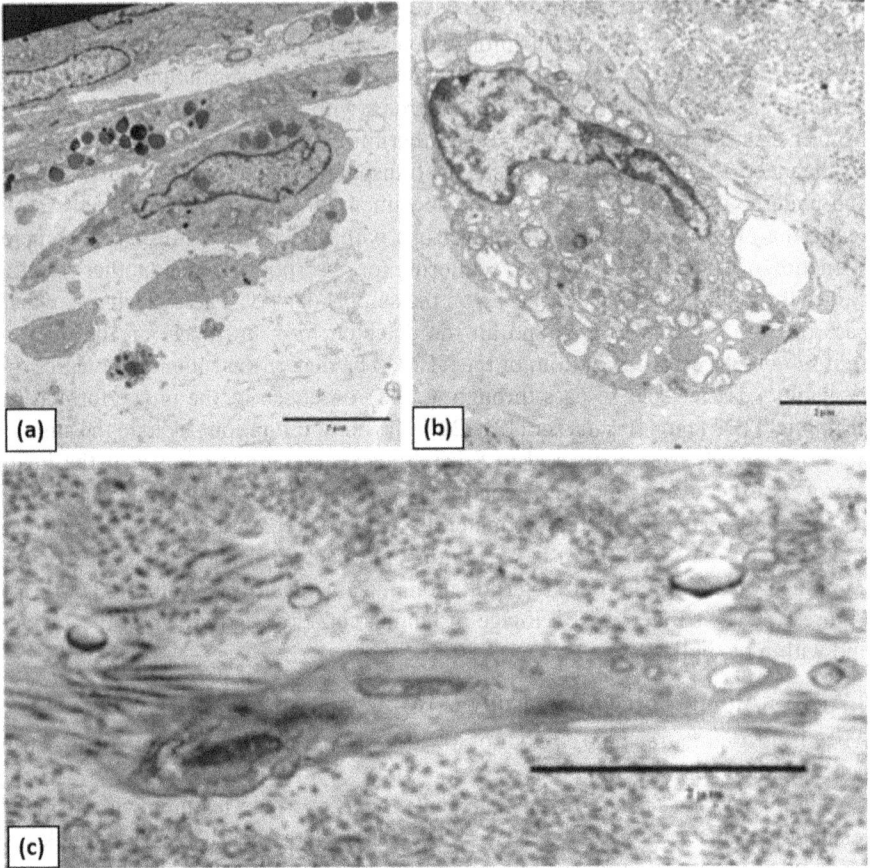

FIGURE 3.3   TEM-BF image showing the morphology of human chondrocytes (grown at the surface and within the bulk): (a) unmodified bacterial cellulose, (b) articular cartilage bulk and (c) articular cartilage surface [125].

3.7.2   IN-VITRO CHARACTERISATION

3.7.2.1   Cytotoxicity Testing

This is a testing technique for determining the cytotoxic effects of a biomaterial in a living organism [127]. It is one of the earliest in-vitro techniques meant for the evaluation of biocompatibility of materials [128,129]. Typical biological endpoints (in cytotoxicity testing) include:

- **Morphological evaluation**: This is performed by using an ultrastructural examination of the cells using either SEM or TEM, depending on the level of accuracy and resolution (required in terms of morphology), and microscopy parameters field of view and depth of field.

- **Cell viability and proliferation assays**: Common examples include Alamar blue assay, 3-(4,5 dimethylthiazol-2-yl)-2,5-diphenyltetrazolium bromide assay, bromodeoxyuridine incorporation assay, 3H-thymidine incorporation assay, and DNA or protein analysis.
- **Cell function assays**: These involve measurement of the release of inflammatory markers, glutathione determination, heat-shock protein and apoptosis assay.

3.7.2.2   Haemocompatibility Testing

This is a testing method to analyse the adverse effects (e.g., thrombosis, haemolysis and platelet activation) and blood–biomaterial interaction [129]. One of the primary issues associated with haemocompatibility is the absence of adequate standards for anticoagulation. As a result, it is a difficult task to classify a particular biomaterial as either haemocompatible or non-haemocompatible [130]. Parameters such as physical and chemical features, experimental conditions, stability of the materials and aspects of feasibility are important factors in haemocompatibility analysis.

3.7.2.3   Genotoxicity and Carcinogenicity Testing

These are meant to study the genotoxic effect (e.g. change in DNA, gene mutation and modifications in chromosome) and the carcinogenic effects of an implant on a living organism [131]. Micronucleus assay, Ames test and comet assay have been used to determine the genotoxic effects of nanomaterials, among which the Ames test and comet assay are known for being quick (in terms of detecting deoxyribonucleic acid (DNA) damage) and also for their simplicity and low cost [130].

3.7.2.4   Reverse Transcription-Polymerase Chain Reaction (RT-PCR)

This method is used for identifying and comparing the levels of messenger-ribonucleic acid (mRNA) and the surface proteins [127]. PCR can be carried out as (i) real-time PCR and (ii) end-point PCR [128]. End-point PCR is a low-cost technique and requires low-cost equipment. Measurement of gene expression is the main role of end-point PCR [127].

3.7.3   In-vivo Characterisation

3.7.3.1   Sensitisation, Irritation and Toxicity Tests

Sensitisation may be described as an intensification in immune response and hindered hypersensitive response to a biomaterial (in a living organism), which otherwise may result in skin irritation and local inflammation on the skin [129]. This may be a highly time-taking process as it needs a film of chemical agent (in a saline solution) to be retained on the skin followed by monitoring of the effects of a particular biomaterial over time [130]. Murine local lymph node assay and Buehler and guinea pig maximisation are examples of sensitisation testing. The other common in-vivo tests for determining the extent of irritation caused by the biomaterials in animals are intracutaneous reactivity, subacute systemic toxicity, chronic toxicity tests and subchronic systemic toxicity [132].

3.7.3.2 Implantation Testing

In this process, the pathological influences (ranging from macroscopic to microscopic levels) of biomaterials are assessed by implanting materials into the connective tissue, animal bone or muscle by which the functioning and structure of tissues are understood [130]. This may be used to determine tissue necrosis and cell proliferation, apoptosis, collagen deposition, thrombus formation and endothelialisation. Both short- and long-term testing may be used to determine the instant and late response of the tissue to the implant [131].

3.7.3.3 Biodegradation Test

Several degradable biomaterials may discharge degradation products (commonly impurities and corrosion products) to the adjacent tissues and even the organs (which may be distant). In-vivo biodegradation tests have an important role in investigating the effects of biodegradation of biomaterials on living tissues [132]. Biological and tissue responses in a living organism may be identified using histological analysis [130].

3.8 SUMMARY AND FUTURE OUTLOOKS: FROM THE AUTHORS' VIEWPOINT

At present, there is a sufficient amount of information on the different AM-based fabrication techniques for all three different types of biomaterials (viz. metallic biomaterials, bioceramics and biopolymers and co-polymers) as discussed in Sections 3.2–3.6. Hence, it is reasonable to infer that there is a good amount of information on the process parameters involved in different AM-based techniques for the fabrication of biomaterials. Besides, there are a huge number of reports on the fabrication of different biomaterials using different AM-based techniques getting published frequently. However, the missing aspect in all the present reports is a proper understanding of the microstructure in biomaterials, which is important to engineer the biocompatibility (especially the mechanical biocompatibility) of biomaterials. As briefly mentioned in the Introduction section (Section 3.1), mechanical biocompatibility (between tissues/bones and a biomaterial) is essential to prevent micro-injuries, cell damage, inflammation, necrosis, etc. [133–137]. The aforementioned mechanical biocompatibility is hugely influenced by the microstructure of the bio-implant. Although a number of recent reports have been aimed towards addressing the corrosion and wear resistance and also the tensile, compressive and flexural properties for a number of different biomaterials, a systematic correlation between the microstructure and the aforementioned properties is missing in the present reports.

In the recent decade, a correlative approach towards microstructural characterisation has been widely employed for correlating the structural information with the local chemistry of especially nanosised features in metallic materials. The pre-requisite for such characterisation mainly involves careful sample preparation (which may sometimes be time-consuming) [138]. However, these techniques involve a huge amount of investment and may sometimes lack consistency of experimental results. Moreover, owing to the complexity of structures and of sample preparation in bioceramics and biopolymers (and co-polymers), there is hardly any report (to date) on the correlative characterisation of these materials. In addition, only a few groups have reported the characterisation of biomaterials at an atomic scale using the atom probe tomography (APT) technique in the present decade [139–144]. Hence, correlative microscopy may be used as a potential tool for correlating the wide range of interesting properties shown by the biomaterials (fabricated using different AM-based techniques) with both structural and chemical information in their microstructure. This is necessary to establish a systemic structure–property correlation in these materials, which is the least understood in the context of biomaterials.

REFERENCES

1. J. de Krijger, C. Rans, B. van Hooreweder, K. Lietaert, B. Pouran, and A. A. Zadpoor, "Effects of applied stress ratio on the fatigue behavior of additively manufactured porous biomaterials under compressive loading," *Journal of the Mechanical Behavior of Biomedical Materials*, vol. 70, pp. 7–16, Jun. 2017, doi: 10.1016/j.jmbbm.2016.11.022.
2. M. Afshar, A. P. Anaraki, H. Montazerian, and J. Kadkhodapour, "Additive manufacturing and mechanical characterization of graded porosity scaffolds designed based on triply periodic minimal surface architectures," *Journal of the Mechanical Behavior of Biomedical Materials*, vol. 62, pp. 481–494, Sep. 2016, doi: 10.1016/j.jmbbm.2016.05.027.
3. R. Pecci, S. Baiguera, P. Ioppolo, R. Bedini, and C. del Gaudio, "3D printed scaffolds with random microarchitecture for bone tissue engineering applications: Manufacturing and characterization," *Journal of the Mechanical Behavior of Biomedical Materials*, vol. 103, p. 103583, Mar. 2020, doi: 10.1016/j.jmbbm.2019.103583.
4. F. Bartolomeu et al., "Predicting the output dimensions, porosity and elastic modulus of additive manufactured biomaterial structures targeting orthopedic implants," *Journal of the Mechanical Behavior of Biomedical Materials*, vol. 99, pp. 104–117, Nov. 2019, doi: 10.1016/j.jmbbm.2019.07.023.
5. N. E. Putra, M. J. Mirzaali, I. Apachitei, J. Zhou, and A. A. Zadpoor, "Multi-material additive manufacturing technologies for Ti-, Mg-, and Fe-based biomaterials for bone substitution," *Acta Biomaterialia*, vol. 109. Acta Materialia Inc, pp. 1–20, Jun. 01, 2020, doi: 10.1016/j.actbio.2020.03.037.
6. V. S. Cheong, P. Fromme, A. Mumith, M. J. Coathup, and G. W. Blunn, "Novel adaptive finite element algorithms to predict bone ingrowth in additive manufactured porous implants," *Journal of the Mechanical Behavior of Biomedical Materials*, vol. 87, pp. 230–239, Nov. 2018, doi: 10.1016/j.jmbbm.2018.07.019.
7. J. Ju et al., "Tribological investigation of additive manufacturing medical Ti6Al4V alloys against Al_2O_3 ceramic balls in artificial saliva," *Journal of the Mechanical Behavior of Biomedical Materials*, vol. 104, p. 103602, Apr. 2020, doi: 10.1016/j.jmbbm.2019.103602.
8. M. Navarro, A. Michiardi, O. Castaño, and J. A. Planell, "Biomaterials in orthopaedics," *Journal of the Royal Society Interface*, vol. 5, no. 27. Royal Society, pp. 1137–1158, Oct. 06, 2008, doi: 10.1098/rsif.2008.0151.
9. Z. Z. Yin et al., "Advances in coatings on biodegradable magnesium alloys," *Journal of Magnesium and Alloys*, vol. 8, no. 1. National Engg. Research Center for Magnesium Alloys, pp. 42–65, Mar. 01, 2020, doi: 10.1016/j.jma.2019.09.008.
10. A. Kania, W. Pilarczyk, and M. M. Szindler, "Structure and corrosion behavior of TiO2 thin films deposited onto Mg-based alloy using magnetron sputtering and sol-gel," *Thin Solid Films*, vol. 701, May 2020, doi: 10.1016/j.tsf.2020.137945.
11. R. Karunakaran, S. Ortgies, A. Tamayol, F. Bobaru, and M. P. Sealy, "Additive manufacturing of magnesium alloys," *Bioactive Materials*, vol. 5, no. 1. KeAi Communications Co., pp. 44–54, Mar. 01, 2020, doi: 10.1016/j.bioactmat.2019.12.004.

12. W. Pompe et al., "Functionally graded materials for biomedical applications," *Materials Science and Engineering A*, vol. 362, no. 1–2, pp. 40–60, Dec. 2003, doi: 10.1016/S0921-5093(03)00580-X.

13. A. Castelão, B. A. R. Soares, C. M. Machado, M. Leite, and A. J. M. Mourão, "Design for AM: Contributions from surface finish, part geometry and part positioning," *Procedia CIRP*, Jan. 2019, vol. 84, pp. 491–495, doi: 10.1016/j.procir.2019.04.247.

14. M. Saha and M. Mallik, "Additive manufacturing of ceramics and cermets: Present status and future perspectives," *Sādhanā*, vol. 46, no. 3, pp. 1–35, Aug. 2021, doi: 10.1007/S12046-021-01685-2.

15. O. Abdulhameed, A. Al-Ahmari, W. Ameen, and S. H. Mian, "Additive manufacturing: Challenges, trends, and applications," *Advances in Mechanical Engineering*, vol. 11, no. 2, Feb. 2019, doi: 10.1177/1687814018822880.

16. B. Durakovic, "Design for additive manufacturing: Benefits, trends and challenges," *Periodicals of Engineering and Natural Sciences*, vol. 6, no. 2, pp. 179–191, Dec. 2018, doi: 10.21533/pen.v6i2.224.

17. A. Gisario, M. Kazarian, F. Martina, and M. Mehrpouya, "Metal additive manufacturing in the commercial aviation industry: A review," *Journal of Manufacturing Systems*, vol. 53. Elsevier B.V., pp. 124–149, Oct. 01, 2019, doi: 10.1016/j.jmsy.2019.08.005.

18. T. D. Ngo, A. Kashani, G. Imbalzano, K. T. Q. Nguyen, and D. Hui, "Additive manufacturing (3D printing): A review of materials, methods, applications and challenges," *Composites Part B: Engineering*, vol. 143. Elsevier Ltd, pp. 172–196, Jun. 15, 2018, doi: 10.1016/j.compositesb.2018.02.012.

19. M. K. Thompson et al., "Design for additive manufacturing: Trends, opportunities, considerations, and constraints," *CIRP Annals - Manufacturing Technology*, vol. 65, no. 2, pp. 737–760, Jan. 2016, doi: 10.1016/j.cirp.2016.05.004.

20. D. R. Calderaro, D. P. Lacerda, and D. R. Veit, "Selection of additive manufacturing technologies in productive systems: A decision support model," *Gestao e Producao*, vol. 27, no. 3, p. 2020, 2020, doi: 10.1590/0104-530x5363-20.

21. J. W. Koo, J. S. Ho, J. An, Y. Zhang, C. K. Chua, and T. H. Chong, "A review on spacers and membranes: Conventional or hybrid additive manufacturing?" *Water Research*, vol. 188. Elsevier Ltd, Jan. 01, 2021, doi: 10.1016/j.watres.2020.116497.

22. M. Touri, F. Kabirian, M. Saadati, S. Ramakrishna, and M. Mozafari, "Additive Manufacturing of biomaterials – The evolution of rapid prototyping," *Advanced Engineering Materials*, vol. 21, no. 2, p. 1800511, Feb. 2019, doi: 10.1002/adem.201800511.

23. E. A. Guzzi and M. W. Tibbitt, "Additive manufacturing of precision biomaterials," *Advanced Materials*, vol. 32, no. 13, p. 1901994, Apr. 2020, doi: 10.1002/adma.201901994.

24. D. Foehring, H. B. Chew, and J. Lambros, "Characterizing the tensile behavior of additively manufactured Ti-6Al-4V using multiscale digital image correlation," *Materials Science and Engineering A*, vol. 724, pp. 536–546, May 2018, doi: 10.1016/j.msea.2018.03.091.

25. B. Barkia et al., "On the origin of the high tensile strength and ductility of additively manufactured 316L stainless steel: Multiscale investigation," *Journal of Materials Science and Technology*, vol. 41, pp. 209–218, Mar. 2020, doi: 10.1016/j.jmst.2019.09.017.

26. S. A. H. Motaman, F. Roters, and C. Haase, "Anisotropic polycrystal plasticity due to microstructural heterogeneity: A multi-scale experimental and numerical study on additively manufactured metallic materials," *Acta Materialia*, vol. 185, pp. 340–369, Feb. 2020, doi: 10.1016/j.actamat.2019.12.003.

27. C. K. Chua, K. F. Leong, and J. An, "Additive manufacturing and 3D printing," *Biomedical Materials*, Springer International Publishing, 2021, pp. 621–652.

28. P. Kingshott, G. Andersson, S. L. McArthur, and H. J. Griesser, "Surface modification and chemical surface analysis of biomaterials," *Current Opinion in Chemical Biology*, vol. 15, no. 5. Elsevier Current Trends, pp. 667–676, Oct. 01, 2011, doi: 10.1016/j.cbpa.2011.07.012.

29. R. Hedayati et al., "Isolated and modulated effects of topology and material type on the mechanical properties of additively manufactured porous biomaterials," *Journal of the Mechanical Behavior of Biomedical Materials*, vol. 79, pp. 254–263, Mar. 2018, doi: 10.1016/j.jmbbm.2017.12.029.

30. H. Rojbani, M. Nyan, K. Ohya, and S. Kasugai, "Evaluation of the osteoconductivity of α-tricalcium phosphate, β-tricalcium phosphate, and hydroxyapatite combined with or without simvastatin in rat calvarial defect," *Journal of Biomedical Materials Research – Part A*, vol. 98 A, no. 4, pp. 488–498, Sep. 2011, doi: 10.1002/jbm.a.33117.

31. P. A. Tran, L. Sarin, R. H. Hurt, and T. J. Webster, "Opportunities for nanotechnology-enabled bioactive bone implants," *Journal of Materials Chemistry*, vol. 19, no. 18, pp. 2653–2659, Apr. 2009, doi: 10.1039/b814334j.

32. J. R. Jones, "Review of bioactive glass: From Hench to hybrids," *Acta Biomaterialia*, vol. 9, no. 1. Elsevier, pp. 4457–4486, Jan. 01, 2013, doi: 10.1016/j.actbio.2012.08.023.

33. H. Plenk, "The role of materials biocompatibility for functional electrical stimulation applications," *Artificial Organs*, vol. 35, no. 3, pp. 237–241, Mar. 2011, doi: 10.1111/j.15 25-1594.2011.01221.x.

34. C. P. Bergmann and A. Stumpf, *Dental ceramics: Microstructure, Properties and Degradation*. Springer, 2013.

35. H. Tian, Z. Tang, X. Zhuang, X. Chen, and X. Jing, "Biodegradable synthetic polymers: Preparation, functionalization and biomedical application," *Progress in Polymer Science (Oxford)*, vol. 37, no. 2. Elsevier Ltd, pp. 237–280, Feb. 01, 2012, doi: 10.1016/j. progpolymsci.2011.06.004.

36. S. K. Prajapati, A. Jain, A. Jain, and S. Jain, "Biodegradable polymers and constructs: A novel approach in drug delivery," *European Polymer Journal*, vol. 120. Elsevier Ltd, p. 109191, Nov. 01, 2019, doi: 10.1016/j.eurpolymj.2019.08.018.

37. A. C. Popa, G. E. Stan, M. Enculescu, C. Tanase, D. U. Tulyaganov, and J. M. F. Ferreira, "Superior biofunctionality of dental implant fixtures uniformly coated with durable bioglass films by magnetron sputtering," *Journal of the Mechanical Behavior of Biomedical Materials*, vol. 51, pp. 313–327, Nov. 2015, doi: 10.1016/j.jmbbm.2015.07.028.

38. K. S. Ødegaard, J. Torgersen, and C. W. Elverum, "Structural and biomedical properties of common additively manufactured biomaterials: A concise review," *Metals*, Vol. 10, p. 1677, Dec. 2020, doi: 10.3390/MET10121677.

39. X. Y. Zhang, G. Fang, and J. Zhou, "Additively manufactured scaffolds for bone tissue engineering and the prediction of their mechanical behavior: A review," *Materials*, vol. 10, no. 1. MDPI AG, p. 50, Jan. 10, 2017, doi: 10.3390/ma10010050.

40. S. v. Dorozhkin, "Bioceramics of calcium orthophosphates," *Biomaterials*, vol. 31, no. 7. pp. 1465–1485, Mar. 2010, doi: 10.1016/j.biomaterials.2009.11.050.

41. V. Biehl, T. Wack, S. Winter, U. T. Seyfert, and J. Breme, "Evaluation of the haemocompatibility of titanium based biomaterials," *Biomolecular Engineering*, vol. 19, no. 2–6, pp. 97–101, Aug. 2002, doi: 10.1016/S1389-0344(02)00016-3.

42. R. Palanivelu, S. Kalainathan, and A. Ruban Kumar, "Characterization studies on plasma sprayed (AT/HA) bi-layered nano ceramics coating on biomedical commercially pure titanium dental implant," *Ceramics International*, vol. 40, no. 6, pp. 7745–7751, 2014, doi: 10.1016/j.ceramint.2013.12.116.

43. C. C. Shih, C. M. Shih, Y. Y. Su, L. H. J. Su, M. S. Chang, and S. J. Lin, "Effect of surface oxide properties on corrosion resistance of 316L stainless steel for biomedical applications," *Corrosion Science*, vol. 46, no. 2, pp. 427–441, 2004, doi: 10.1016/S0010-938X (03)00148-3.

44. M. M. Dewidar, K. A. Khalil, and J. K. Lim, "Processing and mechanical properties of porous 316L stainless steel for biomedical applications," *Transactions of Nonferrous Metals Society of China (English Edition)*, vol. 17, no. 3, pp. 468–473, Jun. 2007, doi: 10.1016/S1003-6326(07)60117-4.

45. F. Kafkas and T. Ebel, "Metallurgical and mechanical properties of Ti-24Nb-4Zr-8Sn alloy fabricated by metal injection molding," *Journal of Alloys and Compounds*, vol. 617, pp. 359–366, Dec. 2014, doi: 10.1016/j.jallcom.2014.07.168.

46. Y. R. Sui, Y. P. Song, S. Q. Lv, Z. W. Wang, B. Yao, and J. H. Yang, "Enhancing of the rapid thermal annealing for the p-type transition in sodium-doped ZnCdO thin films using RF reactive magnetron sputtering synthesis," *Journal of Alloys and Compounds*, vol. 701, pp. 689–697, 2017, doi: 10.1016/j.jallcom.2017.01.141.

47. Y. Okazaki and E. Gotoh, "Comparison of metal release from various metallic biomaterials in vitro," *Biomaterials*, vol. 26, no. 1, pp. 11–21, Jan. 2005, doi: 10.1016/j.biomaterials.2004.02.005.

48. R. C. Starling et al., "Results of the post-U.S. food and drug administration-approval study with a continuous flow left ventricular assist device as a bridge to heart transplantation: A prospective study using the INTERMACS (Interagency Registry for Mechanically Assisted Circulatory Support)," *Journal of the American College of Cardiology*, vol. 57, no. 19, pp. 1890–1898, May 2011, doi: 10.1016/j.jacc.2010.10.062.

49. T. Habijan et al., "The biocompatibility of dense and porous Nickel-Titanium produced by selective laser melting," *Materials Science and Engineering C*, vol. 33, no. 1, pp. 419–426, Jan. 2013, doi: 10.1016/j.msec.2012.09.008.

50. S. Y. Yu and J. R. Scully, "Corrosion and passivity of Ti-13% Nb-13% Zr in comparison to other biomedical implant alloys," *Corrosion (Houston)*, vol. 53, no. 12, pp. 965–976, 1997, doi: 10.5006/1.3290281.

51. M. Geetha, A. K. Singh, R. Asokamani, and A. K. Gogia, "Ti based biomaterials, the ultimate choice for orthopaedic implants - A review," *Progress in Materials Science*, vol. 54, no. 3. pp. 397–425, May 2009, doi: 10.1016/j.pmatsci.2008.06.004.

52. J. Vaithilingam, S. Kilsby, R. D. Goodridge, S. D. R. Christie, S. Edmondson, and R. J. M. Hague, "Functionalisation of Ti6Al4V components fabricated using selective laser melting with a bioactive compound," *Materials Science and Engineering C*, vol. 46, pp. 52–61, Jan. 2015, doi: 10.1016/j.msec.2014.10.015.

53. L. jian CHEN, T. LI, Y. min LI, H. HE, and Y. hua HU, "Porous titanium implants fabricated by metal injection molding," *Transactions of Nonferrous Metals Society of China (English Edition)*, vol. 19, no. 5, pp. 1174–1179, Oct. 2009, doi: 10.1016/S1003-6326(08)60424-0.

54. C. S. S. de Oliveira, S. Griza, M. V. de Oliveira, A. A. Ribeiro, and Mô. B. Leite, "Study of the porous Ti35Nb alloy processing parameters for implant applications," *Powder Technology*, vol. 281, pp. 91–98, Sep. 2015, doi: 10.1016/j.powtec.2015.03.014.

55. J. E. G. González and J. C. Mirza-Rosca, "Study of the corrosion behavior of titanium and some of its alloys for biomedical and dental implant applications," *Journal of Electroanalytical Chemistry*, vol. 471, no. 2, pp. 109–115, Aug. 1999, doi: 10.1016/S0022-0728(99)00260-0.

56. K. v. Rajagopalan, "Molybdenum: An essential trace element in human nutrition," *Annual Review of Nutrition*, vol. 8. pp. 401–427, 1988, doi: 10.1146/annurev.nu.08.070188.002153.

57. W. F. Ho, C. H. Cheng, C. H. Pan, S. C. Wu, and H. C. Hsu, "Structure, mechanical properties and grindability of dental Ti-10Zr-X alloys," *Materials Science and Engineering C*, vol. 29, no. 1, pp. 36–43, Jan. 2009, doi: 10.1016/j.msec.2008.05.004.

58. Y. H. Kwon, H. J. Seol, H. il Kim, K. J. Hwang, S. G. Lee, and K. H. Kim, "Effect of acidic fluoride solution on β titanium alloy wire," *Journal of Biomedical Materials Research - Part B Applied Biomaterials*, vol. 73, no. 2, pp. 285–290, May 2005, doi: 10.1002/jbm.b.30212.

59. H. C. Hsu, C. H. Pan, S. C. Wu, and W. F. Ho, "Structure and grindability of cast Ti-5Cr-xFe alloys," *Journal of Alloys and Compounds*, vol. 474, no. 1–2, pp. 578–583, Apr. 2009, doi: 10.1016/j.jallcom.2008.07.003.

60. E. B. Taddei, V. A. R. Henriques, C. R. M. Silva, and C. A. A. Cairo, "Production of new titanium alloy for orthopedic implants," *Materials Science and Engineering C*, vol. 24, no. 5, pp. 683–687, Nov. 2004, doi: 10.1016/j.msec.2004.08.011.
61. M. Nakagawa, S. Matsuya, T. Shiraishi, and M. Ohta, "Effect of fluoride concentration and pH on corrosion behavior of titanium for dental use," *Journal of Dental Research*, vol. 78, no. 9, pp. 1568–1572, 1999, doi: 10.1177/00220345990780091201.
62. M. Dadfar, M. H. Fathi, F. Karimzadeh, M. R. Dadfar, and A. Saatchi, "Effect of TIG welding on corrosion behavior of 316L stainless steel," *Materials Letters*, vol. 61, no. 11–12, pp. 2343–2346, May 2007, doi: 10.1016/j.matlet.2006.09.008.
63. Q. Chen and G. A. Thouas, "Metallic implant biomaterials," *Materials Science and Engineering R: Reports*, vol. 87. Elsevier Ltd, pp. 1–57, 2015, doi: 10.1016/j.mser.2014.10.001.
64. A. Fukuda et al., "Osteoinduction of porous Ti implants with a channel structure fabricated by selective laser melting," *Acta Biomaterialia*, vol. 7, no. 5, pp. 2327–2336, May 2011, doi: 10.1016/j.actbio.2011.01.037.
65. Q. Chen, S. Liang, and G. A. Thouas, "Elastomeric biomaterials for tissue engineering," *Progress in Polymer Science*, vol. 38, no. 3–4. Elsevier Ltd, pp. 584–671, 2013, doi: 10.1016/j.progpolymsci.2012.05.003.
66. N. Kurgan, "Effect of porosity and density on the mechanical and microstructural properties of sintered 316L stainless steel implant materials," *Materials and Design*, vol. 55, pp. 235–241, 2014, doi: 10.1016/j.matdes.2013.09.058.
67. K. S. Katti, "Biomaterials in total joint replacement," *Colloids and Surfaces B: Biointerfaces*, vol. 39, no. 3, pp. 133–142, Dec. 2004, doi: 10.1016/j.colsurfb.2003.12.002.
68. C. Xie, "Bio-inspired nanofunctionalisation of biomaterial surfaces: A review," *Biosurface and Biotribology*, vol. 5, no. 3. Institution of Engineering and Technology, pp. 83–92, Sep. 01, 2019, doi: 10.1049/bsbt.2019.0009.
69. L. E. Murr, S. M. Gaytan, E. Martinez, F. Medina, and R. B. Wicker, "Next generation orthopaedic implants by additive manufacturing using electron beam melting," *International Journal of Biomaterials*, 2012, doi: 10.1155/2012/245727.
70. M. Niinomi, "Recent metallic materials for biomedical applications," *Metallurgical and Materials Transactions A*, vol. 33, no. 3, pp. 477–486, Mar. 2002, doi: 10.1007/s11661-002-0109-2.
71. C. Schmidleithner, S. Malferrari, R. Palgrave, D. Bomze, M. Schwentenwein, and D. M. Kalaskar, "Application of high resolution DLP stereolithography for fabrication of tricalcium phosphate scaffolds for bone regeneration," *Biomedical Materials (Bristol)*, vol. 14, no. 4, p. 45018, Jun. 2019, doi: 10.1088/1748-605X/ab279d.
72. H. P. Tang, G. Y. Yang, W. P. Jia, W. W. He, S. L. Lu, and M. Qian, "Additive manufacturing of a high niobium-containing titanium aluminide alloy by selective electron beam melting," *Materials Science and Engineering A*, vol. 636, pp. 103–107, Jun. 2015, doi: 10.1016/j.msea.2015.03.079.
73. R. Wauthle et al., "Additively manufactured porous tantalum implants," *Acta Biomaterialia*, vol. 14, pp. 217–225, Mar. 2015, doi: 10.1016/j.actbio.2014.12.003.
74. R. Wauthle et al., "Revival of pure titanium for dynamically loaded porous implants using additive manufacturing," *Materials Science and Engineering C*, vol. 54, pp. 94–100, Sep. 2015, doi: 10.1016/j.msec.2015.05.001.
75. H. J. Rack and J. I. Qazi, "Titanium alloys for biomedical applications," *Materials Science and Engineering C*, vol. 26, no. 8, pp. 1269–1277, Sep. 2006, doi: 10.1016/j.msec.2005.08.032.
76. X. Y. Zhang, G. Fang, and J. Zhou, "Additively manufactured scaffolds for bone tissue engineering and the prediction of their mechanical behavior: A review," *Materials*, vol. 10, no. 1. MDPI AG, p. 50, Jan. 10, 2017, doi: 10.3390/ma10010050.

77. S. R. Dutta, D. Passi, P. Singh, and A. Bhuibhar, "Ceramic and non-ceramic hydroxy-apatite as a bone graft material: A brief review," *Irish Journal of Medical Science*, vol. 184, no. 1. Springer-Verlag London Ltd, pp. 101–106, Mar. 01, 2015, doi: 10.1007/s11845-014-1199-8.

78. M. H. Fathi, A. Hanifi, and V. Mortazavi, "Preparation and bioactivity evaluation of bone-like hydroxyapatite nanopowder," *Journal of Materials Processing Technology*, vol. 202, no. 1–3, pp. 536–542, Jun. 2008, doi: 10.1016/j.jmatprotec.2007.10.004.

79. S. B. H. Farid, *Bioceramics: For Materials Science and Engineering*. Elsevier, 2018.

80. H. Rojbani, M. Nyan, K. Ohya, and S. Kasugai, "Evaluation of the osteoconduc-tivity of α-tricalcium phosphate, β-tricalcium phosphate, and hydroxyapatite com-bined with or without simvastatin in rat calvarial defect," *Journal of Biomedical Materials Research – Part A*, vol. 98 A, no. 4, pp. 488–498, Sep. 2011, doi: 10.1002/jbm.a.33117.

81. M. N. Rahaman, "Bioactive ceramics and glasses for tissue engineering," in *Tissue Engineering Using Ceramics and Polymers*: Second Edition, Elsevier Inc., 2014, pp. 67–114.

82. V. Sollazzo et al., "Zirconium oxide coating improves implant osseointegration in vivo," *Dental Materials*, vol. 24, no. 3, pp. 357–361, Mar. 2008, doi: 10.1016/j.dental.2007.06.003.

83. R. S. Pillai, M. Frasnelli, and V. M. Sglavo, "HA/β-TCP plasma sprayed coatings on Ti substrate for biomedical applications," *Ceramics International*, vol. 44, no. 2, pp. 1328–1333, Feb. 2018, doi: 10.1016/j.ceramint.2017.08.113.

84. Y. Wang et al., "Osteoblastic cell response on fluoridated hydroxyapatite coatings," *Acta Biomaterialia*, vol. 3, no. 2, pp. 191–197, Mar. 2007, doi: 10.1016/j.actbio.2006.10.002.

85. A. Sola, D. Bellucci, V. Cannillo, and A. Cattini, "Bioactive glass coatings: A review," *Surface Engineering*, vol. 27, no. 8. Taylor & Francis, pp. 560–572, Sep. 2011, doi: 10.1179/1743294410Y.0000000008.

86. T. L. A. Ae, S. S. Alameer, A. E. Thekra, I. Ae, A. Y. Alhijazi, and A. M. Geetha, "In vivo studies of the ceramic coated titanium alloy for enhanced osseointegration in den-tal applications," Springer, doi: 10.1007/s10856-008-3479-1.

87. G. Mitteramskogler et al., "Light curing strategies for lithography-based additive manu-facturing of customized ceramics," *Additive Manufacturing*, vol. 1, pp. 110–118, Oct. 2014, doi: 10.1016/j.addma.2014.08.003.

88. Z. Liu et al., "Additive manufacturing of hydroxyapatite bone scaffolds via digital light processing and in vitro compatibility," *Ceramics International*, vol. 45, no. 8, pp. 11079–11086, Jun. 2019, doi: 10.1016/j.ceramint.2019.02.195.

89. P. F. Manicone, P. Rossi Iommetti, and L. Raffaelli, "An overview of zirconia ceram-ics: Basic properties and clinical applications," *Journal of Dentistry*, vol. 35, no. 11. Elsevier, pp. 819–826, Nov. 01, 2007, doi: 10.1016/j.jdent.2007.07.008.

90. B. Zhang et al., "Porous bioceramics produced by inkjet 3D printing: Effect of print-ing ink formulation on the ceramic macro and micro porous architectures control," *Composites Part B: Engineering*, vol. 155, pp. 112–121, Dec. 2018, doi: 10.1016/j.compositesb.2018.08.047.

91. B. Lechner et al., "Additive manufacturing of bioactive glasses and silicate bioceramics thermal shock behavior of high temperature ceramics View project CD-Laboratory for photo polymers in digital and restorative dentistry view project additive manufacturing of bioactive glasses and silicate bioceramics," *Article in Journal of Ceramic Science and Technology*, pp. 6–8, 2015, doi: 10.4416/JCST2015-00001.

92. C. Shuai, Z. Mao, Z. Han, S. Peng, and Z. Li, "Fabrication and characterization of cal-cium silicate scaffolds for tissue engineering," *Journal of Mechanics in Medicine and Biology*, vol. 14, no. 4, Jul. 2014, doi: 10.1142/S0219519414500493.

93. E. Vorndran et al., "3D powder printing of β-tricalcium phosphate ceramics using dif-ferent strategies," *Advanced Engineering Materials*, vol. 10, no. 12, pp. B67–B71, Dec. 2008, doi: 10.1002/adem.200800179.

94. R. Felzmann et al., "Lithography-based additive manufacturing of cellular ceramic structures," in *Advanced Engineering Materials*, Dec. 2012, vol. 14, no. 12, pp. 1052–1058, doi: 10.1002/adem.201200010.

95. X. Liu and P. X. Ma, "Polymeric scaffolds for bone tissue engineering," *Annals of Biomedical Engineering*, vol. 32, no. 3, pp. 477–486, Mar. 2004, doi: 10.1023/B:ABM E.0000017544.36001.8e.

96. K. Jha, R. Kataria, J. Verma, and S. Pradhan, "Potential biodegradable matrices and fiber treatment for green composites: A review," *AIMS Materials Science*, vol. 6, no. 1. AIMS Press, pp. 119–138, 2019, doi: 10.3934/matersci.2019.1.119.

97. A. Banerjee, K. Chatterjee, and G. Madras, "Enzymatic degradation of polymers: A brief review," *Materials Science and Technology (United Kingdom)*, vol. 30, no. 5. Maney Publishing, pp. 567–573, 2014, doi: 10.1179/1743284713Y.0000000503.

98. H. Jia, S. Y. Gu, and K. Chang, "3D printed self-expandable vascular stents from bio-degradable shape memory polymer," *Advances in Polymer Technology*, vol. 37, no. 8, pp. 3222–3228, Dec. 2018, doi: 10.1002/adv.22091.

99. Y. K. Yeon et al., "New concept of 3D printed bone clip (polylactic acid/hydroxyapatite/silk composite) for internal fixation of bone fractures," *Journal of Biomaterials Science, Polymer Edition*, vol. 29, no. 7–9, pp. 894–906, Jun. 2018, doi: 10.1080/09205063.2017.1384199.

100. Z. Z. Zhang et al., "Role of scaffold mean pore size in meniscus regeneration," *Acta Biomaterialia*, vol. 43, pp. 314–326, Oct. 2016, doi: 10.1016/j.actbio.2016.07.050.

101. M. Vert, "Polymeric biomaterials: Strategies of the past vs. strategies of the future," *Progress in Polymer Science (Oxford)*, vol. 32, no. 8–9. Pergamon, pp. 755–761, Aug. 01, 2007, doi: 10.1016/j.progpolymsci.2007.05.006.

102. S. Singh and S. Ramakrishna, "Biomedical applications of additive manufacturing: Present and future," *Current Opinion in Biomedical Engineering*, vol. 2. Elsevier B.V., pp. 105–115, Jun. 01, 2017, doi: 10.1016/j.cobme.2017.05.006.

103. J. Kim and T. S. Creasy, "Selective laser sintering characteristics of nylon 6/clay-reinforced nanocomposite," *Polymer Testing*, vol. 23, no. 6, pp. 629–636, Sep. 2004, doi: 10.1016/j.polymertesting.2004.01.014.

104. J. Edgar and S. Tint, "'Additive manufacturing technologies: 3D printing, rapid proto-typing, and direct digital manufacturing', 2nd Edition," *Johnson Matthey Technology Review*, vol. 59, no. 3, pp. 193–198, Aug. 2015, doi: 10.1595/205651315x688406.

105. J. M. Sobral, S. G. Caridade, R. A. Sousa, J. F. Mano, and R. L. Reis, "Three-dimensional plotted scaffolds with controlled pore size gradients: Effect of scaffold geometry on mechanical performance and cell seeding efficiency," *Acta Biomaterialia*, vol. 7, no. 3, pp. 1009–1018, Mar. 2011, doi: 10.1016/j.actbio.2010.11.003.

106. J. Korpela, A. Kokkari, H. Korhonen, M. Malin, T. Narhi, and J. Seppalea, "Biodegradable and bioactive porous scaffold structures prepared using fused deposition modeling," *Journal of Biomedical Materials Research - Part B Applied Biomaterials*, vol. 101, no. 4, pp. 610–619, May 2013, doi: 10.1002/jbm.b.32863.

107. B. Cullity and S.R. Stock, *Elements of X-ray Diffraction*, Pearson; 3rd edition (6 March 2001).

108. P. Yu, A. Jonker, and M. Gruber, "Molecular basis of protein structure in proanthocyan-idin and anthocyanin-enhanced Lc-transgenic alfalfa in relation to nutritive value using synchrotron-radiation FTIR microspectroscopy: A novel approach," *Spectrochimica Acta - Part A: Molecular and Biomolecular Spectroscopy*, vol. 73, no. 5, pp. 846–853, Sep. 2009, doi: 10.1016/j.saa.2009.04.006.

109. T. S. Sampath Kumar, "Physical and chemical characterization of biomaterials," in *Characterization of Biomaterials*, Elsevier Inc., 2013, pp. 11–47.

110. S. Kassi, K. Didriche, C. Lauzin, X.D.G.D.E Vaernewijckb, A. Rizopoulos, and M. Herman, "Demonstration of cavity enhanced FTIR spectroscopy using a femtosecond laser absorption source," *Spectrochimica Acta - Part A: Molecular and Biomolecular Spectroscopy*, vol. 75, no. 1, pp. 142–145, Jan. 2010, doi: 10.1016/j.saa.2009.09.058.

111. M. Omidi et al., "Characterization of biomaterials," in *Biomaterials for Oral and Dental Tissue Engineering*, Elsevier Inc., 2017, pp. 97–115.

112. S. Ahuja and S. Scypinski, *Handbook of Modern Pharmaceutical Analysis,* vol. 10, 2010, Academic Press, USA.

113. L. O. F. de Araujo, O. Barreto, A. A. M. de Mendonça, and R. França, "Assessment of the degree of conversion in light-curing orthodontic resins with various viscosities," *Applied Adhesion Science*, vol. 3, no. 1, pp. 1–7, Dec. 2015, doi: 10.1186/s40563-015-0055-z.

114. J. Durner, J. Obermaier, M. Draenert, and N. Ilie, "Correlation of the degree of conversion with the amount of elutable substances in nano-hybrid dental composites," *Dental Materials*, vol. 28, no. 11, pp. 1146–1153, Nov. 2012, doi: 10.1016/j.dental.2012.08.006.

115. D. Bazin et al., "Diffraction techniques and vibrational spectroscopy opportunities to characterise bones," *Osteoporosis International*, vol. 20, no. 6, pp. 1065–1075, Jun. 2009, doi: 10.1007/s00198-009-0868-3.

116. H. G. Brittain, *Characterization of Pharmaceutical Compounds in the Solid State*, vol. 10, no. C. Academic Press, 2011.

117. S. Bose, S. Vahabzadeh, and A. Bandyopadhyay, "Bone tissue engineering using 3D printing," *Materials Today*, vol. 16, no. 12. Elsevier, pp. 496–504, Dec. 01, 2013, doi: 10.1016/j.mattod.2013.11.017.

118. K. Ikemura, K. Ichizawa, Y. Jogetsu, and T. Endo, "Synthesis of a novel camphorquinone derivative having acylphosphine oxide group, characterization by UV-VIS spectroscopy and evaluation of photopolymerization performance," *Dental Materials Journal*, vol. 29, no. 2, pp. 122–131, 2010, doi: 10.4012/dmj.2009-026.

119. D. E. Newbury and N. W. M. Ritchie, "Is scanning electron microscopy/energy dispersive X-ray spectrometry (SEM/EDS) quantitative?" *Scanning*, vol. 35, no. 3, pp. 141–168, May 2013, doi: 10.1002/sca.21041.

120. S. Zaefferer, "On the formation mechanisms, spatial resolution and intensity of backscatter Kikuchi patterns," *Ultramicroscopy*, vol. 107, no. 2–3, pp. 254–266, 2007, doi: 10.1016/j.ultramic.2006.08.007.

121. S. Zaefferer and N. N. Elhami, "Theory and application of electron channelling contrast imaging under controlled diffraction conditions," *Acta Materialia*, vol. 75, pp. 20–50, Aug. 2014, doi: 10.1016/j.actamat.2014.04.018.

122. I. Gutierrez-Urrutia and D. Raabe, "Influence of Al content and precipitation state on the mechanical behavior of austenitic high-Mn low-density steels," *Scripta Materialia*, vol. 68, no. 6, pp. 343–347, Mar. 2013, doi: 10.1016/j.scriptamat.2012.08.038.

123. S. Zaefferer, "New developments of computer-aided crystallographic analysis in transmission electron microscopy," *Journal of Applied Crystallography*, vol. 33, no. 1, pp. 10–25, 2000, doi: 10.1107/S0021889899010894.

124. D. Williams and C. Carter, *Transmission Electron Microscopy. A Textbook for Materials Science*. Springer, 2009, Accessed: Sep. 27, 2020. [Online].

125. A. Svensson et al., "Bacterial cellulose as a potential scaffold for tissue engineering of cartilage," *Biomaterials*, vol. 26, no. 4, pp. 419–431, Feb. 2005, doi: 10.1016/j.biomaterials.2004.02.049.

126. G. Haugstad, *Atomic Force Microscopy: Understanding Basic Modes and Advanced Applications*. 2012, Wiley.

127. H. Reza Rezaie, H. Beigi Rizi, M. M. Rezaei Khamseh, and A. Öchsner, "Primary information about biomaterials," *Advanced Structured Materials*, vol. 123, Springer, 2020, pp. 1–30.

128. J. Park and R. S. Lakes, *Biomaterials: An Introduction*. 2007, Third Edition, Springer.

129. A. Rosengren, L. Faxius, N. Tanaka, M. Watanabe, and L. M. Bjursten, "Comparison of implantation and cytotoxicity testing for initially toxic biomaterials," *Wiley Online Library*, vol. 75, no. 1, pp. 115–122, Oct. 2005, doi: 10.1002/jbm.a.30431.

130. M. Robinson, T. Nusair, E. Fletcher, H. R.- Toxicology, and undefined 1990, "A review of the Buehler guinea pig skin sensitization test and its use in a risk assessment process for human skin sensitization," Elsevier, Accessed: Jun. 12, 2021. [Online]. Available: https://www.sciencedirect.com/science/article/pii/0300483X90900126.

131. B. Ratner, A. Hoffman, F. Schoen, and J. Lemons, *Biomaterials Science: An Introduction to Materials in Medicine,* Second Edition, Academic Press USA, 2004.

132. M. Razavi et al., "Nanobiomaterials in periodontal tissue engineering," in *Nanobiomaterials in Hard Tissue Engineering: Applications of Nanobiomaterials,* Elsevier Inc., 2016, pp. 323–351.

133. E. Mazza and A. E. Ehret, "Mechanical biocompatibility of highly deformable biomedical materials," *Journal of the Mechanical Behavior of Biomedical Materials,* vol. 48. Elsevier Ltd, pp. 100–124, Aug. 01, 2015, doi: 10.1016/j.jmbbm.2015.03.023.

134. L. E. Flynn and K. A. Woodhouse, "Burn dressing biomaterials and tissue engineering," in *Biomedical Materials,* Springer International Publishing, 2021, pp. 537–580.

135. T. Barbin et al., "3D metal printing in dentistry: An in vitro biomechanical comparative study of two additive manufacturing technologies for full-arch implant-supported prostheses," *Journal of the Mechanical Behavior of Biomedical Materials,* vol. 108, p. 103821, Aug. 2020, doi: 10.1016/j.jmbbm.2020.103821.

136. P. Karimipour-Fard, A. H. Behravesh, H. Jones-Taggart, R. Pop-Iliev, and G. Rizvi, "Effects of design, porosity and biodegradation on mechanical and morphological properties of additive-manufactured triply periodic minimal surface scaffolds," *Journal of the Mechanical Behavior of Biomedical Materials,* vol. 112, p. 104064, Dec. 2020, doi: 10.1016/j.jmbbm.2020.104064.

137. K. B. Putra, X. Tian, J. Plott, and A. Shih, "Biaxial test and hyperelastic material models of silicone elastomer fabricated by extrusion-based additive manufacturing for wearable biomedical devices," *Journal of the Mechanical Behavior of Biomedical Materials,* vol. 107, p. 103733, Jul. 2020, doi: 10.1016/j.jmbbm.2020.103733.

138. M. Mallik and M. Saha, *Carbon-Based Nanocomposites: Processing, Electronic Properties and Applications,* Springer, 2021, pp. 97–122.

139. G. Sundell, C. Dahlin, M. Andersson, and M. Thuvander, "The bone-implant interface of dental implants in humans on the atomic scale," *Acta Biomaterialia,* vol. 48, pp. 445–450, Jan. 2017, doi: 10.1016/j.actbio.2016.11.044.

140. W. Xiaoyue, L. Brian, S. Furqan, P. Anders, and G. Kathryn, "Atomic-scale osseointegration in human revealed by atom probe tomography," *Frontiers in Bioengineering and Biotechnology,* vol. 4, 2016, doi: 10.3389/conf.fbioe.2016.01.00768.

141. X. Wang, R. M. S. Schofield, M. H. Nesson, and A. Devaraj, "Atomic elemental tomography of heavy element biomaterials," *Journal of Insect Physiology,* vol. 49, no. 1, p. 31, 2021, doi: 10.1017/S1431927617004068.

142. S. il Baik, D. Isheim, and D. N. Seidman, "Systematic approaches for targeting an atom-probe tomography sample fabricated in a thin TEM specimen: Correlative structural, chemical and 3-D reconstruction analyses," *Ultramicroscopy,* vol. 184, pp. 284–292, Jan. 2018, doi: 10.1016/j.ultramic.2017.10.007.

143. B. Gault, M. P. Moody, J. M. Cairney, and S. P. Ringer, "Specimen preparation," in *Springer Series in Materials Science,* vol. 160, Springer Science and Business Media Deutschland GmbH, 2012, pp. 71–110.

144. M. E. Greene, T. J. Prosa, J. A. Panitz, D. J. Larson, and T. F. Kelly, "Development of atom probe tomography for biological materials," *Microscopy and Microanalysis,* vol. 15, no. SUPPL. 2, pp. 582–583, Jul. 2009, doi: 10.1017/S1431927609098511.

4 Cellulose – A Sustainable Material for Biomedical Applications

N. Vignesh and K. Chandraraj
Indian Institute of Technology Madras

S.P. Suriyaraj
PSG College of Technology Coimbatore

R. Selvakumar
PSG Institute of Advanced Studies Coimbatore

CONTENTS

4.1 INTRODUCTION

Cellulose is the most abundantly available natural biopolymer on earth. The interesting properties of cellulose make it highly suitable for versatile applications in diverse fields. Cellulose is predominantly available in renewable biomass resources like plants, woods, agricultural residues, energy crops, etc. Recent works on cellulose have highlighted its extraction from other attractive resources like bacteria, algae,

DOI: 10.1201/9781003286806-4

tunicates, etc. [1]. Though cellulose is a simple polysaccharide consisting of glucose monomers linked by the β (1–4) linkage, it exists as strong and recalcitrant fibers with high tensile strength and ductility. The structured organization of cellulose in the form of bundles of microfibers imparts high crystallinity. The linear chains of cellulose are assembled into microfibers through numerous intermolecular and intramolecular hydrogen bonding networks. Moreover, cellulose chains are stacked in parallel directions thereby making the structure highly ordered and resilient [2]. Interestingly, cellulose is structurally anisotropic due to the orientations of hydroxyl and hydrophobic groups along the equatorial and axial directions respectively [3]. The native form of cellulose consists of uniaxial and parallel arrangement of cellulose microfibrils and it is termed polymorph I. In the plant cell wall, cellulose is distributed with amorphous components like lignin and hemicellulose. Moreover, the cellulose microfibers are stacked in the form of layers and the lignin and hemicellulose act as adhesive components holding the cellulose fibers tightly. Besides, the presence of amorphous components interferes with the ordered structure of cellulose [4]. As a result, the supramolecular structure of cellulose consists of alternating crystalline and amorphous domains depending on the cellulose polymorph. Cellulose polymorph II is present in the amorphous domain and it consists of cellulose chains stacked in the antiparallel direction with disordered hydrogen bonding [1]. Apart from the exquisite structural integrity of cellulose, it is associated with other promising features like biocompatibility, biodegradability, low toxicity,etc. Considering the widespread availability and potential features of cellulose, it is the most preferred source for the production of various biomaterials and nanocomposites to meet some of the indispensable challenges in biomedical research [5]. Different forms of cellulose like bacterial cellulose (BC), cellulose nanofibrils (CNFs), cellulose nanocrystals (CNCs) and cellulose derivatives have been produced commercially. Besides, they have been extensively used to develop interesting nanostructures like hydrogels, aerogels and membranes for biomedical applications (Table 4.1). The production of cellulosic materials is associated with overwhelming advantages like renewability and sustainability [6]. The following sections describe the production of various forms of cellulosic materials and their potential applications in biomedical research.

4.2 CELLULOSIC MATERIALS

4.2.1 BACTERIAL CELLULOSE

BC is naturally synthesized by Gram-negative bacteria such as *Gluconacetobacter*, *Agrobacterium*, *Rhizobium*, *Pseudomonas* and *Alcaligenes* and secreted in the form of a pellicle or mat in the extracellular medium [23]. The cultivation of *Gluconacetobacter xylinum* in the Hestrin–Schramm (HS) medium containing glucose, peptone, yeast extract, Na_2HPO_4 and citric acid is sufficient to produce BC. In addition, the production of BC is carried out using other carbon sources such as maltose, fructose, mannitol, xylose, sucrose and galactose [24]. The nanostructure of BC can be varied by altering the culturing conditions (Figure 4.1a). For instance, the growth of *Komagataeibacter xylinus* under static conditions produces BC in the

TABLE 4.1

Cellulose and Cellulose-Based Derivatives for Biomedical Applications

Type of Cellulose	Cellulose Source	Method of Preparation	Applications	References
Bacterial cellulose (BC)	Komagataeibacter xylinus	Microbial synthesis in corn steep liquor with a fructose medium	BC hydrogel cross-linked with dextran showed accelerated wound healing in vivo and skin maturation	[7]
	Acetobacter xylinum	Microbial synthesis in corn steep liquor	A BC/poly(2-hydroxyethyl methacrylate) composite prepared by in situ ultraviolet radical polymerization was compatible with mouse mesenchymal stem cells	[8]
	Gluconacetobacterxylinus	Microbial synthesis in a Hestrin–Schramm medium	A calcium-filled BC hydrogel prepared by in vitro bio-mineralization was an efficient scaffold for bone tissue engineering	[9]
	BC pellicle	Solvent exchange treatment	An ionic conductor was fabricated using BC and polymerizable deep eutectic solvents for detecting body movements	[10]
Cellulose nanocrystal (CNC)	Microcrystalline cellulose	Acid hydrolysis, ion-exchange and ultrasonic treatments	Incorporation of CNC and reduced graphene oxide in a polylactic acid film produced an antibacterial wound dressing material	[11]
	Cotton fiber	Acid hydrolysis and surface cationization	Metal ion (Ca^{2+}) cross-linking of cationic CNC and sodium alginate produced a double membrane hydrogel for the sustained release of human epidermal growth factor	[12]
	Cotton Whatman ashless filter aid	Acid hydrolysis and magnetic co-extrusion	An injectable CNC hydrogel was produced by cross-linking with poly(oligoethylene glycol methacrylate) for subcutaneous drug delivery	[13]
	Bleached softwood pulp	Acid hydrolysis and high-pressure homogenization	Tannic acid-coated CNC was cross-linked with polyacrylic acid to produce a self-adhesive ionic hydrogel for detecting human body movements	[14]

(Continued)

TABLE 4.1 (*Continued*)
Cellulose and Cellulose-Based Derivatives for Biomedical Applications

Type of Cellulose	Cellulose Source	Method of Preparation	Applications	References
Cellulose nanofibril (CNF)	Bleached hardwood Kraft pulp	TEMPO oxidation and room temperature homogenization	Incorporation of mercaptopyrimidine-conjugated gold nanoclusters into TEMPO-oxidized CNF for producing antibacterial wound dressing material	[15]
	Basswood	Sodium chlorite bleaching, chemical cross-linking and degassing	CNF extracted from wood was cross-linked with polyacrylamide to produce a strong, anisotropic and conductive hydrogel for nanofluidic applications	[16]
	Softwood pulp	Enzymatic pretreatment, mechanical shearing and high-pressure homogenization	Formulation of a hydrogel ink by cross-linking CNF with tyramine-modified xylan for producing scaffold constructs by 3D printing	[17]
	Softwood pulp	TEMPO oxidation and ultrasonic treatment	3D printing of TEMPO–CNFs and titanium carbide produced flexible fiber for use as a sensitive strain sensor	[18]
Cellulose derivatives	Cellulose acetate	Phase inversion, alkali treatment and covalent immobilization	Production of a resveratrol-immobilized cellulose acetate membrane for facilitating the proliferation of pre-osteoblastic MC3T3-E1 cells and improvement of osseointegration	[19]
	Cellulose sulfate	Orifice polymerization	Sustained release of 5-aminosalicylic acid using a polyphosphate-modified microcapsule containing cellulose sulfate and chitosan hydrochloride	[20]
	Cellulose nitrate	Solvent evaporation and self-assembly	Fabrication of a patterned photonic nitrocellulose array containing silicon dioxide nanoparticles for ultrasensitive detection of nucleic acids	[21]
	Carboxymethyl cellulose	Periodate oxidation and biphasic solvent system	Hydrogel produced by the cross-linking of dialdehyde carboxymethyl cellulose with collagen for supporting the adhesion and proliferation of L929 fibroblasts	[22]

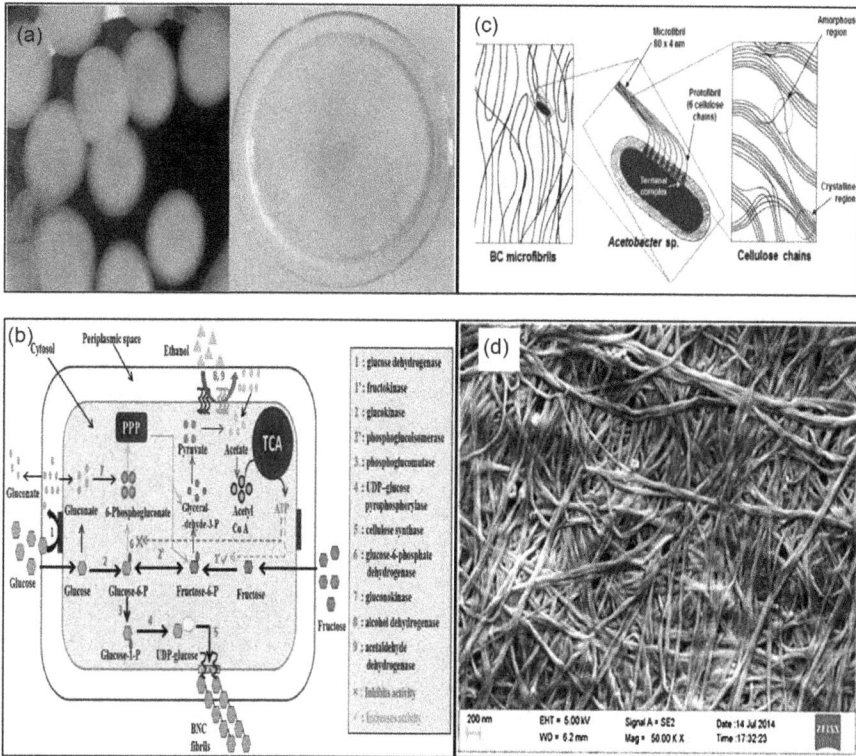

FIGURE 4.1 (a) BC produced in the form of a pellicle (reproduced with copyright permission from the American Chemical Society [26]) and a mat (reproduced with copyright permission from Elsevier[27]), as a result of varying culture conditions. (b) Metabolism for the production of BC in bacteria. (Reproduced with permission from Elsevier [28].)(c) Secretion of protofibrils from bacteria and the formation of BC fibers. (Reproduced with copyright permission from Elsevier [29].)(d) Microstructure of BC viewed by SEM. (Reproduced with copyright permission from Elsevier [28].)

form of a mat. However, BC in the form of a pellicle is obtained under mild agitation of the culture [25].

Unlike cellulose present in plants, BC is associated with high purity (Table 4.2). Furthermore, other interesting features of BC like high hydrophilicity, high crystallinity, high degree of polymerization, high biodegradability and low toxicity complement its facile production process [29].

The synthesis of BC proceeds through a bottom-up approach wherein the glucose monomers taken up by the bacteria are assembled into cellulose through metabolic pathways inside the cell (Figure 4.1b). Initially, glucose is phosphorylated to glucose-6-phosphate by glucokinase. The isomerization of glucose-6-phosphate to glucose-1-phosphate is catalyzed by phosphoglucomutase. Further, glucose-1-phosphate is converted into uridine diphosphate glucose (UDPG) by UDPG pyrophosphorylase. The polymerization of glucose into cellulose is finally catalyzed by cellulose synthase

TABLE 4.2

Overview of the Production Methods and Properties of Cellulosic Materials

Cellulosic material	Production	Morphology	Properties	Challenges	References
Bacterial cellulose	Oxidative fermentation by *Acetobacter* species	Sphere-like pellicle and mat	High crystallinity, high degree of polymerization, high porosity and high purity.	Low productivity. Requires large vessels and continuous aeration.	[30]
Cellulose nanocrystal (CNC)	Hydrolysis by concentrated acids	Rod-shaped nanowhiskers	Highly crystalline, enhanced dispersion in water, reinforcing filler in other polymers.	Low production yield, equipment corrosion and significant water usage.	[31]
Cellulose nanofibril (CNF)	Chemical treatment and mechanical disintegration	Aggregated long fibrils with one dimension at the nanoscale	Presence of both crystalline and amorphous regions, a high aspect ratio and a large surface structure.	High energy demand for fibrillation, significant usage of chemicals and difficulty in the separation of individual fibrils	[32]
Cellulose acetate	Acetylation by acetic acid and acetic anhydride	Electrospun membrane	Porous with a high surface area required for the encapsulation of drugs.	Solubility and biodegradability depend on the degree of substitution.	[33]
Cellulose sulfate	Sulfation by a mixture of sulfuric acid, N,N-dimethyl formamide and isopropyl alcohol	Electrospun membrane	High molecular weight and high degree of sulfation required for the purification of viral particles.	Non-specific sulfation of cellulose and the formation of degradation products.	[34]
Cellulose nitrate	Nitration by nitric acid and dichloromethane	Electrospun membrane	Biocompatible at a low nitrogen content (<12%) with a high surface area required for binding of proteins.	Risk of explosive decomposition during the nitration process.	[35]
Carboxymethyl cellulose	Etherification by sodium hydroxide and monochloroacetic acid	Hydrogel or non-woven sheet	Non-toxic, low immunogenic and water-soluble, with high purity and high biodegradability.	Low mechanical properties and thermal stability.	[36]

through the formation of linear β-1,4-glucan chains [30]. The synthesized cellulose present in the form of protofibrils is secreted across the cell wall through transporters (Figure 4.1c). In the extracellular medium, the secreted protofibrils aggregate into microfibrils, which further organize into a desired nanostructure like a pellicle or mat depending on the culture condition [25].The production of BC is simple, as it requires optimum physical conditions like pH, temperature and aeration for the growth of the bacterial strain. Moreover, the secreted BC is treated with alkali to produce cellulose polymorph II for increasing the pore size, surface area and elasticity of the material [37]. Besides, the elevated porosity of BC facilitates its application as a precursor material for aerogel preparation (Figure 4.1d). To improve the properties of BC, *in situ* modification of its structure has been reported in many studies. Unlike an external chemical treatment, *in situ* modification refers to an alteration in the chemical composition of BC through the supplementation of additives in the growth medium. As a result, the desired components are incorporated into the structure of BC during microbial synthesis [38]. BC conjugates produced using additives such as polyvinyl alcohol, hydroxyapatite, chitosan, heparin and dextrin have been used for developing cardiovascular soft tissue, bone regeneration scaffold, antimicrobial membrane, anticoagulant wound dressing material and blood transfusion membrane respectively [29]. Eventhough BC is associated with intriguing properties and environmentally friendly production, the requirements of a large vessel, continuous aeration and longer process time are the major limitations hindering the commercial feasibility (Table 4.2).

4.2.2 Cellulose Nanocrystals

The highly crystalline form of cellulose produced by acid hydrolysis is termed CNC. The generation of CNCs through successive hydrolysis of amorphous regions enhances the crystallinity and mechanical properties of cellulose [39]. CNCs are observed as small nanowhiskers using microscopic imaging. Most of the CNCs are derived from plants through the separation of cellulose from heterogeneous components like hemicellulose and lignin (Figure 4.2a).

Initial steps of cellulose extraction include alkali treatment and bleaching. Further, the cellulose hydrolysis is carried out using concentrated acid under mild conditions to breakdown the cellulose chains into CNCs [44]. During the hydrolysis of cellulose by strong inorganic sulfuric acid, negatively charged sulfate groups are introduced into cellulose. As a result, the prepared CNCs do not aggregate due to electrostatic repulsion (Figure 4.2b). The good dispersion of sulfated CNCs in solution facilitates its use as a reinforcing polymer in various composite materials [45]. The preparation of CNCs is carried out using other inorganic acids like hydrochloric acid, phosphoric acid, nitric acid, hydrobromic acid, etc. CNCs have a small aspect ratio due to the depolymerization of the cellulose fibers by strong acids (Table 4.2). However, the CNCs are covalently modified during the acid treatment [32]. As a result, it is associated with interesting properties for producing composite hydrogel materials with both hydrophobic and hydrophilic polymers. Another interesting property of CNCs is their self-assembly. Above the critical concentration, the randomly dispersed CNCs in solution show coordinated orientation and structured arrangement with the

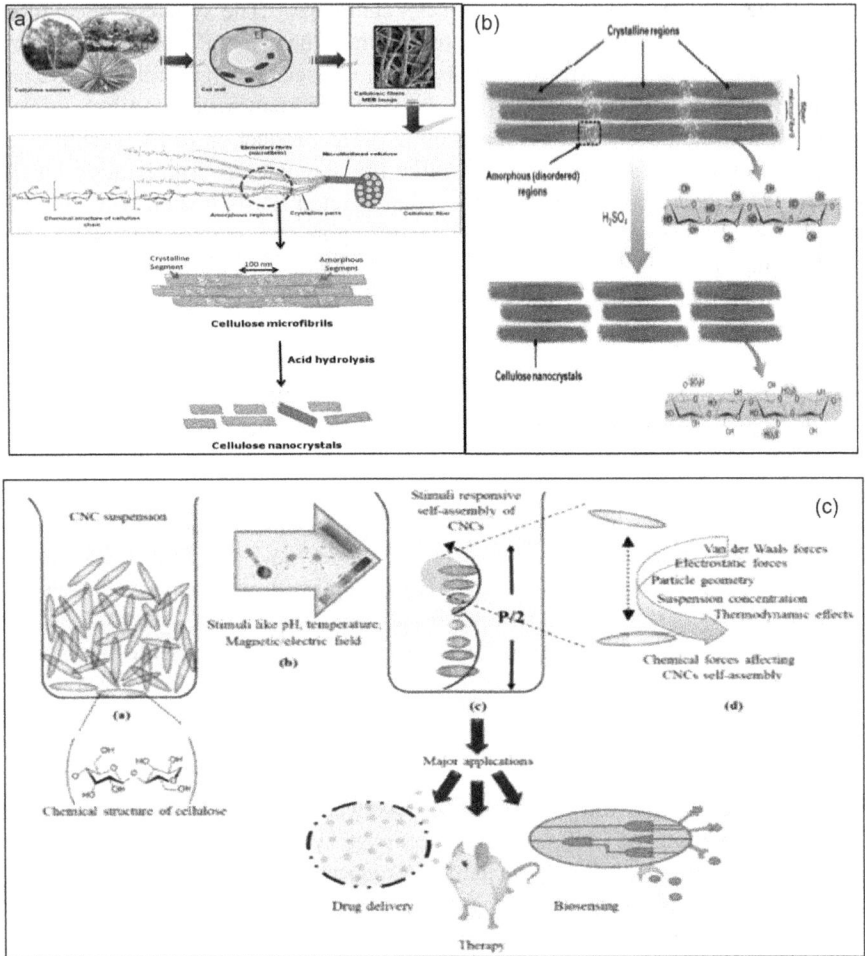

FIGURE 4.2 (a) Mechanism of CNC production from plant biomass. (Reproduced with copyright permission from Elsevier [40,41].)(b) Introduction of sulfate groups in the CNCs during hydrolysis using sulfuric acid. (Reproduced with copyright permission from the American Chemical Society [42].)(c) Phenomenon of self-assembly of CNCs in response to external stimuli. (Reproduced with copyright permission from Elsevier [43].)

application of heat, electric current, magnetic field,etc. (Figure 4.2c). This behavior is mainly attributed to the presence of intrinsic factors in CNCs such as surface properties, polarizability, charge and magnetic dipole[43]. The self-assembly of CNCs is potentially investigated as an attractive principle for the delivery of susceptible drugs. Moreover, it is used for the fabrication of smart biosensors with enhanced detection of enzymes and antibodies [46]. Eventhough CNCs have been used as renewable reinforcement fillers in polymer matrices, the surface modification of cellulose by strong acids reduces its compatibility for biomedical applications (Table 4.2). Besides, the production of CNCs involves major limitations like equipment corrosion, large water usage, low production yield, etc. [31]. However, few of these problems have been addressed by replacing strong inorganic acids with environmentally friendly solvents like ionic liquids, deep eutectic solvents, organic acids, etc. [32].

4.2.3 CELLULOSE NANOFIBRILS

Unlike CNCs, CNFs refer to cellulosic materials consisting of long fibrils with one dimension atleast at the nanoscale. The fibrils are associated with both amorphous and crystalline regions and hence they are less crystalline as compared to CNCs [32]. On the contrary, CNFs have a high aspect ratio and a large surface structure (Table 4.2). The preparation of CNFs involves the initial separation of cellulose from other amorphous components like lignin and hemicellulose (Figure 4.3a), followed by the mechanical disintegration of the complex cellulose structure to individual cellulose fibrils [47].

Chemical treatments such as alkali treatment, bleaching, sodium sulfite pulping and organosolv extraction have been carried out to remove lignin [52]. In the case of agricultural crops such as rice straw, corn stover and sugarcane bagasse, cellulose isolation has been carried out by alkali treatment using sodium hydroxide and bleaching using sodium chlorite [53]. However, highly recalcitrant wood biomass demands extensive delignification by processes such as sulfite pulping and organosolv extraction in addition to the alkali and bleaching treatments [54]. After the complete removal of lignin, the resulting biomass consists of compactly packed cellulose fibers. The breakdown of well-organized cellulose into elementary fibrils requires high mechanical energy. The mechanical disintegration of cellulose is carried out by different methods like high-pressure homogenization, microfluidization, disc refining, etc. [55]. The cellulose suspensions after the fibrillation consist of nanosized fibrils with high affinity and hydrophilicity. As a result, the fibrils show enhanced aggregation and the separation of individual fibrils becomes challenging. To reduce the fibril aggregation and minimize the energy demand for mechanical fibrillation, carboxyl groups are introduced into cellulose through 2,2,6,6-tetramethylpiperidine-1-oxyl radical (TEMPO)-mediated oxidation [56]. The resulting cellulose is obtained as individual fibrils due to the electrostatic repulsion between negatively charged carboxyl groups (Figure 4.3b). In addition, the surface modification of cellulose is carried out by other methods such as amidation and sulfonation [32]. The transmission electron microscopy image of a well-fibrillated CNF extracted from soybean fiber is shown in Figure 4.3c. The CNFs are associated with promising attributes such as biodegradability, biocompatibility, renewability and low toxicity. As compared to CNCs, CNFs have been used independently for the production of different materials like hydrogels, aerogels, membranes, etc. CNFs are cross-linked by metal cations like Ca^{2+}, Zn^{2+}, Cu^{2+}, Al^{3+} and Fe^{3+} to produce flexible and strong hydrogels, as seen in Figure 4.3d. These hydrogels have been shown to be associated with improved elasticity [51]. Although CNFs have been widely utilized in the fabrication of several biomaterials, the quest for an environmentally friendly and cost-effective production is unresolved (Table 4.2). The current CNF production process involves energy-intensive mechanical disintegration [32]. Nevertheless, the mechanical fibrillation of cellulose is combined with methods such as TEMPO oxidation, enzymatic hydrolysis and high-intensity sonication to reduce the energy demand and generate a high yield of CNFs [55].

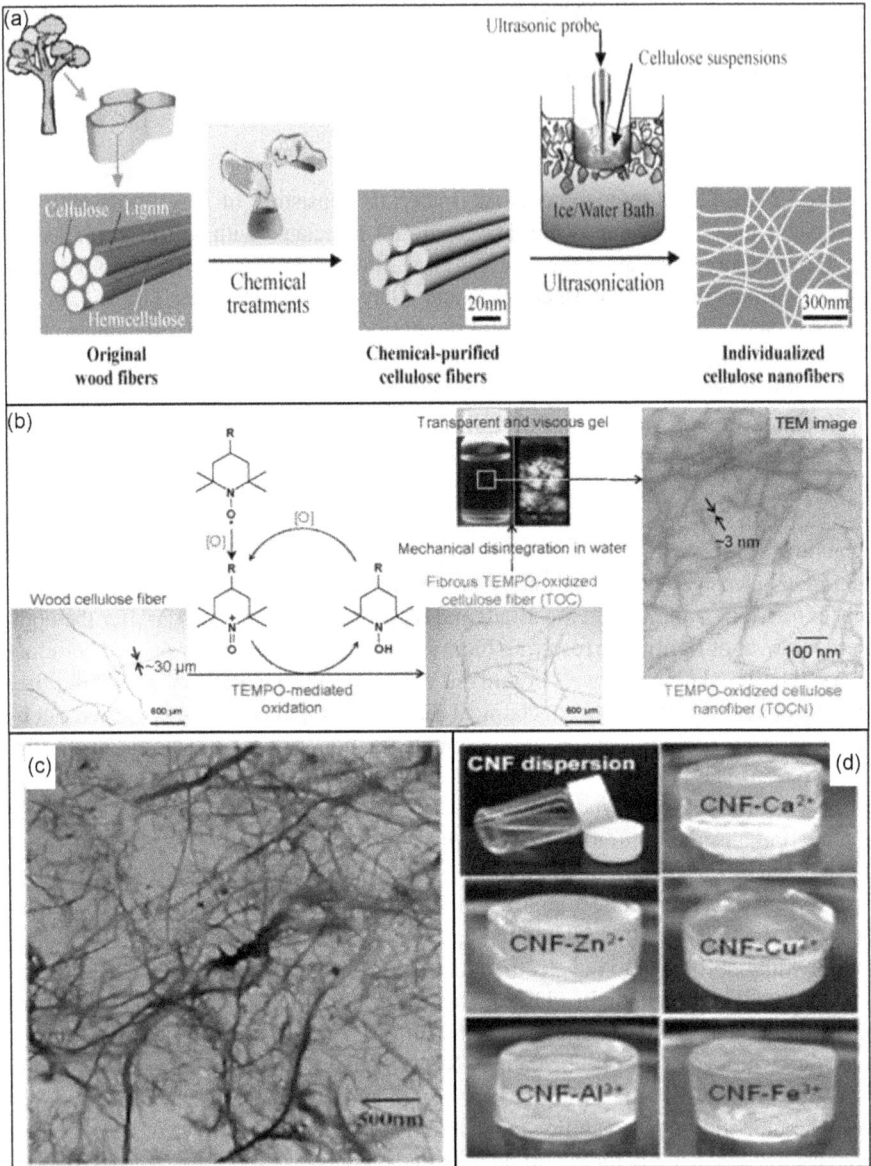

FIGURE 4.3 (a) Schematic showing the isolation of CNFs from poplar wood. (Reproduced with copyright permission from Elsevier [48].)(b) Separation of CNFs by TEMPO oxidation. (Reproduced with copyright permission from Elsevier[49].)(c) Microstructure of CNFs viewed by transmission electron microscopy.(Reproduced with copyright permission from Elsevier [50].)(d) Formation of a CNF-based hydrogel by ion cross-linking. (Reproduced with copyright permission from the American Chemical Society [51].)

4.2.4   Cellulose Derivatives

Cellulose derivatives come under the group of soluble cellulose polymers. These are associated with properties like biocompatibility, biodegradability and low toxicity similar to CNCs and CNFs. However, cellulose is converted to different products like cellulose acetate, cellulose sulfate, cellulose nitrate and carboxymethyl cellulose using chemical treatments (Table 4.2). The degree of substitution and derivatization of cellulose depends on the process conditions [57]. Cellulose acetate is produced by acetylation of cellulose using acetic anhydride in the presence of sulfuric acid as a catalyst [33]. Cellulose acetate has been combined with hydroxyapatite to synthesize a composite membrane by the electrospinning process (Figure 4.4a). The composite has also been used as a hemodialysis membrane [58].

The introduction of sulfate groups in cellulose through treatments using sulfuric acid and other cosolvents such as N,N-dimethylformamide and isoamyl alcohol produces cellulose sulfate with innate antiviral and anticoagulant properties [63]. Cellulose sulfate has been cross-linked with gelatin to produce a scaffold (Figure 4.4b) for the regeneration of nerve tissue [60]. Cellulose nitrate is another derivative produced by the electrophilic attack of NO_2^+ ions on the hydroxyl groups of cellulose. The nitration of cellulose is catalyzed by the mixture of nitric acid and dichloromethane [35]. Cellulose nitrate membranes immobilized with antibodies and nucleic acids have been used for the detection of specific biomolecules (Figure 4.4c) and the diagnosis of infectious diseases [61]. Carboxymethyl cellulose (CMC) is synthesized by the etherification process using the combination of sodium hydroxide and monochloroacetic acid [64]. CMC is majorly recommended as the ideal material for biomedical applications due to its non-toxicity and low immunogenicity. CMC has been shown to induce osteogenic differentiation (Figure 4.4d) and provide the platform for the *in vivo* regeneration of bone tissue [62]. Despite many advantages associated with the applications of cellulose derivatives, the production process involves the use of toxic chemicals and acids (Table 4.2). Moreover, the derivatization of cellulose involves numerous side reactions leading to the generation of a variety of byproducts [57].

4.3   BIOMEDICAL APPLICATION

4.3.1   Drug Delivery System

Drug administration into the human body requires suitable carriers for the controlled delivery of a drug to the target tissue. The drug-loading vehicle should not only bind and release the drug but also protect it from unfavorable environments like low pH, proteases, immune system, etc. Also, the delivery system needs to be biocompatible and biodegradable to nullify harmful immunogenic reactions like inflammation, complement activation, etc. [65]. The polymers produced by synthetic reactions are associated with problems like cytotoxicity, non-biodegradability and increased rejection by the immune system. Cellulose-based materials are considered ideal alternatives to synthetic polymers for the development of drug-loading carriers (Table 4.3). Different types of cellulose have been used for the production of hydrogels, membranes, etc. to encapsulate the biologically active molecules [32]. The composite hydrogel

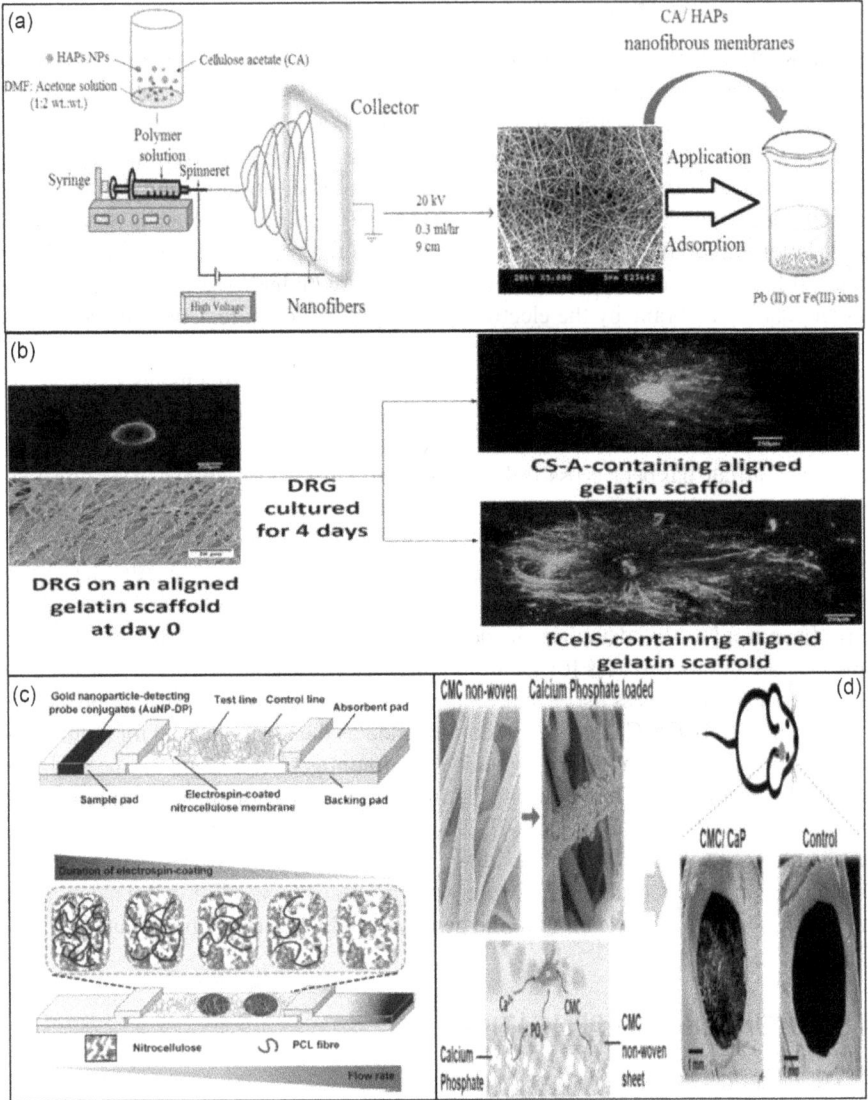

FIGURE 4.4 (a) Production of a cellulose acetate hydroxyapatite composite membrane by electrospinning. (Reproduced with copyright permission from Elsevier [59].)(b) Growth of dorsal root ganglion representing neurite development on a cellulose sulfate (fCelS)–gelatin composite scaffold. (Reproduced with copyright permission from Elsevier [60].)(c) Fabrication of a nitrocellulose membrane coated with polycaprolactone and gold nanoparticles for lateral flow assay. (Reproduced with copyright permission from Elsevier [61].)(d) Regeneration of bone tissue *in vivo* using a calcium phosphate-loaded carboxymethyl cellulose non-woven sheet. (Reproduced with copyright permission from Elsevier [62].)

TABLE 4.3

Reported Studies on the Production of Different Cellulose-Based Products and Their Biomedical Applications

Cellulosic Material	Conjugate Ion/Polymer	Product	Function	Application	Reference
Bacterial cellulose (BC)	Chitosan	Antimicrobial membrane	Inhibition of *Staphylococcus aureus* and *Escherichia coli*	Wound dressing	[68]
	Hydroxyapatite	3D scaffold	Regeneration of bone tissue	Tissue engineering	[69]
	Alginate	Transdermal patch	Loading of tetracycline, ibuprofen and diclofenac	Drug delivery	[29]
	Polymerizable deep eutectic solvents	Ionic hydrogel	Detection of body movements	Wearable sensor	[10]
Cellulose nanocrystal (CNC)	Polyvinyl alcohol	Hydrogel	Fabrication of contact lens	Ophthalmic drug delivery	[70]
	Alginate	Double membrane hydrogel	Sustained release of antibiotic ceftazidime hydrate	Drug delivery	[12]
	Poly(oligoethylene glycol methacrylate)	3D scaffold	Development of cartilage tissue	Tissue engineering	[13]
	Polyacrylic acid	Chiral nematic film	Detection of moisture and relative humidity	Wearable sensor	[71]
Cellulose nanofibril (CNF)	Silver and copper ions	Antibacterial hydrogels	Inhibition of wound pathogens	Wound dressing	[9]
	Sodium alginate	pH-sensitive hydrogel	Release of probiotics in the intestinal fluid	Drug delivery	[66]
	Calcium ion and polydopamine	Hydrogel loaded with tetracycline hydrochloride	Treatment of damaged skin *in vivo*	Wound dressing	[72]
	Gelatin methacrylamide	Hydrogel ink	3D printing of human nose	Tissue engineering	[17]
Cellulose acetate	Gliadin	Core–shell nanostructure	Encapsulation of drug ibuprofen	Drug delivery	[73]
Cellulose sulfate	Chitosan hydrochloride	Microcapsules	Encapsulation of 5-aminosalicylic acid	Drug delivery	[20]
Cellulose nitrate	Polycaprolactone	Electrospun membrane	Detection of antibodies and oligonucleotides	Biosensor	[61]
Carboxymethyl cellulose	Silver chloride and zinc oxide nanostructures	Hydrogel	Growth of new fibroblast cells and wound healing	Wound dressing	[74]

consisting of TEMPO-oxidized CNFs and sodium alginate has been reported to show pH-sensitive release of probiotics (Figure 4.5a). The polymer–drug interaction is strong at pH less than 4.0 and the release of the drug has been reported to be faster at the physiological pH. As a result, oral drugs susceptible to breakdown at low pH inside the gastrointestinal tract can be safely administered using the composite hydrogel [66]. On the other hand, the drugs sensitive to thermal degradation at 37°C can be encapsulated using TEMPO-oxidized CNFs and poly(N-isopropylacrylamide) (PNIPAM). The polymer–polymer interactions at 35°C form a boundary layer around the drug, as seen in Figure 4.5b. Interestingly, this layer diminishes at a temperature below 25°C for the sustained release of the drug [67].

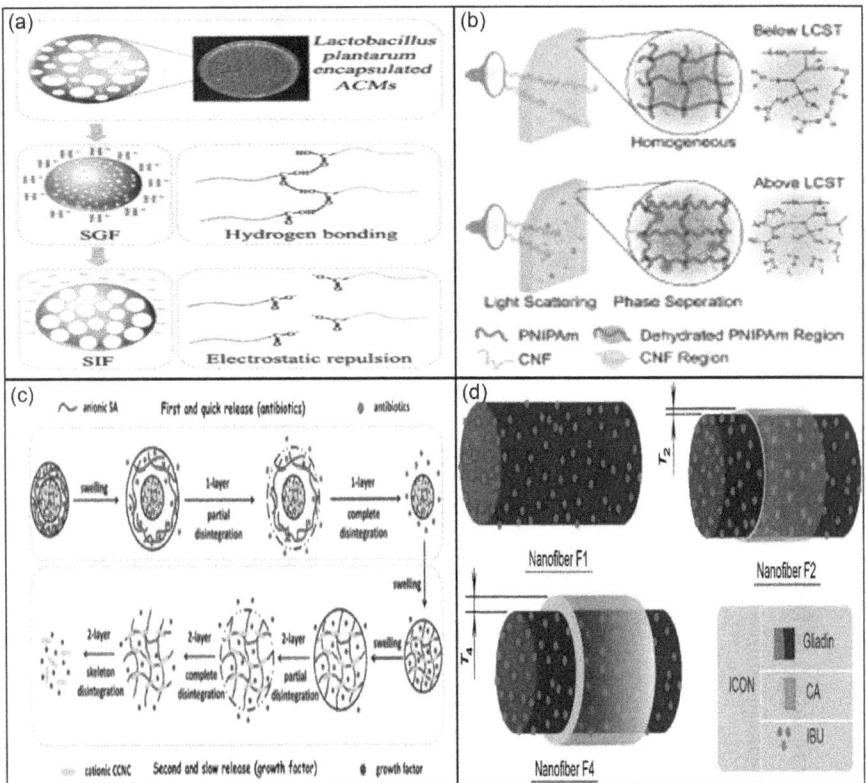

FIGURE 4.5   (a) Release of probiotics from the CNF–sodium alginate composite hydrogel in response to pH of the gastrointestinal fluid. (Reproduced with copyright permission from the American Chemical Society [66].)(b) Light scattering experiment indicating temperature-sensitive interaction of CNFs with poly(N-isopropylacrylamide). (Reproduced with copyright permission from Elsevier [67].)(c) Sustained release of the drug ceftazidime hydrate from the double membrane hydrogel containing cationic CNCs and anionic alginate. (Reproduced with copyright permission from the American Chemical Society [12].)(d) Novel core–shell nanostructures representing cellulose acetate and a drug–protein composite fabricated by triaxial electrospinning. (Reproduced with copyright permission from Elsevier [73].)

In the case of CNCs, stimuli-responsive hydrogels have been prepared owing to their self-assembly property. The CNCs present in hydrogels also influence the sustained release of drugs [43]. The double membrane hydrogel fabricated using cationic CNCs and anionic alginate has been reported to show a two-step sustained release of drug ceftazidime hydrate (Figure 4.5c). In the initial step, the disintegration of the outer alginate hydrogel promotes the rapid release of the drug in the first 3 days. However, the cationic CNCs containing the inner hydrogel degrades slowly thereby extending the drug release upto 12 days [12]. On the other hand, the derivatives of cellulose have been widely used in the manufacture of drug-loading membranes. Novel core–shell nanostructures containing drug–protein composites and cellulose acetate have been used for the encapsulation of the ibuprofen–gliadin mixture (Figure 4.5d). The interactions between the cellulose acetate and the drug mixture have been shown to enhance the therapeutic agent release upto 43 hours and prevent the initial burst release [73].

4.3.2 Wound Dressing Material

Human skin is the major barrier protecting vital body functions from the external environment. The skin itself functions as a filter for maintaining the levels of water and salt, excretes toxins and shields the body from harmful ultraviolet radiation. An injury to the skin as a result of burns and cuts increases the risk of infection and forms the site for the entry of pathogens and other harmful toxins from the surrounding environment [75]. A wound dressing material ideally targets the protection of the wound site and promotes wound healing. It also forms a barrier against microbial infection and facilitates the exchange of gases and the maintenance of moisture. During the wound healing process, the regeneration of new tissue occurs in different stages such as clot formation, granulation, proliferation of endothelial and fibroblast cells and blood vessel formation (Figure 4.6a).

The use of a synthetic and less cytocompatible material for wound dressing is associated with the major risk of wound enlargement and severe inflammation. Cellulose has been considered as a safe and highly biocompatible material for preparing different wound dressing materials like membranes, transdermal patches, etc. (Table 4.3). Besides, cellulose materials have been shown to support cell adhesion and facilitate further growth and proliferation [32]. BC has been reported to promote epithelialization and tissue regeneration in diabetic foot wounds [29]. However, the lack of antimicrobial property limited the usage of BC for the treatment of chronic wounds, burns, etc. Nevertheless, BC-based antimicrobial composites have been reported by cross-linking BC with other polymers like chitosan and alginate [29,68]. Moreover, a silver-containing BC composite has been shown to be a promising wound dressing material (Figure 4.6b) due to its antibacterial activity against *Escherichia coli*, *Staphylococcus aureus*, *Klebsiella pneumoniae*, *Bacillus subtilis* and *Pseudomonas aeruginosa* [77]. In the case of CNFs, metal cation cross-linked hydrogels have been used as wound dressing materials [32]. Also, CNF hydrogels have been combined with other ionic polymers to develop multiresponsive composite materials [78]. For instance, a composite hydrogel consisting of Ca^{2+} cross-linked CNF and polydopamine (PDA) has been loaded with tetracycline hydrochloride to treat the damaged

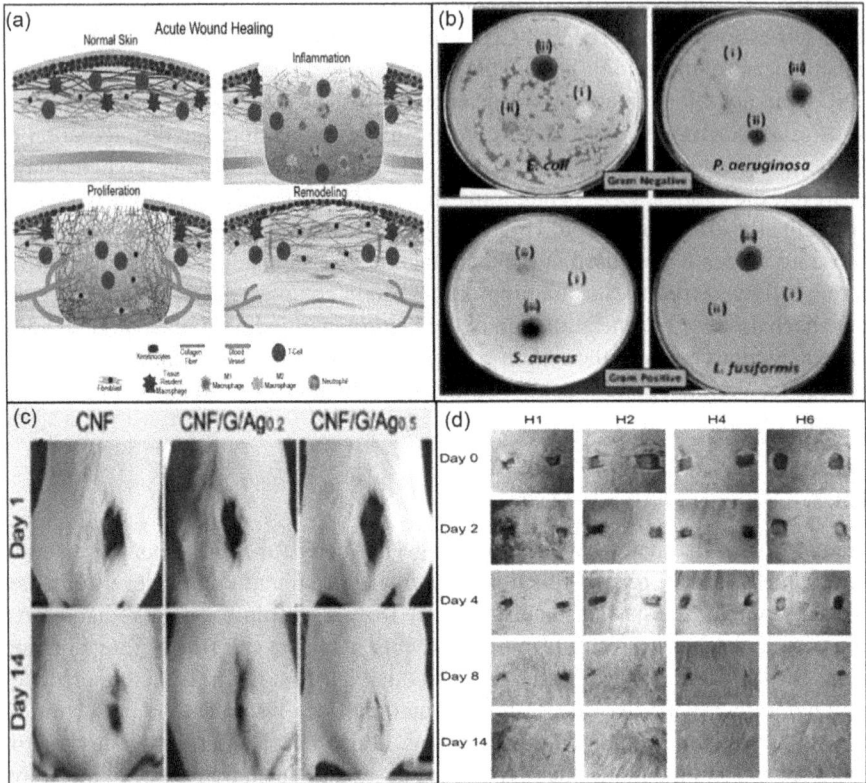

FIGURE 4.6 (a) Stages of the wound healing process. (Reproduced with copyright permission from Elsevier [76].)(b) Antibacterial activities of graphene oxide and a silver nanoparticle-coated BC wound dressing material against Gram-positive and Gram-negative bacteria. (Reproduced with copyright permission from the American Chemical Society [77].)(c) Effect of a nanocomposite hydrogel containing CNFs, gelatin and aminated silver nanoparticles on the wound size reduction. (Reproduced with copyright permission from Elsevier [72].)(d) Progressive healing of the wound upon application of a carboxymethyl cellulose hydrogel containing silver chloride and zinc oxide nanostructures. (Reproduced with copyright permission from the American Chemical Society [74].)

skin *in vivo* (Figure 4.6c) and enhance wound healing [72]. Among the cellulose derivatives, CMC has been majorly used for the fabrication of wound dressing materials due to its high biocompatibility (Figure 4.6d). Acceleration of wound healing and growth of new fibroblast cells have been reported for the CMC hydrogel embedded with silver chloride and zinc oxide nanostructures [74].

4.3.3 Tissue Engineering Scaffold

The problems of organ failure, bone degeneration, kidney and liver dysfunction and skin trauma require the transplantation of regenerated tissues to maintain the vital functions of the body. Often, the transplantation of organs from a donor to a recipient is associated with the major risk of graft rejection. However, the development of scaf-folds for the regeneration of the damaged tissue is a promising solution to minimize the host versus graft reaction [29]. Moreover, materials required for constructing the tissue scaffolds need to be highly biocompatible and provide a favorable environment for cell adhesion, proliferation and differentiation (Figure 4.7a).

In addition, the scaffolds should undergo natural biodegradation inside the body to eliminate the need for surgical removal [78]. Cellulose-based hydrogels produced using CNFs and CNCs have been increasingly used as scaffolds for tissue engineer-ing (Table 4.3). Moreover, cellulosic materials have been shown to be associated with highly hydrated 3D porous structures that are analogous to biological tissues [32]. Also, the microenvironment present in the cellulose-based hydrogel is similar to the extracellular matrix (ECM) and it facilitates gas transport, metabolite exchange and new blood vessel formation [83].In recent works on tissue regeneration for organ repair and replacement, biological scaffolds have been fabricated by the 3D printing technology. In the process of 3D printing, the hydrogels are used as bioinks and the specialized structures are constructed through computer-aided extrusion [32]. For instance, hydrogel in the shape of the human nose has been printed by using CNFs and gelatin methacrylamide as the composite bioink [84]. Interestingly, the hydrogel produced by cross-linking 80% CNFs and 20% alginate has been used for printing the human ear (Figure 4.7b). Moreover, the CNF-based hydrogels have been bio-printed with the human chondrocytes to regenerate the auricular cartilage tissue [85]. Apart from the nanocellulose extracted from plants, BC has also been extensively investigated to produce different 3D structures for the regeneration of ophthalmic, bone and skeletal tissue grafts [29]. The porous scaffold matrix (Figure 4.7c) syn-thesized using surface phosphorylated BC, calcium phosphate and hydroxyapatite has been used for the regeneration of bone tissue [81]. Interestingly, a temporary bone substituent prepared using BC and calcium phosphate has been loaded with a cellulosic enzyme to induce natural biodegradation of the composite after the bone regeneration [86]. Other interesting applications of BC include the development of artificial blood vessel implants, heart valves, cardiovascular stents, etc. [29]. As a result of the moldable nature of BC, it has been used to produce small-diameter blood vessels to replace the atherosclerotic arteries (Figure 4.7d).

4.3.4 Wearable Sensor

Modern-day devices for monitoring health and human activities have been fabricated in a smarter and user-friendly fashion. An ideal material for making smart sensors should be associated with high flexibility, high reproducibility, high sensitivity, etc. [87]. Cellulose has been widely used for the production of smart sensors due to its flexible surface chemistry, high elasticity, tunable properties, low thermal expansion, anisotropy, biodegradability, etc. [78]. Moreover, cellulose provides the mechani-cal support for the integration of numerous organic and inorganic compounds with special properties like electrical conductivity and energy storage (Table 4.3). Also, it forms the base material for the fabrication of multifunctional composite sensors [88]. In addition, cellulose produced in the form of CNFs and CNCs has been used for the development of various multidimensional structures like microfibers, yarns,

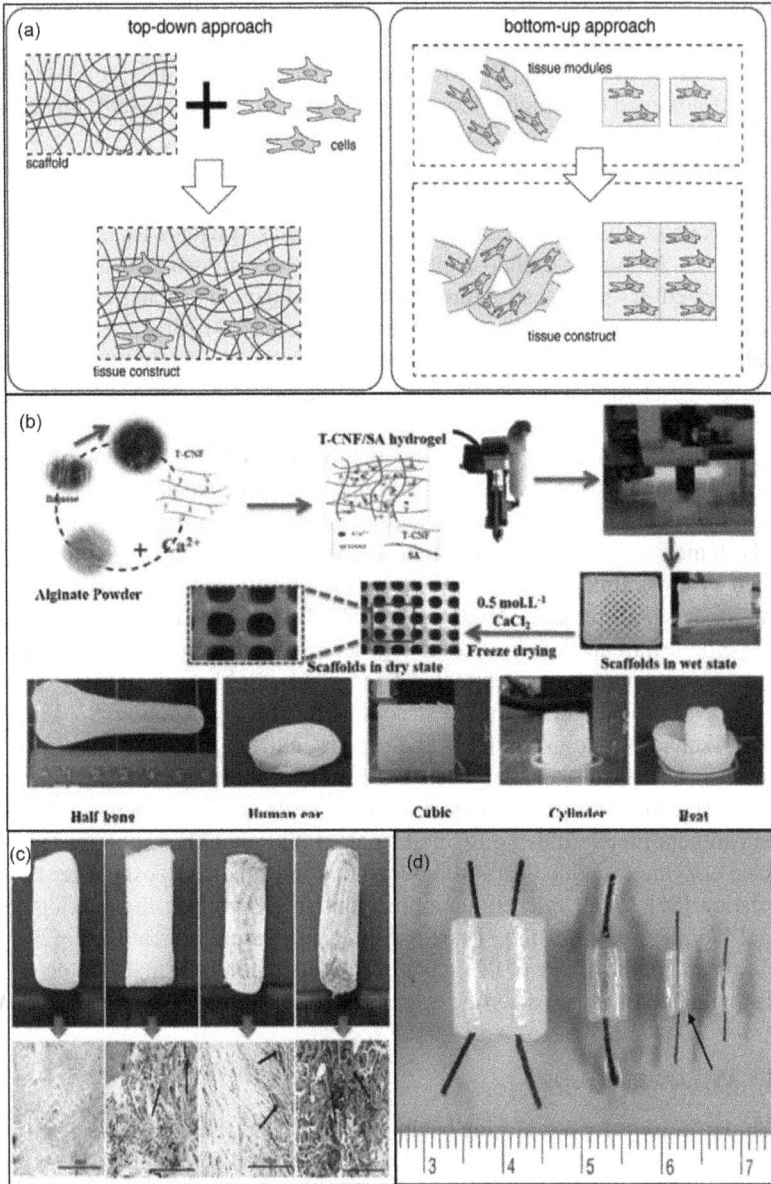

FIGURE 4.7 (a) Different approaches underlying the construction of scaffolds for tissue engineering. (Reproduced with copyright permission from Elsevier [79].)(b) Development of scaffolds from the CNF–sodium alginate composite hydrogel by the 3D printing technology. (Reproduced with copyright permission from the American Chemical Society [80].) (c) Photographs showing the scaffolds produced from BC and the proliferation of human bone marrow stromal cells. (Reproduced with copyright permission from Elsevier [81].)(d) Fabrication of artificial blood vessels from BC for microsurgery. (Reproduced with copyright permission from Elsevier [82].)

films, hydrogels, aerogels, sponges, foams, etc. for increasing the versatility of the sensing materials [89]. A self-healable pressure sensor fabricated using a polypyrrole (PPy)-coated PVA/CNC nanocomposite film (Figure 4.8a) has been shown to sense tiny scale movements in the body such as finger bending, swallowing and wrist pulse [90]. A multilayered sensor for monitoring the human perspiration rate has been constructed by the sequential deposition of polyacrylonitrile (PAN) and CNFs over polyethylene terephthalate (PET) (Figure 4.8b). The sensor's sensitivity to ions and dissolved salts in the sweat has been improved through the incorporation of gold nanoparticles (Au NPs) [91]. In the case of fabrication of a wireless skin sensor, polyacrylic acid (PAA) has been covalently linked with tannic acid-coated CNCs (Figure 4.8c). This self-adhesive,strain-sensitive sensor has been reported to detect both large-scale movements (e.g. bending of joints) and tiny scale motions (e.g. pulse and breathing) [14].

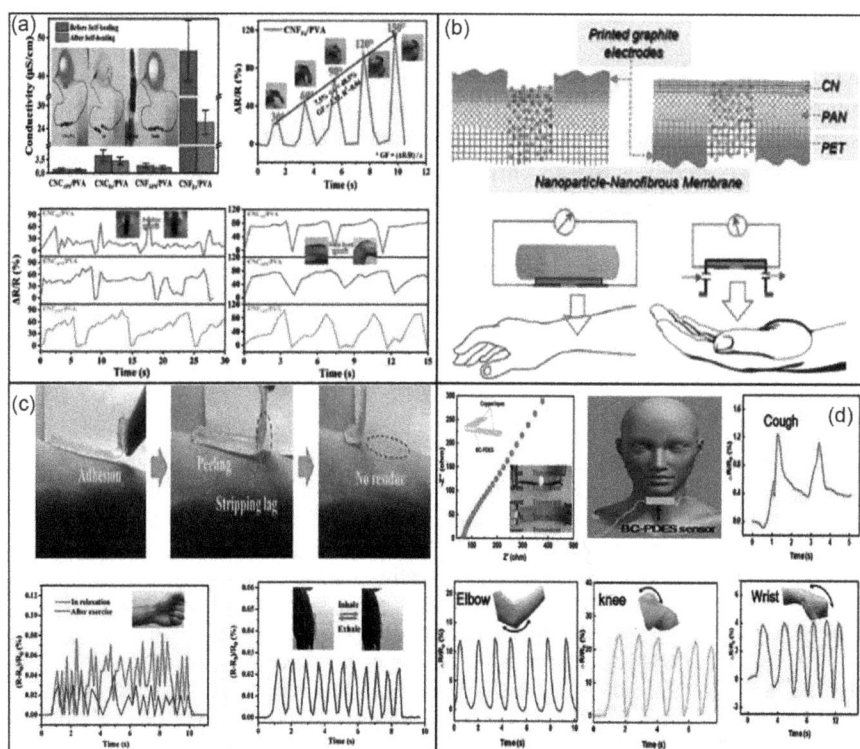

FIGURE 4.8 (a) A self-healable conductive skin sensor produced using nanocellulose and polyvinyl alcohol. (Reproduced with copyright permission from the American Chemical Society [90].)(b) Multilayered sweat sensor fabricated through electrospinning of CNFs, polyacrylonitrile and polyethylene terephthalate. (Reproduced with copyright permission from the American Chemical Society [91].) (c) A self-adhesive and strain-sensitive nanocomposite consisting of tannic acid-coated CNCs and polyacrylic acid for detecting tiny scale body movements. (Reproduced with copyright permission from the American Chemical Society [14].) (d) A multifunctional ionic hydrogel produced from BC for monitoring joint and throat movements. (Reproduced with copyright permission from the American Chemical Society [10].)

Interestingly, high-performance wearable sensors have also been produced using BC (Figure 4.8d). A multifunctional ionic hydrogel made up of BC and polymerizable deep eutectic solvents has been used as an ultrasensitive and mechanically robust sensor to examine the full range of bodily movements like limb motions, throat vibrations and other biophysical activities [10].

4.4 CONCLUSION

Cellulose is one of the most extensively available biopolymers with intriguing properties for producing renewable materials. Different types of cellulosic materials like CNF, CNC, BC and cellulose derivatives have been widely used for preparing hydrogels, membranes and scaffolds for various biomedical applications. Also, cellulose has been combined with biodegradable and cytocompatible polymers for fabricating multifunctional composite materials. Stimuli-responsive *in vivo* drug release is one of the interesting properties of the cellulosic materials for increasing the stability, bioavailability and efficacy of essential drugs. In the regeneration of tissues for organ transplantation, cellulosic materials loaded with cellulolytic enzymes have been used as naturally biodegradable scaffolds. Interestingly, wearable and portable sensors for monitoring vital body activities have been fabricated using cellulose-based materials. However, cellulosic materials are associated with both pros and cons depending on the methods applied for the production and surface modification of cellulose. Nevertheless, the exceptional biocompatibility of cellulose and the sustainable production of versatile cellulose-based materials make key contributions to the advancements in healthcare.

REFERENCES

1. Ioelovich, M. Y. (2016). Models of supramolecular structure and properties of cellulose. *Polymer Science Series A*, *58*(6), 925–943.
2. McNamara, J. T., Morgan, J. L., &Zimmer, J. (2015). A molecular description of cellulose biosynthesis. *Annual Review of Biochemistry*, *84*, 895–921.
3. Medronho, B., & Lindman, B. (2014). Competing forces during cellulose dissolution: From solvents to mechanisms. *Current Opinion in Colloid & Interface Science*, *19*(1), 32–40.
4. Saba, N., & Jawaid, M. (2017). Recent advances in nanocellulose-based polymer nanocomposites. In Mohammad Jawaid, Sami Boufi, & Abdul Khalil H.P.S. (Eds.) Cellulose-Reinforced Nanofibre Composites (pp. 89–112). Woodhead Publishing.
5. Jorfi, M., & Foster, E. J. (2015). Recent advances in nanocellulose for biomedical applications. *Journal of Applied Polymer Science*, *132*(14), 1–19.
6. Gopi, S., Balakrishnan, P., Chandradhara, D., Poovathankandy, D., & Thomas, S. (2019). General scenarios of cellulose and its use in the biomedical field. *Materials Today Chemistry*, *13*, 59–78.
7. Lin, S. P., Kung, H. N., Tsai, Y. S., Tseng, T. N., Hsu, K. D., & Cheng, K. C. (2017). Novel dextran modified bacterial cellulose hydrogel accelerating cutaneous wound healing. *Cellulose*, *24*(11), 4927–4937.
8. Hobzova, R., Hrib, J., Sirc, J., Karpushkin, E., Michalek, J., Janouskova, O., & Gatenholm, P. (2018). Embedding of bacterial cellulose nanofibers within PHEMA hydrogel matrices: Tunable Stiffness composites with potential for biomedical applications. *Journal of Nanomaterials*, *2018*.

9. Basu, P., Saha, N., Alexandrova, R., Andonova-Lilova, B., Georgieva, M., Miloshev, G., & Saha, P. (2018). Biocompatibility and biological efficiency of inorganic calcium filled bacterial cellulose based hydrogel scaffolds for bone bioengineering. *International Journal of Molecular Sciences*, *19*(12), 3980.

10. Wang, M., Li, R., Feng, X., Dang, C., Dai, F., Yin, X.,...Qi, H. (2020). Cellulose nano-fiber-reinforced ionic conductors for multifunctional sensors and devices. *ACS Applied Materials & Interfaces*, *12*(24), 27545–27554.

11. Pal, N., Dubey, P., Gopinath, P., & Pal, K. (2017). Combined effect of cellulose nanocrys-tal and reduced graphene oxide into poly-lactic acid matrix nanocomposite as a scaffold and its anti-bacterial activity. *International Journal of Biological Macromolecules*, *95*, 94–105.

12. Lin, N., Gèze, A., Wouessidjewe, D., Huang, J., & Dufresne, A. (2016). Biocompatible double-membrane hydrogels from cationic cellulose nanocrystals and anionic alginate as complexing drugs codelivery. *ACS Applied Materials & Interfaces*, *8*(11), 6880–6889.

13. De France, K. J., Badv, M., Dorogin, J., Siebers, E., Panchal, V., Babi, M.,...Hoare, T. (2019). Tissue response and biodistribution of injectable cellulose nanocrystal compos-ite hydrogels. *ACS Biomaterials Science & Engineering*, *5*(5), 2235–2246.

14. Shao, C., Wang, M., Meng, L., Chang, H., Wang, B., Xu, F.,...Wan, P. (2018). Mussel-inspired cellulose nanocomposite tough hydrogels with synergistic self-healing, adhe-sive, and strain-sensitive properties. *Chemistry of Materials*, *30*(9), 3110–3121.

15. Wang, P., Yin, B., Dong, H., Zhang, Y., Zhang, Y., Chen, R.,...Jiang, Q. (2020). Coupling biocompatible au nanoclusters and cellulose nanofibrils to prepare the antibacterial nanocomposite films. *Frontiers in Bioengineering and Biotechnology*, *8*, 986.

16. Kong, W., Wang, C., Jia, C., Kuang, Y., Pastel, G., Chen, C.,...Hu, L. (2018). Muscle-Inspired highly anisotropic, strong, ion-conductive hydrogels. *Advanced Materials*, *30*(39), 1801934.

17. Markstedt, K., Escalante, A., Toriz, G., & Gatenholm, P. (2017). Biomimetic inks based on cellulose nanofibrils and cross-linkable xylans for 3D printing. *ACS Applied Materials & Interfaces*, *9*(46), 40878–40886.

18. Cao, W. T., Ma, C., Mao, D. S., Zhang, J., Ma, M. G., & Chen, F. (2019). MXene-reinforced cellulose nanofibril inks for 3D-printed smart fibres and textiles. *Advanced Functional Materials*, *29*(51), 1905898.

19. Pandele, A. M., Neacsu, P., Cimpean, A., Staras, A. I., Miculescu, F., Iordache, A.,...Toader, O. D. (2018). Cellulose acetate membranes functionalized with resveratrol by covalent immobilization for improved osseointegration. *Applied Surface Science*, *438*, 2–13.

20. Su, T., Wu, Q. X., Chen, Y., Zhao, J., Cheng, X. D., & Chen, J. (2019). Fabrication of the polyphosphates patched cellulose sulfate-chitosan hydrochloride microcapsules and as vehicles for sustained drug release. *International Journal of Pharmaceutics*, *555*, 291–302.

21. Chi, J., Ma, B., Dong, X., Gao, B., Elbaz, A., Liu, H., & Gu, Z. (2018). A bio-inspired photonic nitrocellulose array for ultrasensitive assays of single nucleic acids. *Analyst*, *143*(19), 4559–4565.

22. Yang, H., Shen, L., Bu, H., & Li, G. (2019). Stable and biocompatible hydrogel com-posites based on collagen and dialdehyde carboxymethyl cellulose in a biphasic solvent system. *Carbohydrate Polymers*, *222*, 114974.

23. Chawla, P. R., Bajaj, I. B., Survase, S. A., & Singhal, R. S. (2009). Microbial cellulose: Fermentative production and applications. *Food Technology and Biotechnology*, *47*(2), 107–124.

24. Zhang, H., Chen, C., Zhu, C. H. U. N. L. I. N., & Sun, D. (2016). Production of BC by Acetobacter xylinum: Effects of carbon/nitrogen-ratio on cell growth and metabolite production. *Cellulose Chemistry and Technology*, *50*, 997–1003.

25. Wang, J., Tavakoli, J., & Tang, Y. (2019). BC production, properties and applications with different culture methods–A review. *Carbohydrate Polymers*, *219*, 63–76.
26. Hu, Y., Catchmark, J. M., & Vogler, E. A. (2013). Factors impacting the formation of sphere-like bacterial cellulose particles and their biocompatibility for human osteoblast growth. *Biomacromolecules*, *14*(10), 3444–3452.
27. Yang, G., Xie, J., Hong, F., Cao, Z., & Yang, X. (2012). Antimicrobial activity of silver nanoparticle impregnated bacterial cellulose membrane: Effect of fermentation carbon sources of bacterial cellulose. *Carbohydrate Polymers*, *87*(1), 839–845.
28. Dubey, S., Sharma, R. K., Agarwal, P., Singh, J., Sinha, N., & Singh, R. P. (2017). From rotten grapes to industrial exploitation: Komagataeibacter europaeus SGP37, a microfactory for macroscale production of bacterial nanocellulose. *International Journal of Biological Macromolecules*, *96*, 52–60.
29. Picheth, G. F., Pirich, C. L., Sierakowski, M. R., Woehl, M. A., Sakakibara, C. N., de Souza, C. F.,…de Freitas, R. A. (2017). BC in biomedical applications: A review. *International Journal of Biological Macromolecules*, *104*, 97–106.
30. Moniri, M., Boroumand Moghaddam, A., Azizi, S., Abdul Rahim, R., Bin Ariff, A., Zuhainis Saad, W.,…Mohamad, R. (2017). Production and status of BC in biomedical engineering. *Nanomaterials*, *7*(9), 257.
31. Xie, H., Du, H., Yang, X., & Si, C. (2018). Recent strategies in preparation of cellulose nanocrystals and cellulose nanofibrils derived from raw cellulose materials. *International Journal of Polymer Science*, *2018*, 1–26.
32. Du, H., Liu, W., Zhang, M., Si, C., Zhang, X., & Li, B. (2019). Cellulose nanocrystals and cellulose nanofibrils based hydrogels for biomedical applications. *Carbohydrate Polymers*, *209*, 130–144.
33. Cheng, H. N., Dowd, M. K., Selling, G. W., & Biswas, A. (2010). Synthesis of cellulose acetate from cotton byproducts. *Carbohydrate Polymers*, *80*(2), 449–452.
34. Strätz, J., Liedmann, A., Heinze, T., Fischer, S., & Groth, T. (2020). Effect of sulfation route and subsequent oxidation on derivatization degree and biocompatibility of cellulose sulfates. *Macromolecular Bioscience*, *20*(2), 1900403.
35. Li, L., & Frey, M. (2010). Preparation and characterization of cellulose nitrate-acetate mixed ester fibers. *Polymer*, *51*(16), 3774–3783.
36. Singh, V., Joshi, S., & Malviya, T. (2018). Carboxymethyl cellulose-rosin gum hybrid nanoparticles: An efficient drug carrier. *International Journal of Biological Macromolecules*, *112*, 390–398.
37. Hsieh, Y. C., Yano, H., Nogi, M., & Eichhorn, S. J. (2008). An estimation of the Young's modulus of BC filaments. *Cellulose*, *15*(4), 507–513.
38. Gao, M., Li, J., Bao, Z., Hu, M., Nian, R., Feng, D.,…Zhang, H. (2019). A natural in situ fabrication method of functional BC using a microorganism. *Nature Communications*, *10*(1), 1–10.
39. Lu, P., & Hsieh, Y. L. (2010). Preparation and properties of cellulose nanocrystals: Rods, spheres, and network. *Carbohydrate Polymers*, *82*(2), 329–336.
40. Lavoine, N., Desloges, I., Dufresne, A., & Bras, J. (2012). Microfibrillated cellulose– Its barrier properties and applications in cellulosic materials: A review. *Carbohydrate Polymers*, *90*(2), 735–764.
41. Reddy, M. M., Vivekanandhan, S., Misra, M., Bhatia, S. K., & Mohanty, A. K. (2013). Biobased plastics and bionanocomposites: Current status and future opportunities. *Progress in Polymer Science*, *38*(10–11), 1653–1689.
42. Domingues, R. M., Gomes, M. E., & Reis, R. L. (2014). The potential of cellulose nanocrystals in tissue engineering strategies. *Biomacromolecules*, *15*(7), 2327–2346.
43. Ganguly, K., Patel, D. K., Dutta, S. D., Shin, W. C., & Lim, K. T. (2020). Stimuli-responsive self-assembly of cellulose nanocrystals (CNCs): Structures, functions, and biomedical applications. *International Journal of Biological Macromolecules*, *155*, 456–469.

44. Ng, H. M., Sin, L. T., Tee, T. T., Bee, S. T., Hui, D., Low, C. Y., & Rahmat, A. R. (2015). Extraction of cellulose nanocrystals from plant sources for application as reinforcing agent in polymers. *Composites Part B: Engineering, 75*, 176–200.
45. Kargarzadeh, H., Ahmad, I., Abdullah, I., Dufresne, A., Zainudin, S. Y., & Sheltami, R. M. (2012). Effects of hydrolysis conditions on the morphology, crystallinity, and thermal stability of cellulose nanocrystals extracted from kenaf bast fibers. *Cellulose, 19*(3), 855–866.
46. Aziz, T., Ullah, A., Fan, H., Ullah, R., Haq, F., Khan, F. U.,...Wei, J. (2021). Cellulose nanocrystals applications in health, medicine and catalysis. *Journal of Polymers and the Environment, 29*, 2062–2071.
47. Feng, Y. H., Cheng, T. Y., Yang, W. G., Ma, P. T., He, H. Z., Yin, X. C., & Yu, X. X. (2018). Characteristics and environmentally friendly extraction of cellulose nanofibrils from sugarcane bagasse. *Industrial Crops and Products, 111*, 285–291.
48. Chen, W., Yu, H., Liu, Y., Chen, P., Zhang, M., & Hai, Y. (2011). Individualization of cellulose nanofibers from wood using high-intensity ultrasonication combined with chemical pretreatments. *Carbohydrate Polymers, 83*(4), 1804–1811.
49. Isogai, A., & Bergström, L. (2018). Preparation of cellulose nanofibers using green and sustainable chemistry. *Current Opinion in Green and Sustainable Chemistry, 12*, 15–21.
50. Wang, B., & Sain, M. (2007). Isolation of nanofibers from soybean source and their reinforcing capability on synthetic polymers. *Composites Science and Technology, 67*(-11–12), 2521–2527.
51. Dong, H., Snyder, J. F., Williams, K. S., & Andzelm, J. W. (2013). Cation-induced hydrogels of cellulose nanofibrils with tunable moduli. *Biomacromolecules, 14*(9), 3338–3345.
52. Liu, X., Li, Y., Ewulonu, C. M., Ralph, J., Xu, F., Zhang, Q.,...Huang, Y. (2019). Mild alkaline pretreatment for isolation of native-like lignin and lignin-containing cellulose nanofibers (LCNF) from crop waste. *ACS Sustainable Chemistry & Engineering, 7*(16), 14135–14142.
53. Gu, J., & Hsieh, Y. L. (2017). Alkaline cellulose nanofibrils from streamlined alkali treated rice straw. *ACS Sustainable Chemistry & Engineering, 5*(2), 1730–1737.
54. Zhao, X., Cheng, F., Hu, Y., & Cheng, R. (2021). Facile extraction of cellulose nano-fibrils (Cnfs) from wood using acidic ionic liquid-catalyzed organosolv pretreatment followed by ultrasonic processing. *Journal of Natural Fibers, 18*, 1–12.
55. Santucci, B. S., Bras, J., Belgacem, M. N., da Silva Curvelo, A. A., & Pimenta, M. T. B. (2016). Evaluation of the effects of chemical composition and refining treatments on the properties of nanofibrillated cellulose films from sugarcane bagasse. *Industrial Crops and Products, 91*, 238–248.
56. Fukuzumi, H., Saito, T., & Isogai, A. (2013). Influence of TEMPO-oxidized cellulose nanofibril length on film properties. *Carbohydrate Polymers, 93*(1), 172–177.
57. Heinze, T., & Koschella, A. (2005). Solvents applied in the field of cellulose chemistry: A mini review. *Polímeros, 15*(2), 84–90.
58. Pandele, A. M., Comanici, F. E., Carp, C. A., Miculescu, F., Voicu, S. I., Thakur, V. K., & Serban, B. C. (2017). Synthesis and characterization of cellulose acetate-hydroxyapatite micro and nano compositesmembranes for water purification and biomedical applications. *Vacuum, 146*, 599–605.
59. Hamad, A. A., Hassouna, M. S., Shalaby, T. I., Elkady, M. F., Abd Elkawi, M. A., & Hamad, H. A. (2020). Electrospun cellulose acetate nanofiber incorporated with hydroxyapatite for removal of heavy metals. *International Journal of Biological Macromolecules, 151*, 1299–1313.
60. Menezes, R., Hashemi, S., Vincent, R., Collins, G., Meyer, J., Foston, M., & Arinzeh, T. L. (2019). Investigation of glycosaminoglycan mimetic scaffolds for neurite growth. *Acta Biomaterialia, 90*, 169–178.

61. Yew, C. H. T., Azari, P., Choi, J. R., Li, F., & Pingguan-Murphy, B. (2018). Electrospin-coating of nitrocellulose membrane enhances sensitivity in nucleic acid-based lateral flow assay. *Analytica Chimica Acta*, *1009*, 81–88.
62. Qi, P., Ohba, S., Hara, Y., Fuke, M., Ogawa, T., Ohta, S., & Ito, T. (2018). Fabrication of calcium phosphate-loaded carboxymethyl cellulose non-woven sheets for bone regeneration. *Carbohydrate Polymers*, *189*, 322–330.
63. Rohowsky, J., Heise, K., Fischer, S., & Hettrich, K. (2016). Synthesis and characterization of novel cellulose ether sulfates. *Carbohydrate Polymers*, *142*, 56–62.
64. Mohkami, M., & Talaeipour, M. (2011). Investigation of the chemical structure of carboxylated and carboxymethylated fibers from waste paper via XRD and FTIR analysis. *Bioresources*, *6*(2), 1988–2003.
65. Li, C., Wang, J., Wang, Y., Gao, H., Wei, G., Huang, Y.,…Jin, Y. (2019). Recent progress in drug delivery. *Acta PharmaceuticaSinica B*, *9*(6), 1145–1162.
66. Zhang, H., Yang, C., Zhou, W., Luan, Q., Li, W., Deng, Q.,…Huang, F. (2018). A pH-responsive gel macrosphere based on sodium alginate and cellulose nanofiber for potential intestinal delivery of probiotics. *ACS Sustainable Chemistry & Engineering*, *6*(11), 13924–13931.
67. Sun, X., Tyagi, P., Agate, S., McCord, M. G., Lucia, L. A., & Pal, L. (2020). Highly tunable bioadhesion and optics of 3D printable PNIPAm/cellulose nanofibrils hydrogels. *Carbohydrate Polymers*, *234*, 115898.
68. Wahid, F., Hu, X. H., Chu, L. Q., Jia, S. R., Xie, Y. Y., & Zhong, C. (2019). Development of bacterial cellulose/chitosan based semi-interpenetrating hydrogels with improved mechanical and antibacterial properties. *International Journal of Biological Macromolecules*, *122*, 380–387.
69. Favi, P. M., Ospina, S. P., Kachole, M., Gao, M., Atehortua, L., & Webster, T. J. (2016). Preparation and characterization of biodegradable nano hydroxyapatite–bacterial cellulose composites with well-defined honeycomb pore arrays for bone tissue engineering applications. *Cellulose*, *23*(2), 1263–1282.
70. Åhlén, M., Tummala, G. K., & Mihranyan, A. (2018). Nanoparticle-loaded hydrogels as a pathway for enzyme-triggered drug release in ophthalmic applications. *International Journalof Pharmaceutics*, *536*(1), 73–81.
71. Lu, T., Pan, H., Ma, J., Li, Y., Bokhari, S. W., Jiang, X.,…Zhang, D. (2017). Cellulose nanocrystals/polyacrylamide composites of high sensitivity and cycling performance to gauge humidity. *ACS Applied Materials & Interfaces*, *9*(21), 18231–18237.
72. Liu, Y., Sui, Y., Liu, C., Liu, C., Wu, M., Li, B., & Li, Y. (2018). A physically crosslinked polydopamine/nanocellulose hydrogel as potential versatile vehicles for drug delivery and wound healing. *Carbohydrate Polymers*, *188*, 27–36.
73. Yang, Y., Li, W., Yu, D. G., Wang, G., Williams, G. R., & Zhang, Z. (2019). Tunable drug release from nanofibers coated with blank cellulose acetate layers fabricated using tri-axial electrospinning. *Carbohydrate Polymers*, *203*, 228–237.
74. Mao, C., Xiang, Y., Liu, X., Cui, Z., Yang, X., Yeung, K. W. K.,…Wu, S. (2017). Photo-inspired antibacterial activity and wound healing acceleration by hydrogel embedded with Ag/Ag@ AgCl/ZnO nanostructures. *ACSNano*, *11*(9), 9010–9021.
75. Kamoun, E. A., Kenawy, E. R. S., & Chen, X. (2017). A review on polymeric hydrogel membranes for wound dressing applications: PVA-based hydrogel dressings. *Journal of Advanced Research*, *8*(3), 217–233.
76. Strang, H., Kaul, A., Parikh, U., Masri, L., Saravanan, S., Li, H.,…Balaji, S. (2020). Role of cytokines and chemokines in wound healing. In Debasis Bagchi, Amitava Das, & Sashwati Roy (Eds.) *Wound Healing, Tissue Repair, and Regeneration in Diabetes* (pp. 197–235). Elsevier. Academic Press.

77. Khamrai, M., Banerjee, S. L., Paul, S., Ghosh, A. K., Sarkar, P., & Kundu, P. P. (2019). A mussel mimetic, bioadhesive, antimicrobial patch based on dopamine-modified bacterial cellulose/rGO/Ag NPs: A green approach toward wound-healing applications. *ACS Sustainable Chemistry & Engineering, 7*(14), 12083–12097.
78. Fu, L. H., Qi, C., Ma, M. G., & Wan, P. (2019). Multifunctional cellulose-based hydrogels for biomedical applications. *Journal of Materials Chemistry B, 7*(10), 1541–1562.
79. Tamayol, A., Akbari, M., Annabi, N., Paul, A., Khademhosseini, A., & Juncker, D. (2013). Fiber-based tissue engineering: Progress, challenges, and opportunities. *Biotechnology Advances, 31*(5), 669–687.
80. Abouzeid, R. E., Khiari, R., Beneventi, D., & Dufresne, A. (2018). Biomimetic mineralization of three-dimensional printed alginate/TEMPO-oxidized cellulose nanofibril scaffolds for bone tissue engineering. *Biomacromolecules, 19*(11), 4442–4452.
81. Huang, Y., Wang, J., Yang, F., Shao, Y., Zhang, X., & Dai, K. (2017). Modification and evaluation of micro-nano structured porous bacterial cellulose scaffold for bone tissue engineering. *Materials Science & Engineering. C, Materials for Biological Applications, 75*, 1034–1041.
82. Klemm, D., Schumann, D., Udhardt, U., & Marsch, S. (2001). Bacterial synthesized cellulose—artificial blood vessels for microsurgery. *Progress in Polymer Science, 26*(9), 1561–1603.
83. Moohan, J., Stewart, S. A., Espinosa, E., Rosal, A., Rodríguez, A., Larrañeta, E.,... Domínguez-Robles, J. (2020). Cellulose nanofibers and other biopolymers for biomedical applications. A review. *Applied Sciences, 10*(1), 65.
84. Markstedt, K., Mantas, A., Tournier, I., MartínezÁvila, H., Hagg, D., & Gatenholm, P. (2015). 3D bioprinting human chondrocytes with nanocellulose–alginate bioink for cartilage tissue engineering applications. *Biomacromolecules, 16*(5), 1489–1496.
85. Ávila, H. M., Schwarz, S., Rotter, N., & Gatenholm, P. (2016). 3D bioprinting of human chondrocyte-laden nanocellulose hydrogels for patient-specific auricular cartilage regeneration. *Bioprinting, 1*, 22–35.
86. Hu, Y., Zhu, Y., Zhou, X., Ruan, C., Pan, H., & Catchmark, J. M. (2016). Bioabsorbable cellulose composites prepared by an improved mineral-binding process for bone defect repair. *Journal of Materials Chemistry B, 4*(7), 1235–1246.
87. Wang, P., Hu, M., Wang, H., Chen, Z., Feng, Y., Wang, J.,...Huang, Y. (2020). The evolution of flexible electronics: From nature, beyond nature, and to nature. *Advanced Science, 7*(20), 2001116.
88. Zhou, S., Nyholm, L., Strømme, M., & Wang, Z. (2019). Cladophora cellulose: Unique biopolymer nanofibrils for emerging energy, environmental, and life science applications. *Accounts of Chemical Research, 52*(8), 2232–2243.
89. Dai, L., Wang, Y., Zou, X., Chen, Z., Liu, H., & Ni, Y. (2020). Ultrasensitive physical, bio, and chemical sensors derived from 1-, 2-, and 3-D nanocellulosic materials. *Small, 16*(13), 1906567.
90. Han, L., Cui, S., Yu, H. Y., Song, M., Zhang, H., Grishkewich, N.,...Tam, K. M. C. (2019). Self-healable conductive nanocellulose nanocomposites for biocompatible electronic skin sensor systems. *ACS Applied Materials & Interfaces, 11*(47), 44642–44651.
91. Kang, N., Lin, F., Zhao, W., Lombardi, J. P., Almihdhar, M., Liu, K.,...Zhong, C. J. (2016). Nanoparticle–nanofibrous membranes as scaffolds for flexible sweat sensors. *ACS Sensors, 1*(8), 1060–1069.

5 Magnetic Iron Oxide Nanoparticles for Biomedical Applications

Vikram Hastak, Suresh Bandi,
and Ajeet K. Srivastav
Visvesvaraya National Institute of Technology Nagpur

CONTENTS

DOI: 10.1201/9781003286806-5

5.1   INTRODUCTION

Biocompatible nanoparticle research is one of the most promising branches of nanotechnology where wide spectra of nanoparticles are synthesized for biomedical applications [1]. This entity covers gold nanoparticles, core/shell quantum dots, magnetic nanoparticles, carbon nanoparticles, rare earth nanoparticles, polymers, and liposomes [2]. Apart from this classification, superparamagnetic iron oxide nanoparticles (IONPs, e.g., magnetite and maghemite) find major applications as biocompatible nanoparticles [3–5]. Their biomedical applications include *in-vivo* magnetic resonance imaging (MRI) contrast-enhancing agents [6], magnetic particle imaging (MPI) [7], *in-vitro* bioseparation, targeted *in-vivo* drug delivery [8], and hyperthermia (cancer treatment) [9].

Cornell and Schwertmann [10] reported a vast study on the structure, properties, reactions, occurrences, and uses of eight different forms of iron oxides. However, magnetite (Fe_3O_4) and maghemite (γ-Fe_2O_3) are the widely explored IONPs from the whole classification of iron oxides for biomedical applications. Magnetite possesses an inverse cubic spinel structure with oxygen atoms forming a face-centered cubic lattice and Fe (iron) atoms occupying tetrahedral (Fe^{3+}) and octahedral (Fe^{3+} and Fe^{2+}) sites. In maghemite, Fe^{3+} cations occupy both tetrahedral and octahedral sites leaving some vacant octahedral sites. The structure of maghemite is such that one can pile up three Fe_3O_4 spinels and remove eight Fe atoms from octahedral voids. The Fe and O atomic positions in magnetite and maghemite unit cells are illustrated in Figure 5.1. Based on their size, IONPs are classified into three categories. (i) superparamagnetic IONPs (also referred to as SPIONs) having more than 50 nm hydrodynamic diameter (diameter of the core along with the coating), (ii) ultrasmall superparamagnetic iron oxide nanoparticles (USPIO) having a hydrodynamic diameter of less than 50 nm, and (iii) micron-sized iron oxide nanoparticles (MPIO) [11].

Owing to a broad range of applications served by IONPs, tuning of these structures can be done accordingly by having control over their size [12,13], shape [14,15], and surface [16]. The size of such magnetic nanoparticles falls in the vicinity of a few to hundreds of nanometers. This control over size can resemble the biological tissues

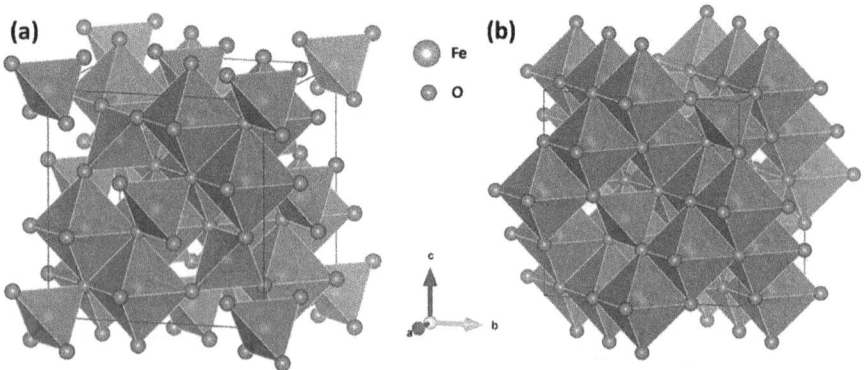

FIGURE 5.1   Crystal structure of (a) magnetite and (b) maghemite showing the atomic positions in their corresponding unit cells.

including proteins (5–50 nm), viruses (20–450 nm), cells (10–100 µm), and genes (10×2–100×2 nm) [17]. These features of IONPs created a path for biomedical applications where they combine with biological entities. IONP-tagged/encapsulated biological molecules (drugs) target certain locations (e.g., sites of malignant tumors) inside the body and can be operated through an external magnetic field gradient [17]. Hyperthermia (heating effect) is a well-known effect that provides an added advantage of desirable energy transfer (i.e., heat producing high temperature inside the body that kills up harmful bacteria and/or viruses [18]).

To shed light on the pathways to synthesize biocompatible IONPs, this chapter tries to put forth the recent progress toward surface functionalization of IONPs for biomedical applications. The chapter begins with reviewing the most frequently practiced synthesis routes. Further, the surface functionalization strategies in view of materials and methods are critically discussed. Finally, the role of functionalized IONPs in various real-time biomedical applications is briefly elaborated.

5.2 SYNTHESIS OF IONPs

Various kinds of synthesis routes exist for the production of IONPs, which are coprecipitation [19], microemulsion [20], sol–gel [21], gas–aerosol technology, sonolysis/ sonochemical [22], hydrothermal/solvothermal [23], microwave irradiation [24], flow injection [25], and electrospray synthesis [26] methods. Some complex purification processes are also employed in addition to the above-mentioned methods, which include ultra-centrifugation [27], magnetic filtration [28], flow field gradient [29], and size exclusion chromatography [30]. Here, we have discussed a few widely practiced synthesis routes.

5.2.1 COPRECIPITATION

It involves the transfer of iron(II) and iron(III) salts (chloride, sulfates, phosphates, or nitrates) into distilled water in appropriate molar ratios followed by the addition of an equivalent stoichiometric amount of a precipitating base (NaOH/NH$_4$OH solution). The process carries the simultaneous operations of magnetic stirring and heating. The usage of inert (preferably nitrogen or argon) gas will result in the formation of magnetite (Fe$_3$O$_4$) nanoparticles while the air atmosphere oxidizes magnetite into maghemite (γ-Fe$_2$O$_3$). The size of superparamagnetic IONPs mainly depend on the molar ratio of iron salts, rate of addition of a precipitating base, and molar concentration of the bases [31]. Magnetite nanoparticles formed through this technique are usually polydisperse with a broad size distribution. Magnetic nanoparticles are kept in the form of a dispersion in an organic stabilizer to ensure stabilization as well as to prevent aggregation. The overall reaction involved in the coprecipitation process can be written as:

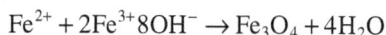

$$Fe^{2+} + 2Fe^{3+} 8OH^{-} \rightarrow Fe_3O_4 + 4H_2O$$

Various modifications in view of materials and methods have been considered to control the shape and size of the IONPs. Wu et al. (2007) reported the coprecipitation of

Fe_3O_4 with high yield and investigated accordingly the variations in various parameters with reference to the reaction temperature [32]. Also, they synthesized 15 nm Fe_3O_4 nanoparticles by an ultrasonic coprecipitation technique utilizing an acidic leaching method to extract high purity iron from iron ore tailings [33]. Hexanoic acid-coated IONPs with diameters in the range of 10–40 nm were synthesized by Petcharoen et al. [34]. The saturation magnetization and electrical conductivity were reported to be 58.72 emu/g and 1.3×10^{-3} S/cm respectively. Mahdavi et al. [35] designed oleic acid-coated magnetite nanoparticles with size ranges of 7.83–9.41 nm and pristine nanoparticles with a maximum size of 16.5 nm. The magnetization behavior of bare and oleic acid-coated Fe_3O_4 showed superparamagnetic behavior with a saturation magnetization of 81.40 and 58.60 emu/g respectively. TG-DTA analysis depicted 2.5% weight loss at 682°C and a maximum of 22% weight loss at 350°C. Kandpal et al. produced magnetite nanoparticles of 20–22 nm, which showed a saturation magnetization of 217.9 emu/g at 301.5°C [36]. The high saturation magnetization values indicate a better crystal spinal structure as compared to the one having lower values.

5.2.2 THERMAL DECOMPOSITION

This method includes the thermal decomposition of organometallic precursors in organic solvents containing surfactants to stabilize the nanoparticles [37]. Iron acetylacetonate ($Fe(acac)_3$), iron cupferronates [$FeCup_3$], or iron carbonyls ($Fe(CO)_5$) are the organometallic compounds generally used in this process [38]. The "cup" in iron cupferronates means N-nitrosophenylhydroxylamine with a chemical formula of $C_6H_5N(-NO)O-$ [39]. Fatty acid (RCOOH) [40], oleic acid ($CH_3(CH_2)_7CH=CH(CH_2)_7COOH$) [41] and hexadecylamine ($CH_3(CH_2)_{14}CH_2NH_2$) [42] are few regularly used surfactants. The size and surface morphology of synthesized IONPs can be controlled by determining the optimum ratios of organometallic precursors, surfactants, and organic solvents. Time, temperature, and aging time also play their roles.

Park et al. [43] controlled the size of IONPs through seed-mediated growth. Further, introducing the gas bubbles by using artificial argon purging or boiling the solvent enhanced the nucleation rate of IONPs over the growth rate [44]. Hyeon et al. replaced expensive and toxic iron pentacarbonyl with cheaper and non-toxic iron chloride during the synthesis of monodispersed IONPs [45]. An iron oleate complex and a surfactant were mixed to form an organic solvent dispersion. Subsequent heat treatment up to the solvent's boiling point formed nearly 40 g of monodisperse IONPs (without considering any size selection process). Jana et al. [40] reported the synthesis of an iron oleate complex through a reaction between ferrous and ferric chlorides with oleic acid followed by their neutralization. Solvent-free synthesis of magnetite nanocubes and nanospheres by thermal decomposition of ferrocene and polyvinyl pyrrolidone (PVP) was reported by Amara et al. [46]. Highly crystalline Fe_3O_4 nanoparticles in the range of 51–85 nm were reported by varying refluxing temperature, amount of solvent, and reaction time [47]. Yu et al. produced superparamagnetic iron oxide nanocrystals of narrow size distribution with 95% reported yield [48].

5.2.3 MICROEMULSION

The isotropic dispersion of two immiscible liquid phases (say water and oil) in the presence of surfactant molecules forms a thermodynamically stable emulsion [49]. These surfactant molecules form a monolayer between the phases such that their hydrophobic tail gets dissolved in one phase (oil) and the hydrophilic head group dissolves in another (water). Bicontinuous microemulsion and spherical/cylindrical micelles (inverse route) can be used to synthesize size and shape-controlled IONPs [50].

The synthesis of monodisperse maghemite nanoparticles by a one-pot microemulsion method was reported by Vidal-Vidal et al. [51]. Darband et al. [52] reported high yields of crystalline and uniformly sized spinel IONPs having mean diameters of about 3, 6, and 9 nm. A capping agent/surfactant namely polyoxyethylene(5)nonylphenylether was used to prevent agglomeration. Okoli et al. reported the synthesis of magnetic IONPs using water-in-oil (W/O) and oil-in-water (O/W) microemulsions for protein separation. Specific surface areas were found to be 147 m^2/g for W/O and 304 m^2/g for O/W. Significant removal and reduction rates of clay particles were observed in IONPs bounded with proteins as compared to uncovered particles [53].

5.2.4 HYDROTHERMAL/SOLVOTHERMAL TREATMENT

In this technique(s), phase separation is a common concept of obtaining IONPs in which the reactions between solid and liquid phases result in the formation of IONPs. The process starts with the preparation of precursor materials where the metal-rich powders/solutions with organic solvents (e.g., ethanol, propanol, etc.) are used as precursors in the solvothermal process. On the other hand, the hydrothermal process demands other chemical solvents instead of organic solvents [54].

Cai et al. reported the facile hydrothermal synthesis of surface-functionalized Fe_3O_4 with polyethylenimine by a one-pot hydrothermal synthesis process. The resulting nanoparticles possessed fine water dispersibility, colloidal stability, and high relaxivity (130–160 m/M.s) with a slight toxicity of 50 μg/mL [55]. Hao and Teja [56] investigated the effects of temperature, the concentration of the precursor, and residence times on the size and morphology of the particles synthesized by this method. With an increase in the precursor concentration, the particle size and distribution increase. Residence time showed a more appreciable impact on the particle size than feed concentration. Particles produced at short residence times were found to be monodispersed. Xu and Teja [57] synthesized polyvinyl alcohol (PVA)-coated IONPs by employing a continuous hydrothermal process. The average particle size was found to be decreasing with an increase in the PVA concentration (residence time being in the order of 2 seconds). However, at a residence time of 10 seconds, the size was independent of PVA concentration. Bonvin et al. [58] combined coprecipitation with hydrothermal methods and produced IONPs that showed better-controlled shape, size, structure, and crystallinity as compared to those obtained using the coprecipitation method. IONPs produced with a combination of coprecipitation and hydrothermal synthesis routes were biocompatible and non-toxic in nature.

5.2.5 AEROSOL/VAPOR TECHNOLOGY

The flame-spray and laser pyrolysis technique comes under this technology. The flame-spray pyrolysis technique involves the mixing of ferric salt and reducing agent in an organic solvent bath and then the resulting aerosol is condensed in a series of reactors followed by evaporation [59]. The size of the particle can be controlled by adjusting the initial droplet size [60]. On the other hand, the laser pyrolysis technique uses a source of laser to heat the iron precursor in gaseous form and produces well-dispersed IONPs [61]. IONPs compatible with various biomedical applications like MRI contrast agents, targeted drug delivery, and cancer treatment can be obtained as silica-spinel IONPs via the spray drying process [62]. However, apart from the above context, this method is not usually preferred as the resulting size distribution is broad and cannot be made compatible for usage.

5.3 SPECIAL FEATURES OF IONPs

5.3.1 SUPERPARAMAGNETISM

Superparamagnetism property is the zero residual magnetization behavior of materials after removal of the external magnetic field on them. A similar kind of behavior was observed in IONPs even at smaller dimensions in the range of a few nanometers. It provides a unique advantage of stability and dispersion of IONPs upon removal of the magnetic field. The magnetic properties of nanoparticles are usually governed by the finite size and surface effects. There are two principal diameters D_{sp} (superparamagnetic limit) and D_{sd} (single-domain limit), on the basis of which magnetic properties differ. For $D < D_{sp}$, particles exhibit superparamagnetism (i.e., zero coercivity); for $D_{sd} < D < D_{sp}$, particles are ferromagnetic and beyond D_{sd}, they are paramagnetic in nature [63].

Single-domain particle is the one with uniformly magnetized and aligned spins in a single direction. The smaller nanoparticles possess high coercivity because the absence of domain walls offers a magnetization reversal effect by the spin rotation. Also, an anisotropy in shape shows a major influence on coercivity [64].

The size of the domain particle is given by equation (5.1) [65],

$$D_c \approx 18 \frac{\sqrt{AK_{eff}}}{\mu_0 M^2} \tag{5.1}$$

where D_c is the critical diameter of the domain particle, A is the exchange constant, K_{eff} is the anisotropy constant, μ_0 is the vacuum permeability, and M is the saturation magnetization.

Superparamagnetic limit [66] refers to the behavior of a single-domain particle that is well isolated. When the particle size decreases, magnetic anisotropy gets dominated by thermal energy kT, which results in fast magnetic moments inside the particle. This limit is referred to as a superparamagnetic limit having no/zero hysteresis. Neel and Brown derived a general expression for the relaxation time of particle moment as given in equation (5.2),

$$\tau = \tau_0 \exp\left(\frac{K_{eff}V}{kT}\right) \qquad (5.2)$$

where $\tau_0 \sim 10^{-9}$ s.

The superparamagnetic systems take a shorter relaxation time for the magnetization reversal. The system that takes more time is in a "blocked state". The differential temperature between both states is called the "blocking temperature". The magnetic property of nanoparticles can be measured with the help of a superconducting quantum interference device (SQUID) magnetometer, vibrating sample magnetometer (VSM), etc.

5.3.2 SELF-ASSEMBLY

The specific interfacial surface area of the nanoparticles increases with the decrease in particle size, which leads to breaking of symmetry, uneven atomic coordination, and changes in the band structure. These ultimately result in the exchange of anisotropy between surfaces and core surfaces. Therefore, the agglomeration of nanoparticles could be prevented through suitable functionalization strategies. However, self-assembly in magnetic nanoparticles is often useful and economical as it serves to manipulate their spatial arrangement. Various morphological self-assembled patterns evolve due to surface functionalization, interparticle interactions, and method of fabrication. Also, the surface coatings have been shown remarkable improvements in the bioactivity of nanoparticles [63]. IONPs are mainly subjected to two types of coatings, viz., magnetically inert surface coatings and magnetic surface coatings (Section 5.4).

5.3.3 CYTOTOXIC BEHAVIOR AND ANTIBACTERIAL ACTIVITY

The capability of being toxic to various cells and efficacy of activity against various bacteria are called cytotoxicity and antibacterial effect respectively. Prior to the usage of IONPs for biomedical applications, their cytotoxicity and antibacterial effect need to be investigated. It is advantageous to be toxic to harmful cells but at the same time, it should not harm any healthy cells. Usually, cell viability assays/methods will be used for measuring the cytotoxicity of IONPs against organ-specific cancer and normal human cell lines. Dead cell staining trypan blue, tritium-labeled thymidine uptake, 51Cr method, LDH (lactate dehydrogenase) assay, and enzyme-based MTT & WST are some of the cell viability testing methods in practice. Various cell lines have been used for determining *in-vitro* cytotoxicity of IONPs.

Soenen et al. [67] demonstrated for the first time the evaluation of core size (using electron microscopy), hydrodynamic radius, and zeta potential (using electrophoretic mobility measurements) of IONPs. In addition, they investigated the type of stabilization, coating, colloidal stability, and potential aggregation of IONPs in physiological saline and in a serum-containing cell medium. Using PC12 (rat phenochromocytoma) cells, quantitative and qualitative measurements of cell viability were assessed through LDH assays. Cell staining was investigated with a fluorescent viability agent, MTT, and trypan blue. Neurite outgrowth (differentiation of neuron cells) was induced by stimulating cells with NGF (nerve growth factor), preparing a stock solution of 1 mg/mL in sterile DMSO (dimethyl sulfoxide) [67]. In response to the cytotoxicity of IONPs, one can stabilize and functionalize nanoparticles and make them compatible for use.

Antibacterial activity is an activity possessed by IONPs to suppress the growth of bacteria. According to the bacterial classification, there are two categories, namely Gram-positive and Gram-negative. The classification is based on the results (positive/negative) of the Gram stain test. For the microbial testing of IONPs, ten pathogenic bacteria were used. The name list is as follows: (1) *Staphylococcus aureus* (MTCC 144), (2) *Shigella flexneri* (lab isolate), (3) *Bacillus licheniformis* (MTCC 7425), (4) *Bacillus brevis* (MTCC 7404), (5) *Vibrio cholerae* (MTCC 3904), (6) *Pseudomonas aeruginosa* (MTCC 1034), (7) *Streptococcus aureus* (lab isolate), (8) *Staphylococcus epidermidis* (MTCC 3615), (9) *Bacillus subtilis* (MTCC 7164), and (10) *Escherichia coli* (MTCC 1089) [68]. In the above-mentioned list, 1, 3, 4, 7, 8, and 9 bacterial species are Gram-positive as they have shown positive results in the Gram stain test and the rest (2, 5, 6, and 10) are Gram-negative as they have not retained crystal violet in the Gram staining test. It was reported that IONPs showed better bactericidal activity against Gram-positive bacteria as compared to Gram-negative bacteria. The interaction between IONPs and bacteria is shown in Figure 5.2.

5.4 SURFACE FUNCTIONALIZATION OF IONPs

IONPs agglomerate as they have the tendency for self-assembly, which leads to the breakdown of certain useful properties. Therefore, surface stabilization of IONPs in terms of utility, synthesis, and storage is a major concern to achieve colloidal stability and to prevent agglomeration [69]. Stabilization of the surface of nanoparticles is also essential for biomedical applications of IONPs as it demands targeting and further functionalization (with biological drugs, etc.). Normally, the coatings that are incorporated on the nanoparticle surfaces are dispersants. The adsorption and desorption tendencies of a dispersant depend on the interactions of the filtration [70]. The coatings for IONPs are classified by magnetic behavior, that is, magnetically inert and magnetic surface coatings, and by the nature of the coating material, that is, polymeric

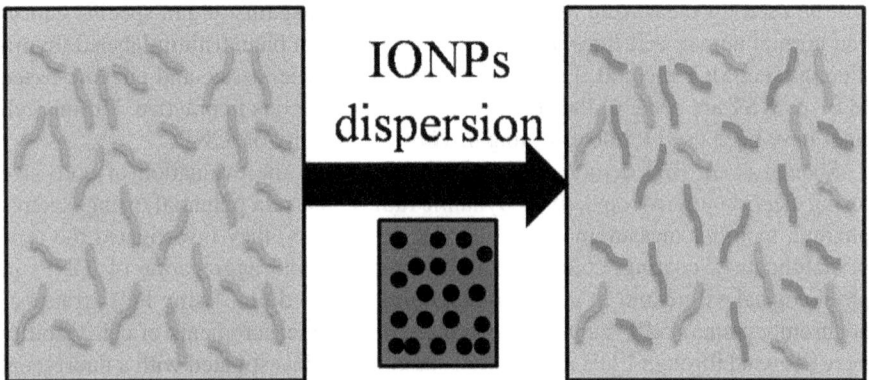

FIGURE 5.2 Interaction between IONPs and bacteria (red stains show bactericidal effects).

coatings and non-polymeric coatings. Amstad et al. [70] explained the structure of surface-functionalized IONPs in four components, namely core (IONPs), anchors (the functional group of low affinity with the nanoparticles giving rise to reversible dispersant adsorption), spacer (low molecular weight surfactant for imparting stability), and functionalities (drugs or biomaterials to be coated which are optional) [70]. The structures of surface-functionalized IONPs can be categorized into core–shell, mosaic, shell–core, shell–core–shell, and dumbbell shapes, which are shown in Figure 5.3 [71]. However, for the usage of IONPs in the biomedical field, the core–shell structure often serves better.

For achieving efficient therapeutic and targeting capability, functionalization involving attachment of IONPs with an amine group (–NH$_2$) and a carboxylic group (–COOH) is given principal importance. However, it imparts multiple synthesis steps as well as the wider size distribution of nanoparticles, which would rather be detrimental for biomedical applications. These effects can be reduced by optimizing processing parameters wherein the *in-situ* functionalization procedure acquired more attention [72].

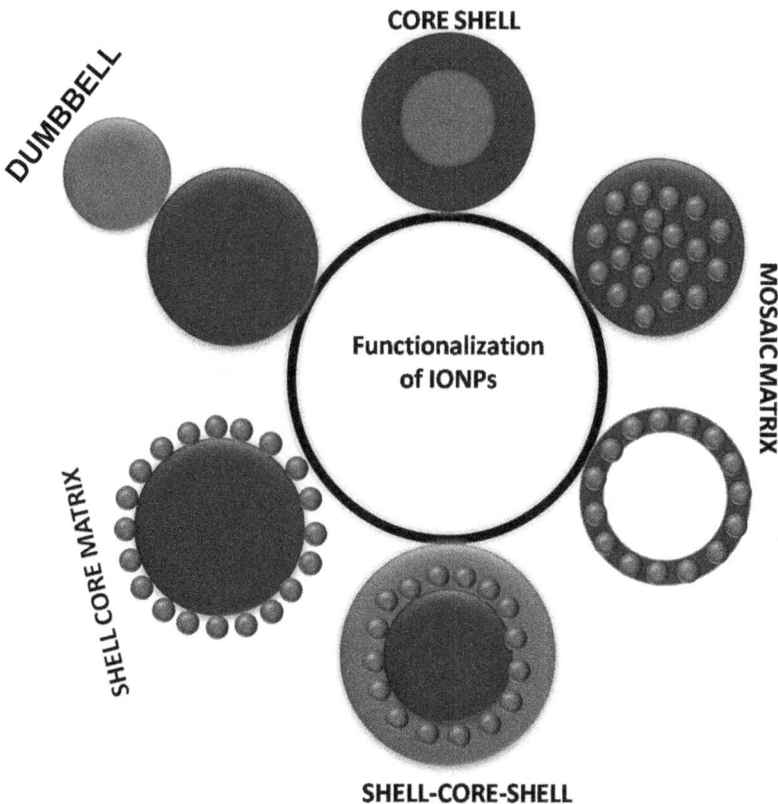

FIGURE 5.3 Different structures of surface-functionalized IONPs. The brown-colored sphere represents IONPs, and gray and blue/gray spheres are surface coatings.

5.4.1   BASED ON THE MAGNETIC BEHAVIOR OF A
SURFACE-FUNCTIONALIZING MATERIAL

5.4.1.1   Magnetically Inert

There exists a net reduction in the magnetization of nanoparticles at the surface in reference to the bulk magnetization due to the presence of a magnetic dead layer and canted spins and/or spin-glass-like behavior on the surface of the particle [73]. The magnetic anisotropy of particles increases with decreasing particle size due to surface effects [74].

Energy anisotropy contributions of both bulk and surface anisotropies could be represented as

$$K_{\text{eff}} = K_v + \frac{6}{D} K_s \qquad (5.3)$$

where K_{eff} = anisotropy constant,
K_v = volume anisotropy,
K_s = surface anisotropy, and
D = diameter of nanoparticles.

The correlation to be established among the influences of surface coatings on the magnetic property of nanoparticles is complex. However, silica-coated magnetic IONPs showed a clear influence on their magnetic properties in terms of the thickness of the inert silica layer. These results were also utilized for manipulating magnetic storage data [75]. It is often observed that magnetic anisotropy increases in the case of applying magnetically inert surface coatings. Thus, the magnetization effect gets reduced, which results in less agglomeration.

5.4.1.2   Magnetically Active

The coating of a magnetic material on magnetic nanoparticles imparts great influence on its magnetic properties. This approach leans toward the formation of magnetic nanocomposites. Thereby, a remarkable feature "exchange bias effect" (shift of hysteresis loop at the interface) occurs [76]. The exchange bias effect generally materializes whenever there exists an interface between the core of a ferromagnetic material and the shell of an antiferromagnetic material or vice versa. Fe_3O_4–CoO (ferrimagnetic–antiferromagnetic) is an example of such a nanocomposite. The exchange bias effect has its advantages in permanent magnets, spintronics, and recording media. Not only are the magnetic properties of nanoparticles influenced by their shape, size distribution, surface effects, and phase morphology, but also there are numerous complications which add up to the contribution.

5.4.2   BASED ON THE NATURE OF A SURFACE-FUNCTIONALIZING MATERIAL

The most commonly used surface coatings over the past decade were some non-polymeric materials like gold and silica as well as polymeric materials like dextran, chitosan, PEG (polyethylene glycol), and PVA [77]. The properties obtained due to these coatings encompass excellent chemical affinity, biocompatibility, non-antigenicity, non-immunogenicity, and protection against plasma proteins (eliminate opsonization) [78]. Recently, ultrasmall IONPs were successfully modified with zwitterionic species (species with two or more functional groups attached such that at least two of them are oppositely charged and the overall charge is balanced). These IONPs were found to possess reduced toxicity, enhanced biocompatibility, and reduced formation of protein corona [79]. The functionalization can be carried out with natural coating agents like human serum albumin (HAS), which also proved to be efficiently reliable in the case of thermal therapy [80].

5.4.2.1 Polymeric Materials

Polymers often provide better surface functionalization for colloidal stability. In addition, they also impart significantly enhanced biomedical properties [81,82]. The approaches to coat polymers include *in-situ* (during synthesis) and post-synthesis methods [83]. Figure 5.4 shows some polymeric materials that can be coated on Fe_3O_4 nanoparticles. Furthermore, these coatings are classified as follows.

5.4.2.1.1 *Polyethylene Glycol*

PEG, being a biocompatible (approved by USFDA, United States Food and Drug Administration) [84] polymer, raises the count of circulating nanoparticles in blood per second. Thus, it was used in targeted drug delivery applications. PEG was also helpful for increasing the efficiency of the internalization of nanoparticles [85]. In addition,

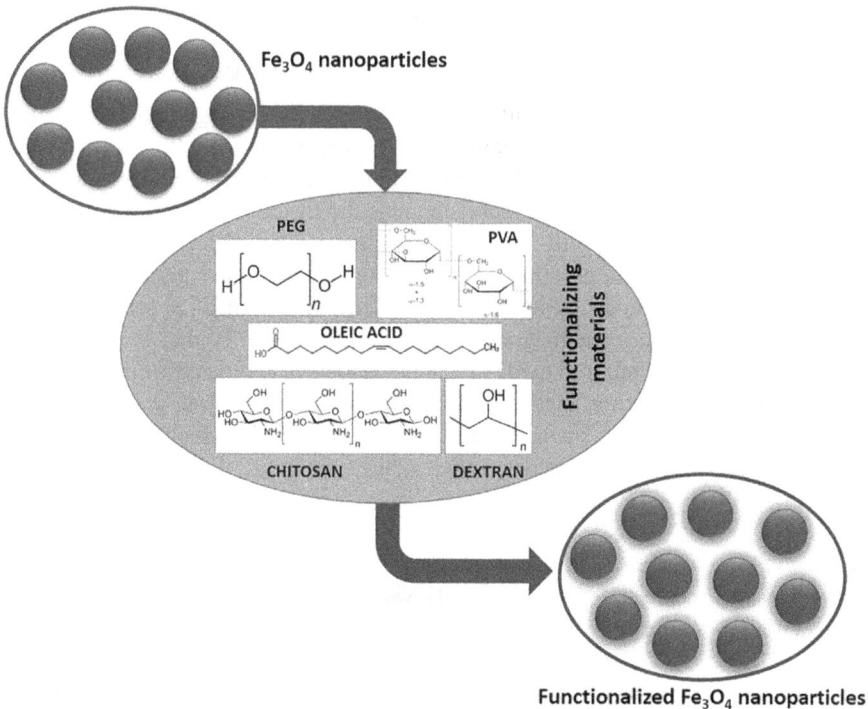

FIGURE 5.4 Various polymeric materials for surface functionalization of IONPs.

their stability in the physiological saline solution was remarkable [86]. PEG-coated IONPs can be synthesized using two methods: imparting PEG coating during synthesis (*in situ*) of IONPs or after the synthesis (*ex-situ*). Dispersion results in the latter case were much better than those of the former [87]. *In-situ* PEG-coated Fe_3O_4 can be synthesized via a coprecipitation technique by using premixed ferric salts of sulfate and PEG [88]. Secondly, the PEG solution can be added to Fe_3O_4 suspension using a two-step approach [89]. Photo-polymerization reactions can also be used for preparing PEG hydrogel-coated IONPs [90]. The limitations of PEG coating were non-biodegradability and misfit behavior toward standard metabolic clearance.

5.4.2.1.2 Polyvinyl Alcohol

PVA marked its suitability because of its biocompatibility, hydrophilic nature, low toxicity, and capability to prevent agglomeration [86]. Coating with PVA leads to the formation of monodispersed IONPs having excellent thermomechanical properties like high modulus of elasticity, crystallinity, and strength [91]. It makes IONPs less sensitive toward a high water content, which tends to reduce the elastic modulus. Thus, it makes these particles compatible for drug delivery [92]. Pardoe et al. [93] carried out a coprecipitation reaction to synthesize IONPs with PVA coating. Mahmoudi et al. used a two-step approach in which IONPs were obtained by precipitation of iron salts under an argon atmosphere followed by addition of PVA solution in ratios of 2:1 (polymer to iron) for 30 minutes, at 3600 rpm and 35°C. PVA-coated IONPs can be synthesized by numerous methods by controlling the reaction time, temperature, amount of PVA, and rate of stirring [94].

5.4.2.1.3 Chitosan

The principle characteristics of chitosan are non-toxicity, biodegradability, alkalinity, biocompatibility, and hydrophilicity [86]. The structure of chitosan is quite similar to that of cellulose. Chitosan does not exhibit water solubility under neutral pH conditions, but it becomes water-soluble in an acidic medium due to the protonation effect. It also has the capability to absorb toxic materials (antimicrobial in nature). Moreover, it is suitable for protein purification due to its adhesive properties. Hence, IONPs coated with chitosan have numerous applications in medical science including *in-vivo* drug delivery and magnetic bioseparation [95,96]. Paul et al. [97] carried out the synthesis of 12 nm iron oxide magnetic nanoparticles coated with chitosan by a controlled coprecipitation method. Shagholani et al. synthesized chitosan-coated IONPs followed by some surface modifications with PVA, which showed a zeta potential value with low protein absorption [98].

5.4.2.1.4 Dextran

Dextran is biocompatible and non-degradable in the human body. It degrades when exposed to an enzyme called dextranase. However, it is non-toxic to the human body as this enzyme is not synthesized by the human body cells [99]. Fundamental applications of IONPs coated with dextran were MRI and cancer treatment therapy [100]. However, the weak bond offered by dextran with the IONP surface is the main disadvantage that limits some critical applications. It also creates an adverse effect on compound tolerance, which slowly influences the infusion [101]. Josephson et al. [102]

suggested that a monolayer of IONPs coated with dextran increases the intracellular magnetic labeling at different target cells. IONPs can be treated with epichlorohydrin to preclude dextran dissociation. The particles are often treated with ammonia for surface functionalization for easy attachment with the target sites. Jafari et al. reported the use of IONPs coated with dextran as a contrast agent in breast cancer therapy [103].

5.4.2.2 Non-polymeric Materials

5.4.2.2.1 Silica

Silica prevents the aggregation of nanoparticles, improves chemical stability, and reduces the toxicity of nanoparticles. The reduction in toxicity increases their biocompatibility. Thus, silica was a widely used material for the functionalization of IONPs [71]. The hydrophilic structure of silica helps to bind various biological ligands. Silica-coated IONPs are used for various applications, viz., biolabeling, bioseparation, catalysts, and ferrofluids [104]. However, it is difficult to obtain a uniform thickness of silica coating on IONPs. This unevenness of coating thickness leads to the development of an irregular magnetic field and uneven heating in hyperthermia (cancer therapy) [105]. However, Santra et al. demonstrated that the DNA molecule can be attached successfully onto the surface of silica-coated IONPs [106].

5.4.2.2.2 Gold

Coating of gold on magnetic nanoparticles was first reported by Lin et al. [107]. Gold has been used to protect the cores of IONPs from oxidation. Gold-coated magnetic IONPs show a high affinity to absorb light because of the high colloidal stability between gold and IONPs. On the other hand, it also causes attenuation in the magnetic properties of IONPs. Liang et al. proposed that the biosensing system for human alpha thrombin consists of gold-coated IONPs [108]. IONPs were synthesized by the coprecipitation method and gold coating was carried out by iterative reduction of $HAuCl_4$ (chloroauric acid) onto dextran-coated Fe_3O_4 nanoparticles. The result proved the capability to detect human alpha thrombin [109].

5.4.2.2.3 Oleic Acid

Normally, oleic acid ($C_{18}H_{34}O_2$) behaves as a capping agent by forming a protective monolayer that strongly bonds with IONPs and gives monodispersed and highly uniform nanoparticles [110]. Park et al. reported that oleic acid was hydrophobic in nature, which is not a suitable property for biomedical applications. Hydrophilic coatings can be imparted using polymers or α-cyclodextrin [45]. The layer of oleic acid covering nanoparticles was not covalently bonded with the surface due to high ionic strength and pH conditions. Thus, their interactions were hindered. IONPs covered with an oleic acid layer show two-electron spin resonance signal (ESR) characterized by transmission electron microscopy, ferromagnetic resonance, and electron paramagnetic resonance (FMR, EPR). Oleic acid also controls the shape and size of IONPs and prevents them from agglomeration. Fourier-transform infrared spectroscopy revealed the adsorption mechanism of oleic acid by characterizing pure oleic acid and comparing the results with Fe_3O_4 composites coated with oleic acid [111].

5.5 IONPs AS A BIOMEDICAL DEVICE

Devising IONPs for biomaterial applications comprises two steps, one is tagging of IONPs with biological entities and the second one is the separation of tagged IONPs from unwanted biomaterials. Usually, surface modification must be carried out prior to the labeling/tagging/binding of magnetic IONPs with biological entities. Surface modification develops compatibility between IONPs and biological entities. The surface modification process is carried out by coating magnetic IONPs with biocompatible molecules like PVA, dextran (complex branch 'glucan' which is a polysaccharide made up of several molecules of glucose), and phospholipids. Magnetic particles coated with agents had the tolerance to avoid allergy (also referred to as immunospecific agents) and were successfully targeted to get bound to biological entities, which include RBCs, Golgi vesicles, lung cancer cells, bacteria, and urological cancer cells [17].

After the successful preparation of tagged particles/entities, they should be separated from the unwanted biomaterials via magnetic separation (which is a fluid-based device). There are two approaches to this separation. In the first approach, a magnet is brought in contact with the wall of a container, which contains a stagnant solution of unwanted biomaterials and magnetically tagged biomaterials. Due to the magnetization effect, the IONPs tagged with biomaterials get attached to the container walls and it allows the removal of the supernatant containing unwanted biomaterials [112]. Figure 5.5 illustrates the separation of magnetically tagged biomaterials in a stagnant solution.

Unlike the first approach, the second one treats a continuous flow of solutions. The external magnetic field fixed in-between the flow catches biomaterials tagged with IONPs and leaves the rest. So, the container column is often packed with steel wool, which grabs the tagged biomaterials. Recovery of magnetically tagged biomaterials can be accomplished by field removal and flushing the container with water [113]. The process is shown in Figure 5.6.

5.6 IONPs IN BIOMEDICAL APPLICATIONS

Iron oxides are more preferred than other competing oxides for biomedical applications due to their inherent non-toxic behavior [70,114]. The idea behind using superparamagnetic materials is that they can be easily magnetized (temporarily) in the presence of an external magnetic field and further recovered through demagnetization by removing the field. In addition, they are biodegradable, biocompatible, magnetic, and heat-medicated therapeutic (which is extremely useful for the treatment of lung cancer, targeted drug delivery, and cystic fibrosis) agents [115,116] (Figure 5.7). As explained earlier, the biomedical applications of IONPs rely on their surface characteristics. Thus, a better understanding of interactions between the nanoparticle surface and the biomolecules is required. Deng and Gao showed the nature of such interactions on the basis of certain parameters affecting cytotoxicity, cellular uptake, intracellular degradation, and protein adsorption of various nanoparticles [117]. Surface modifications in magnetic nanoparticles can be designed advantageous to stimuli-responsive pH, enzyme, redox, thermal, and optical-based biomedical applications including imaging, drug delivery, and hyperthermia [118]. Some important biomedical applications are explained as follows.

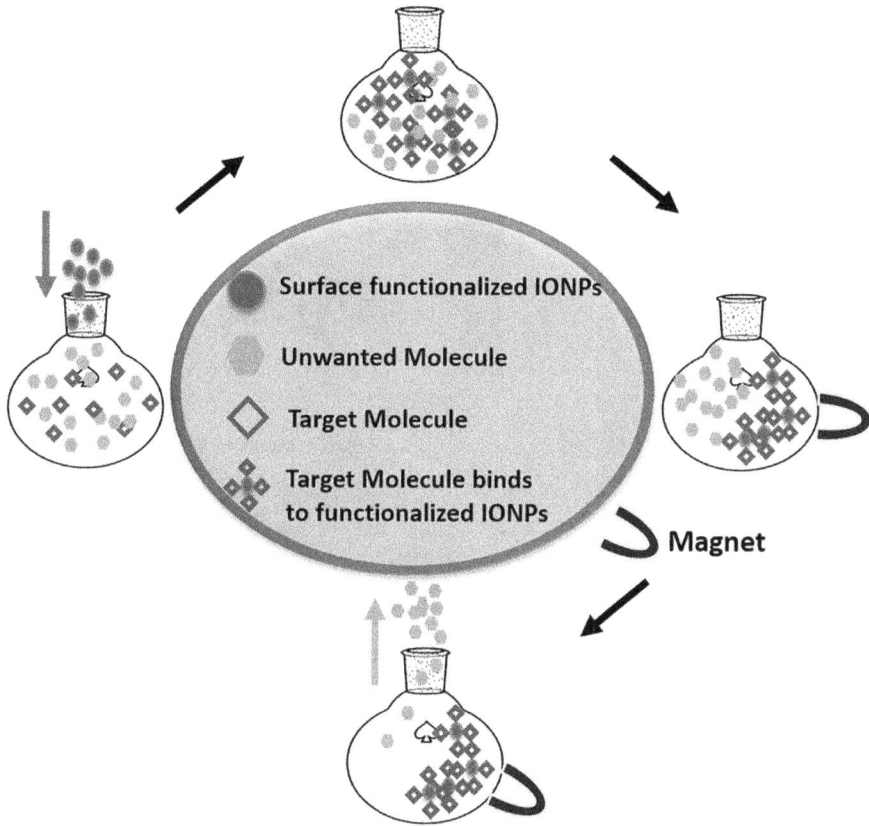

FIGURE 5.5   Magnetic separation of magnetically tagged biomaterials in a stagnant solution.

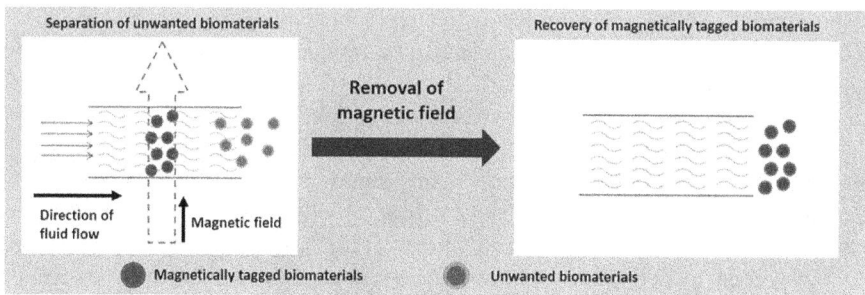

FIGURE 5.6   Magnetic separation of magnetically tagged biomaterials from liquid flow.

5.6.1   Magnetic Resonance Imaging

MRI is a widely used technique in the field of biomedical engineering to obtain visuals of internal body parts to detect the damages and their root cause. MRI uses a powerful magnetic field that interacts with the human body's protons. Currently, several

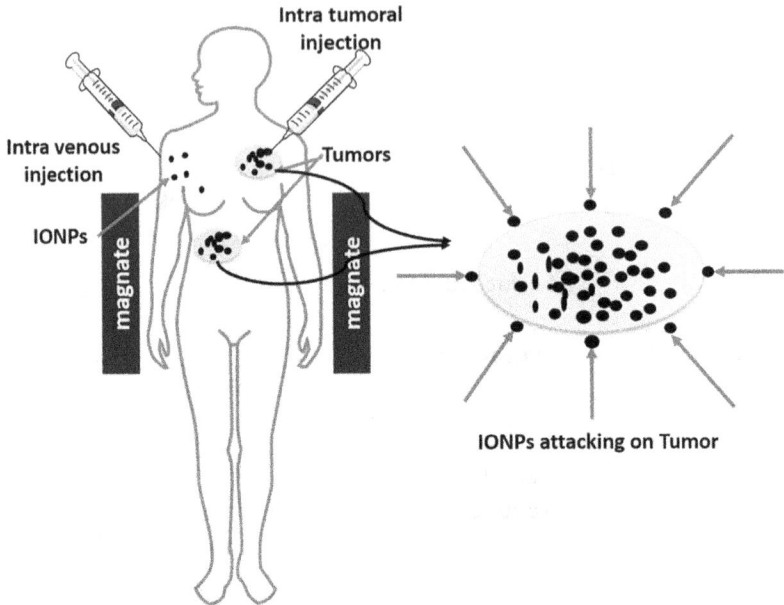

FIGURE 5.7 Schematic representation of a heat-mediated therapeutic treatment using IONPs.

imaging methods based on molecular, functional, and morphological models like positron emission tomography (PET), single-photon emission computed tomography (SPECT), computed tomography (CT), photoacoustic tomography (PAT), fluorescence molecular tomography (FMT), and X-ray-based computed tomography (CT) are also available [119], but MRI only possesses high spatial resolution (100 μm). However, the sensitivity of MRI is lower than SPECT and bioluminescence.

The contrast in MRI images arises from different signal intensities of different volume elements. Paramagnetic metals including lanthanide, magnevist, omniscan, eovist, ferumoxides, and resovist are some of the well-known contrast agents. IONPs smaller than 4 nm which behave primarily paramagnetic in nature are also used as a contrast agent in MRI. MRI is the most effective and safest non-invasive technique for stem cell tracking in living bodies. The enhancement in the functioning of superparamagnetic nanomaterials-based contrast agents can be achieved through proper understanding of various relaxation mechanisms including Neel and Brownian relaxations associated with different processing parameters [120]. Nedyalkova et al. also provided a computational modeling-based study of the essential properties and nature of IONPs for MRI and other biomedical applications [121]. Commercially, superparamagnetic IONPs with transfection agents (TAs) have been applied in the labeling of stem cells. In addition, IONPs are used in clinical applications for brain tumors in MRI [122].

5.6.2 Magnetic Particle Imaging (MPI)

MPI is the latest medical quantitative imaging technique at a level of millimeter resolution, which was first introduced by Gleich and Weizenecker in 2005 [123]. It is a non-invasive, tomographic, and 3D dynamic biomedical imaging technique used to visualize the distribution of superparamagnetic iron IONPs in tissue organs. The direct addition of nanoscale magnetic molecular probes (NMP) makes MPI more sensitive than MRI [124]. The signal of MPI is generated due to the magnetization effect of nanoparticles [125]. There are numerous applications of MPI including cardiovascular imaging, sentinel lymph node biopsy (SLNB), cancer targeting, and cell tracking in the living bodies [126,127]. Despite the stem cells, MPI was also used to monitor blood circulation by operating IONPs labeled with red blood cells. There are two types of relaxation mechanisms involved in the MPI process, one is Brownian rotation and the second is Neel rotation. The transition frequencies of Neel and Brownian motion are dependent on the nanoparticle size, anisotropy, and viscosity of the medium. In addition, the magnetization behavior of large diameter particles is anisotropic in nature [128].

5.6.3   IN-VITRO BIOSEPARATION

Functionalization for cell or *in-vitro* protein separation is an important application of IONPs. The expensive liquid chromatography systems are replaced by magnetic separation techniques where all the purification steps take place in a single test tube [129]. Charged bipyridinium carboxylic acids and biotin-coated magnetic nanoparticles have been used for affinity isolation of avidin protein [130]. Also, IONPs are coated with various functional groups such as $-OH$, $-SH$, or $-NH_2$ through surface exchange reactions [131] or by coprecipitation of iron (II/III) salts in the presence of organic capping groups [132]. Silica coating was performed through two steps: (i) formation of silica by hydrolysis and condensation of the sol–gel precursor (Stober process) [133] and (ii) coating of silica on the crystal core confined by micelles [134]. The separation of proteins from the mixture can also be carried out with magnetoliposomes, which are magnetic nanoparticles coated with phospholipids [83].

5.6.4   TARGETED IN-VIVO DRUG DELIVERY

The main objective of drug delivery is to diminish the extent of cytotoxic drugs that enter into the body and to control the dosage by directly targeting harmed tissues. Targeting the right position and deep level are two main advantages of magnetic nanoparticles used in drug delivery. A drug delivery vehicle is commonly used for drug delivery purposes [135]. The loading of magnetic nanoparticles with a conjugating ligand or antibodies is the first and foremost step. The targeting of drug-loaded magnetic particles is later carried out with the help of the magnetic field generated by magnetic sources. This magnetic field-driven drug targeting is referred to as an intravascular injection in which magnetic nanoparticles are transported through the blood to the target site with the help of the magnetic field. The targeting particle should possess certain features for effective retention at the target. The applied magnetic force should overcome the blood drag force. According to the Stokes law, the drag force is directly proportional to the diameter of the veins and the velocity of the blood. On the other hand, the magnetic force varies in proportion to the blood capillary size (typically varying in the range of 5–10 μm). So the deviation of magnetic nanoparticles from the target site can be subjected to a start in response to magnetic field gradient variation [136]. Finally, the particles should be in the nanorange and the magnetic field should be applied through superconducting magnets for obtaining good results. This technique requires materials having desirable magnetization with zero coercivity, that is, superparamagnetic materials. Such superparamagnetic behavior can be obtained from single-domain nanoparticles. IONPs of magnetite (Fe_3O_4) and maghemite (γ-Fe_2O_3) are the most useful materials in the field of biomedical applications. The large magnetic saturation behavior shown by magnetite makes it more efficient for this usage over maghemite.

Nanoconjugates made of two antibody fragments proved fruitful for being utilized in cell targeting. The internalization of IONPs was first targeted to JC (John Cunningham) virus oncoprotein, T antigen, for non-invasive detection of gene expression in the cell. JC virus is the human polyomavirus that damages the myelin sheath of neurons in the nervous systems in the name of progressive multifocal leukoencephalopathy (PML) disease. More than 80% of the population is infected with this JC virus. The most predominant cure for this virus is a ^{125}I-labeled antibody coupled with CLIO (cross-linked iron oxide) nanoparticles. To accomplish this coupling, sulfo-SMCC (sul fosuccinimidyl-4-[N-maleimidomethyl] cyclohexane-1-carboxylate) had to be reacted with CLIO-NH_2 to form maleimido-NPs. At the same time, the antibody separates into two monovalent halves by reacting with a 2-mercaptoethylamine (2-MEA) solution. The reaction was accompanied by heating and column purification in addition to pre-equilibrating the same with PBS (phosphate-buffered saline) and EDTA (ethylene diamine tetra acetic acid). The final step was the coupling of maleimido-NPs with antibody fragments to produce Ab-CLIO (antibody-CLIO) nanoconjugates [137]. Kohler et al. proposed the use of a biostable methotrexate-immobilized IONP drug carrier in real-time monitoring of drug delivery through MRI [8]. Gallo et al. reported an increment of 100–400 times of oxantrazole levels in the brain by incorporation of magnetic nanospheres than those obtained after solution dosage. The above works were a few examples of the success of magnetic nanoparticles in drug delivery [138].

In cancer therapy, the addition of cytokines with magnetic nanoparticles controls the release of drugs. It was observed that antitumor type1 (T_{h1}) lymphocyte had shown effective response because of its cytotoxic behavior. Its response was characterized by the help of the production of interferon-gamma. Nowadays, cancer immunotherapy is a very active and crucial field to design a new antitumor device. Treatment through antitumor immune response not only removes the primary tumor but also eliminates the neoplastic cell [139]. The recent development in this field manipulated the adaptive immune response to control the development of tumors despite their elimination [140]. It has been found that interferon-gamma was an effective cytokine for tumor elimination. The first trial was performed with epirubicin-coated magnetic particles. After the injection process, a magnetic field was created closer to the tumor for 45 min for efficient targeted drug delivery [141].

5.6.5 HYPERTHERMIA

It is a kind of cancer treatment in which the temperature of the body is increased to above its normal. This whole process can be considered as a destructive metabolism in which certain malignant tissues and tumors are subjected to heat to break down. An external magnetic field applied to a magnetic fluid causes energy release due to hysteresis loss, which finally leads to the increase in temperature of nanoparticles. This localized increase in temperature damages unwanted cells as they cannot survive at a temperature higher than 41°C. The quantification of the heating ability of magnetic nanoparticles is determined using the term 'specific absorption rate (SAR),' which is the heat dissipation rate per unit mass of magnetic nanoparticles. The efficiency of nanoparticles lies in the increased SAR value and reduced overall dosage [58]. IONPs are best suited for their use in magnetic fluid hyperthermia as it requires nanoparticles with optimized biocompatibility and size and efficient heating ability, while being economical and easy to synthesize [142].

In the late 1950s, Gilchrist et al. (1957) used nanoparticles of γ-Fe_2O_3 (ranging from 20 to 100 nm) in the magnetic field of 1.2 MHz intensity to target and heat various tissue samples [143]. In 1957, for the destruction of metastasis in the lymph node, radiofrequency is used to inject magnetic nanoparticles into a dog body. Magnetic nanoparticles possess a unique property that a small amount of their usage can generate heat close to the target point. The concept of intracellular hyperthermia was obtained with the use of FeO(OH) and Fe_3O_4 in the size range of 3–6 nm [144]. Ferrofluids for hyperthermia cancer treatment were investigated for the first time by Jordan et al. in 1993 [145]. Nowadays, hyperthermia mostly relies on magnetic hyperthermia because of the biocompatibility and susceptibility of magnetic nanoparticles (magnetite and maghemite) [146]. Various types of magnetic materials with different strengths, different frequencies of magnetic fields, incorporation of different encapsulations, and particle delivery were also observed from the literature [147,148].

5.7   CONCLUSIONS AND FUTURE PERSPECTIVE

There had been wide research in the field of biomedical applications, which increased the demand for IONPs to larger extents. The size, shape, and distributions are the crucial parameters for their *in-vivo* and *in-vitro* biomedical applications. The controlled shape and size distribution of IONPs is still a limiting factor to utilize their full potential and they need to be optimized depending on their synthesis route and involved conditions. Surface functionalization has emerged as a potential strategy to mitigate such issues by giving IONPs sufficient stability and subsequently improving their performance. There are issues related to the coupling of ligands, which results in higher hydrodynamic sizes of the functionalized IONPs. Zeta potential measurements could be performed for IONPs before and after the functionalization to tackle such egresses. In addition, surface properties such as the surface charge of IONPs should be considered in functionalization strategies, which significantly affect the interaction with biological systems.

Despite the huge potentiality for IONPs in biomedical applications, there exist a few challenges, which are as follows. (i) The magnetic particles tested on animals (reptiles, rabbits, etc.) may not resemble the same behavior on human bodies. (ii) Precision scaling up is quite difficult: As soon as the drugs attached to IONPs are released, their control is no longer possible. (iii) The toxic behavior of most of the magnetic carriers limits their use. (iv) It is often observed that IONPs accumulate at the target and give rise to the embolization of the blood vessels being targeted. The water dispensability and stability of high quality are also major issues but these can be controlled by having control over certain parameters [149]. Keeping the above-mentioned points in mind, the design and stability of IONPs should be better tuned as per the suitable applications.

ACKNOWLEDGMENT

AKS thankfully acknowledges the financial support by SERB-DST (ECR/2016/001081).

REFERENCES

1. De Crozals G, Bonnet R, Farre C, Chaix C. 2016. Nanoparticles with multiple properties for biomedical applications: A strategic guide. *Nano Today* Elsevier Ltd; 11:435–63.
2. Nazarenus M, Zhang Q, Soliman MG, del Pino P, Pelaz B, Carregal-Romero S, et al. 2014. In vitro interaction of colloidal nanoparticles with mammalian cells: What have we learned thus far? *Beilstein J Nanotechnol* 5:1477–90.
3. Deng J, He J, Zheng J-S, Terakawa S, Huang H, Fang L-C, et al. 2013. Preparation and application of amino- and dextran-modified superparamagnetic iron oxide nanoparticles. *Part Sci Technol* 31:241–7.
4. Hastak V, Bandi S, Kashyap S, Singh S, Luqman S, Lodhe M, et al. 2018. Antioxidant efficacy of chitosan/graphene functionalized superparamagnetic iron oxide nanoparticles. *J Mater Sci Mater Med* Springer US; 29:154.
5. Bandi S, Hastak V, Pavithra CLP, Kashyap S, Singh DK, Luqman S, et al. 2019. Graphene/chitosan-functionalized iron oxide nanoparticles for biomedical applications. *J Mater Res* Cambridge University Press; 34:3389–99.
6. Macher T, Totenhagen J, Sherwood J, Qin Y, Gurler D, Bolding MS, et al. 2015. Ultrathin iron oxide nanowhiskers as positive contrast agents for magnetic resonance imaging. *Adv Funct Mater* 25:490–4.
7. Tomitaka A, Arami H, Gandhi S, Krishnan KM. 2015. Lactoferrin conjugated iron oxide nanoparticles for targeting brain glioma cells in magnetic particle imaging. *Nanoscale Royal Soc Chem*; 7:16890–8.
8. Kohler N, Sun C, Fichtenholtz A, Gunn J, Fang C, Zhang M. 2006. Methotrexate-immobilized poly(ethylene glycol) magnetic nanoparticles for MR imaging and drug delivery. *Small* 2:785–92.
9. Laurent S, Dutz S, Häfeli UO, Mahmoudi M. 2011. Magnetic fluid hyperthermia: Focus on superparamagnetic iron oxide nanoparticles. *Adv Colloid Interface Sci* Elsevier B.V.; 166:8–23.
10. Cornell RM, Schwertmann U. 2004. *The Iron Oxides: Structure, Properties, Reactions, Occurences and Uses.* Wiley, ISBN 978-3-527-60644-3. Weinheim, FRG: Wiley-VCH Verlag GmbH & Co. KGaA.
11. Laurent S, Bridot J-L, Elst L Vander, Muller RN. 2010. Magnetic iron oxide nanoparticles for biomedical applications. *Future Med Chem* 2:427–49.
12. Baldi G, Bonacchi D, Innocenti C, Lorenzi G, Sangregorio C. 2007. Cobalt ferrite nanoparticles: The control of the particle size and surface state and their effects on magnetic properties. *J Magn Magn Mater* 311:10–6.
13. Mi X, Tong M, Cai J, Su H, Liu S, Ma Y, et al. 2017. Facile synthesis of superparamagnetic iron oxide nanoparticles with tunable size: From individual nanoparticles to nanoclusters. *Micro Nano Lett* 12:749–53.

14. Song Q, Zhang ZJ. 2004. Shape control and associated magnetic properties of spinel cobalt ferrite nanocrystals. *J Am Chem Soc* 126:6164–8.
15. Palchoudhury S, Xu Y, Rushdi A, Holler RA, Bao Y. 2012. Controlled synthesis of iron oxide nanoplates and nanoflowers. *Chem Commun* 48:10499.
16. Kucheryavy P, He J, John VT, Maharjan P, Spinu L, Goloverda GZ, et al. 2013. Superparamagnetic iron oxide nanoparticles with variable size and an iron oxidation state as prospective imaging agents. *Langmuir* 29:710–6.
17. Pankhurst QA, Connolly J, Jones SK, Dobson J. 2003. Applications of magnetic nanoparticles in biomedicine. *J Phys D Appl Phys* 36:R167–81.
18. Salunkhe AB, Khot VM, Pawar SH. 2014. Magnetic hyperthermia with magnetic nanoparticles: A status review. *Curr Top Med Chem* 14:572–94.
19. Martinez-Mera I, Espinosa-Pesqueira ME, Perez-Hernandez R, Arenas-Alatorre J. 2007. Synthesis of magnetite (Fe_3O_4) nanoparticles without surfactants at room temperature. *Mater Lett* 61:4447–51.
20. Chin AB, Yaacob II. 2007. Synthesis and characterization of magnetic iron oxide nanoparticles via w/o microemulsion and Massart's procedure. *J Mater Process Technol* 191:235–7.
21. Albornoz C, Jacobo SE. 2006. Preparation of a biocompatible magnetic film from an aqueous ferrofluid. *J Magn Magn Mater* 305:12–5.
22. Kim EH, Lee HS, Kwak BK, Kim BK. 2005. Synthesis of ferrofluid with magnetic nanoparticles by sonochemical method for MRI contrast agent. *J Magn Magn Mater* 289:328–30.
23. Wan J, Chen X, Wang Z, Yang X, Qian Y. 2005. A soft-template-assisted hydrothermal approach to single-crystal Fe_3O_4 nanorods. *J Cryst Growth* 276:571–6.
24. Kijima N, Yoshinaga M, Awaka J, Akimoto J. 2011. Microwave synthesis, character-ization, and electrochemical properties of α-Fe_2O_3 nanoparticles. *Solid State Ionics* Elsevier B.V.; 192:293–7.
25. Salazar-Alvarez G, Muhammed M, Zagorodni AA. 2006. Novel flow injection syn-thesis of iron oxide nanoparticles with narrow size distribution. *Chem Eng Sci* 61: 4625–33.
26. Basak S, Chen DR, Biswas P. 2007. Electrospray of ionic precursor solutions to synthe-size iron oxide nanoparticles: Modified scaling law. *Chem Eng Sci* 62:1263–8.
27. Sjögren CE, Johansson C, NÆvestad A, Sontum PC, Briley-SÆbØ K, Fahlvik AK. 1997. Crystal size and properties of superparamagnetic iron oxide (SPIO) particles. *Magn Reson Imaging* 15:55–67.
28. Babes L, Denizot B, Tanguy G, Le Jeune JJ, Jallet P. 1999. Synthesis of iron oxide nanoparticles used as MRI contrast agents: A parametric study. *J Colloid Interface Sci* 212:474–82.
29. Thurm S, Odenbach S. 2002. Magnetic separation of ferrofluids. *J Magn Magn Mater* 252:247–9.
30. Nunes AC, YU Z-C. 1987. Fractionation of a water-based ferrofluid. *J Magn Magn Mater* 65:265–8.
31. Behera SK. 2011. Enhanced rate performance and cyclic stability of Fe_3O_4–graphene nanocomposites for Li ion battery anodes. *Chem Commun* 47:10371.
32. Wu W, He QG, Hu R, Huang JK, and Chen H. 2007. Preparation and characterization of magnetite Fe_3O_4 nanopowders. *Rare Met Mater Eng* 36:238.
33. Wu S, Sun A, Zhai F, Wang J, Xu W, Zhang Q, et al. 2011. Fe_3O_4 magnetic nanoparti-cles synthesis from tailings by ultrasonic chemical co-precipitation. *Mater Lett* Elsevier B.V.; 65:1882–4.
34. Petcharoen K, Sirivat A. 2012. Synthesis and characterization of magnetite nanopar-ticles via the chemical co-precipitation method. *Mater Sci Eng B Solid-State Mater Adv Technol* Elsevier B.V.; 177:421–7.

35. Mahdavi M, Ahmad MB, Haron MJ, Namvar F, Nadi B, Ab Rahman MZ, et al. 2013. Synthesis, surface modification and characterisation of biocompatible magnetic iron oxide nanoparticles for biomedical applications. *Molecules* 18:7533–48.

36. Kandpal ND, Sah N, Loshali R, Joshi R, Prasad J. 2014. Co-precipitation method of synthesis and characterization of iron oxide nanoparticles. *J Sci Ind Res* 73:87–90.

37. Sun S, Zeng H, Robinson DB, Raoux S, Rice PM, Wang SX, et al. 2004. Monodisperse MFe_2O_4 ($M=Fe$, Co, Mn) nanoparticles. *J Am Chem Soc* 126:273–9.

38. Farrell D, Majetich SA, Wilcoxon JP. 2003. Preparation and characterization of monodisperse Fe nanoparticles. *J Phys Chem* 107:11022–30.

39. Jorg Rockenberger, Erik C. Scher and APA. 1999. A new nonhydrolytic single-precursor approach to surfactant-capped nanocrystals of transition metal oxides. *Mater Sci Eng B Solid-State Mater Adv Technol* 121:11595–6.

40. Jana NR, Chen Y, Peng X. 2004. Size- and shape-controlled magnetic (Cr, Mn, Fe, Co, Ni) oxide nanocrystals via a simple and general approach. *Chem Mater* 16:3931–5.

41. Samia ACS, Hyzer K, Schlueter JA, Qin CJ, Jiang JS, Bader SD, et al. 2005. Ligand effect on the growth and the digestion of Co nanocrystals. *J Am Chem Soc* 127:4126–7.

42. Li Y, Afzaal M, O'Brien P. 2006. The synthesis of amine-capped magnetic (Fe, Mn, Co, Ni) oxide nanocrystals and their surface modification for aqueous dispersibility. *J Mater Chem* 16:2175.

43. Park J, Lee E, Hwang N-M, Kang M, Kim SC, Hwang Y, et al. 2005. One-nanometer-scale size-controlled synthesis of monodisperse magnetic iron oxide nanoparticles. *Angew Chemie Int Ed* 44:2872–7.

44. Lynch J, Zhuang J, Wang T, Lamontagne D, Wu H, Cao YC. 2011. Gas-bubble effects on the formation of colloidal iron oxide nanocrystals. *J Am Chem Soc* 133:12664–74.

45. Park J, An K, Hwang Y, Park J-G, Noh H-J, Kim J-Y, et al. 2004. Ultra-large-scale syntheses of monodisperse nanocrystals. *Nat Mater* 3:891–5.

46. Amara D, Grinblat J, Margel S. 2012. Solventless thermal decomposition of ferrocene as a new approach for one-step synthesis of magnetite nanocubes and nanospheres. *J Mater Chem* 22:2188–95.

47. Eom Y, Abbas M, Noh H, Kim C. 2016. Morphology-controlled synthesis of highly crystalline Fe_3O_4 and $CoFe_2O_4$ nanoparticles using a facile thermal decomposition method. *RSC Adv* Royal Society of Chemistry; 6:15861–7.

48. Yu WW, Falkner JC, Yavuz CT, Colvin VL. 2004. Synthesis of monodisperse iron oxide nanocrystals by thermal decomposition of iron carboxylate salts. *Chem Commun*:2306. doi: 10.1039/B409601K.

49. Langevin D. 1992. Micelles and microemulsions. *Annu Rev Phys Chem* 43:341–69.

50. Solans C, Izquierdo P, Nolla J, Azemar N, Garcia-Celma MJ. 2005. Nano-emulsions. *Curr Opin Colloid Interf Sci* 10:102–10.

51. Vidal-Vidal J, Rivas J, López-Quintela MA. 2006. Synthesis of monodisperse maghemite nanoparticles by the microemulsion method. *Colloids Surf A Physicochem Eng Asp* 288:44–51.

52. Darbandi M, Stromberg F, Landers J, Reckers N, Sanyal B, Keune W, et al. 2012. Nanoscale size effect on surface spin canting in iron oxide nanoparticles synthesized by the microemulsion method. *J Phys D Appl Phys* 45:195001.

53. Okoli C, Sanchez-Dominguez M, Boutonnet M, Järås S, Civera C, Solans C, et al. 2012. Comparison and functionalization study of microemulsion-prepared magnetic iron oxide nanoparticles. *Langmuir* 28:8479–85.

54. Wang X, Zhuang J, Peng Q, Li Y. 2005. A general strategy for nanocrystal synthesis. *Nature* 437:121–4.

55. Cai H, An X, Cui J, Li J, Wen S, Li K, et al. 2013. Facile hydrothermal synthesis and surface functionalization of polyethyleneimine-coated iron oxide nanoparticles for biomedical applications. *ACS Appl Mater Interfaces* 5:1722–31.

56. Hao Y, Teja AS. 2003. Continuous hydrothermal crystallization of α–Fe_2O_3 and Co_3O_4 nanoparticles. *J Mater Res* 2003:415–22.
57. Xu C, Teja AS. 2008. Continuous hydrothermal synthesis of iron oxide and PVA-protected iron oxide nanoparticles. *J Supercrit Fluids* 44:85–91.
58. Bonvin D, Arakcheeva A, Millán A, Piñol R, Hofmann H, Mionić Ebersold M. 2017. Controlling structural and magnetic properties of IONPs by aqueous synthesis for improved hyperthermia. *RSC Adv* 7:13159–70.
59. Pecharroman C, Gonzalezcarreno T, Iglesias JE. 1995. The infrared dielectric properties of maghemite, gamma-Fe_2O_3, from reflectance measurement on pressed powders. *Phys Chem Miner* 22:21–9.
60. González-Carreño T, Morales MP, Gracia M, Serna CJ. 1993. Preparation of uniform ??-Fe_2O_3 particles with nanometer size by spray pyrolysis. *Mater Lett* 18:151–5.
61. Veintemillas-Verdaguer S, Morales MP, Serna CJ. 1998. Continuous production of γ-Fe_2O_3 ultrafine powders by laser pyrolysis. *Mater Lett* 35:227–31.
62. Julián-López B, Boissière C, Chanéac C, Grosso D, Vasseur S, Miraux S, et al. 2007. Mesoporous maghemite–organosilica microspheres: A promising route towards multifunctional platforms for smart diagnosis and therapy. *J Mater Chem* 17:1563–9.
63. Bao Y, Wen T, Samia ACS, Khandhar A, Krishnan KM. 2015. Magnetic nanoparticles: Material engineering and emerging applications in lithography and biomedicine. *J Mater Sci* Springer US; 51:513–53.
64. Sorensen CM. 2002. Chap. 6: Magnetism. *Nanoscale Mater Chem Ed Kenneth J Klabunde* 2002:169–221.
65. Batlle X, Labarta A. 2002. Finite-size effects in fine particles: Magnetic and transport properties. *J Phys D Appl Phys* 35:15-42.
66. Lu AH, Salabas EL, Schüth F. 2007. Magnetic nanoparticles: Synthesis, protection, functionalization, and application. *Angew Chemie - Int Ed* 46:1222–44.
67. Soenen SJ, De Cuyper M, De Smedt SC, Braeckmans K. 2012. Investigating the toxic effects of iron oxide nanoparticles. *Methods Enzymol* Elsevier Inc.; 2012:195–224.
68. Behera SS, Patra JK, Pramanik K, Panda N, Thatoi H. 2012. Characterization and evaluation of antibacterial activities of chemically synthesized iron oxide nanoparticles. *World J Nano Sci Eng* 02:196–200.
69. Yeap SP, Lim JK, Ooi BS, Ahmad AL. 2017. Agglomeration, colloidal stability, and magnetic separation of magnetic nanoparticles: Collective influences on environmental engineering applications. *J Nanoparticle Res* 19:368.
70. Amstad E, Textor M, Reimhult E. 2011. Stabilization and functionalization of iron oxide nanoparticles for biomedical applications. *Nanoscale* 3:2819.
71. Wu W, He Q, Jiang C. 2008. Magnetic iron oxide nanoparticles: Synthesis and surface functionalization strategies. *Nanoscale Res Lett* 3:397–415.
72. Manna PK, Nickel R, Wroczynskyj Y, Yathindranath V, Li J, Liu S, et al. 2018. Simple, hackable size selective amine-functionalized Fe-oxide nanoparticles for biomedical applications. *Langmuir* 34:2748–57.
73. Kodama R. 1999. Magnetic nanoparticles. *J Magn Magn Mater* 200:359–72.
74. Respaud M, Broto JM, Rakoto H, Fert AR, Thomas L, Barbara B, et al. 1998. Surface effects on the magnetic properties of ultrafine cobalt particles. *Phys Rev B* 57:2925–35.
75. Homola AM, Lorenz MR, Mastrangelo CJ, Tilbury TL. 1986. Novel magnetic dispersions using silica stabilized particles. *IEEE Trans Magn* 22:716–9.
76. Nogués J, Sort J, Langlais V, Skumryev V, Suriñach S, Muñoz JS, et al. 2005. Exchange bias in nanostructures. *Phys Rep* 422:65–117.

77. Ling D, Hyeon T. 2013. Chemical design of biocompatible iron oxide nanoparticles for medical applications. *Small* 9:1450–66.
78. Nazli C, Demirer GS, Yar Y, Acar HY, Kizilel S. 2014. Targeted delivery of doxorubicin into tumor cells via MMP-sensitive PEG hydrogel-coated magnetic iron oxide nanoparticles (MIONPs). *Colloids Surf B Biointerf* Elsevier B.V.; 122:674–83.
79. Pombo-García K, Rühl CL, Lam R, Barreto JA, Ang CS, Scammells PJ, et al. 2017. Zwitterionic modification of ultrasmall iron oxide nanoparticles for reduced protein corona formation. *Chempluschem* 82:638–46.
80. Mazario E, Forget A, Belkahla H, Lomas J, Decorse P, Chevillot-Biraud A, et al. 2017. Design and characterization of iron oxide nanoparticles functionalized with HSA protein for thermal therapy. *IEEE Trans Magn* 53:1–1.
81. Lam SJ, Wong EHH, Boyer C, Qiao GG. 2018. Antimicrobial polymeric nanoparticles. *Prog Polym Sci* Elsevier Ltd; 76:40–64.
82. Wu W, Wu Z, Yu T, Jiang C, Kim W-S. 2015. Recent progress on magnetic iron oxide nanoparticles: Synthesis, surface functional strategies and biomedical applications. *Sci Technol Adv Mater* IOP Publishing; 16:023501.
83. Laurent S, Forge D, Port M, Roch A, Robic C, Elst L V, et al. 2008. Magnetic iron oxide nanoparticles: Synthesis, stabilization, vectorization, physicochemical characterizations, and biological applications. *Chem Rev* 108:2064–110.
84. Nazli C, Ergenc TI, Yar Y, Acar HY, Kizilel S. 2012. RGDS-functionalized polyethylene glycol hydrogel-coated magnetic iron oxide nanoparticles enhance specific intracellular uptake by HeLa cells. *Int J Nanomedicine* 7:1903–20.
85. Mahmoudi M, Sant S, Wang B, Laurent S, Sen T. 2011. Superparamagnetic iron oxide nanoparticles (SPIONs): Development, surface modification and applications in chemotherapy. *Adv Drug Deliv Rev* Elsevier B.V.; 63:24–46.
86. Laurent S, Forge D, Port M, Roch A, Robic C, Vander Elst L, et al. 2008. Magnetic iron oxide nanoparticles: Synthesis, stabilization, vectorization, physicochemical characterizations and biological applications. *Chem Rev* 108:2064–110.
87. Kataby G, Ulman a, Prozorov R, Gedanken a. 1998. Coating of amorphous iron nanoparticles by long-chain alcohols. *Langmuir* 14:1512–5.
88. Anbarasu M, Anandan M, Chinnasamy E, Gopinath V, Balamurugan K. 2015. Synthesis and characterization of polyethylene glycol (PEG) coated Fe_3O_4 nanoparticles by chemical co-precipitation method for biomedical applications. *Spectrochim Acta Part A Mol Biomol Spectrosc* Elsevier B.V.; 135:536–9.
89. Masoudi A, Madaah Hosseini HR, Shokrgozar MA, Ahmadi R, Oghabian MA. 2012. The effect of poly(ethylene glycol) coating on colloidal stability of superparamagnetic iron oxide nanoparticles as potential MRI contrast agent. *Int J Pharm* Elsevier B.V.; 433:129–41.
90. Neuberger T, Schöpf B, Hofmann H, Hofmann M, Von Rechenberg B. 2005. Superparamagnetic nanoparticles for biomedical applications: Possibilities and limitations of a new drug delivery system. *J Magn Magn Mater* 293:483–96.
91. Zhang H, Wang Q, Li L. 2009. Dehydration of water-plasticized poly(vinyl alcohol) systems: Particular behavior of isothermal mass transfer. *Polym Int* 58:97–104.
92. Rahman MM, Afrin S, Haque P. 2014. Characterization of crystalline cellulose of jute reinforced poly (vinyl alcohol) (PVA) biocomposite film for potential biomedical applications. *Prog Biomater* 3:23.
93. Pardoe H, Chua-anusorn W, St. Pierre TG, Dobson J. 2001. Structural and magnetic properties of nanoscale iron oxide particles synthesized in the presence of dextran or polyvinyl alcohol. *J Magn Magn Mater* 225:41–6.
94. Khosroshahi ME, Ghazanfari L. 2012. Preparation and rheological studies of uncoated and PVA-coated magnetite nanofluid. *J Magn Magn Mater* Elsevier; 324:4143–6.

95. Agnihotri SA, Mallikarjuna NN, Aminabhavi TM. 2004. Recent advances on chitosan-based micro- and nanoparticles in drug delivery. *J Control Release* 100:5–28.

96. Assa F, Jafarizadeh-Malmiri H, Ajamein H, Vaghari H, Anarjan N, Ahmadi O, et al. 2017. Chitosan magnetic nanoparticles for drug delivery systems. *Crit Rev Biotechnol* 37:492–509.

97. Paul KG, Frigo TB, Groman JY, Groman E V. 2004. Synthesis of ultrasmall superparamagnetic iron oxides using reduced polysaccharides. *Bioconjug Chem* 15:394–401.

98. Shagholani H, Ghoreishi SM, Mousazadeh M. 2015. Improvement of interaction between PVA and chitosan via magnetite nanoparticles for drug delivery application. *Int J Biol Macromol* Elsevier B.V.; 78:130–6.

99. Gupta AK, Gupta M. 2005. Synthesis and surface engineering of iron oxide nanoparticles for biomedical applications. *Biomaterials* 26:3995–4021.

100. Mccarthy JR, Weissleder R. 2009. Multifunctional magnetic nanoparticles for targeted imaging and therapy. *Clio - A J Lit Hist Philos Hist* 60:1241–51.

101. Du L, Chen J, Qi Y, Li D, Yuan C, Lin MC, et al. 2007. Preparation and biomedical application of a non-polymer coated superparamagnetic nanoparticle. *Int J Nanomed* 2:805–12.

102. Josephson L, Tung CH, Moore A, Weissleder R. 1999. High-efficiency intracellular magnetic labeling with novel superparamagnetic-tat peptide conjugates. *Bioconjug Chem* 10:186–91.

103. Jafari A, Salouti M, Shayesteh SF, Heidari Z, Rajabi AB, Boustani K, et al. 2015. Synthesis and characterization of Bombesin-superparamagnetic iron oxide nanoparticles as a targeted contrast agent for imaging of breast cancer using MRI. *Nanotechnology* IOP Publishing; 26:075101.

104. Corr SA, Rakovich YP, Gun'Ko YK. 2008. Multifunctional magnetic-fluorescent nanocomposites for biomedical applications. *Nanoscale Res Lett* 3:87–104.

105. Ding HL, Zhang YX, Wang S, Xu JM, Xu SC, Li GH. 2012. $Fe_3O_4@SiO_2$ core/shell nanoparticles: The silica coating regulations with a single core for different core sizes and shell thicknesses. *Chem Mater* 24:4572–80.

106. Santra S, Tapec R, Theodoropoulou N, Dobson J, Hebard A, Tan W. 2001. Synthesis and characterization of silica-coated iron oxide nanoparticles in microemulsion: The effect of nonionic surfactants. *Langmuir* 17:2900–6.

107. Lin J, Zhou W, Kumbhar A, Wiemann J, Fang J, Carpenter EE, et al. 2001. Gold-coated iron (Fe@Au) nanoparticles: Synthesis, characterization, and magnetic field-induced self-assembly. *J Solid State Chem* 159:26–31.

108. Liang G, Cai S, Zhang P, Peng Y, Chen H, Zhang S, et al. 2011. Magnetic relaxation switch and colorimetric detection of thrombin using aptamer-functionalized gold-coated iron oxide nanoparticles. *Anal Chim Acta* Elsevier B.V.; 689:243–9.

109. Mohammad F, Balaji G, Weber A, Uppu RM, Kumar CSSR. 2010. Influence of gold nanoshell on hyperthermia of super paramagnetic iron oxide nanoparticles (SPIONs). *J Phys Chem C Nano Inter* 114:19194–201.

110. Zhang L, He R, Gu HC. 2006. Oleic acid coating on the monodisperse magnetite nanoparticles. *Appl Surf Sci* 253:2611–7.

111. Du, B, Li, J, Wang, F, Yao W, and Yao S. 2015. Influence of monodisperse Fe_3O_4 nanoparticle size on electrical properties of vegetable oil-based nanofluids. *J Nanomater* 2015:560352–61.

112. Owen CS. 1983. Cell Separation; Chapter 8: Magnetic cell sorting, *Elsevier.* 2:127-44.

113. Rheinländer T, Kötitz R, Weitschies W, Semmler W. 2000. Magnetic fractionation of magnetic fluids. *J Magn Magn Mater* 219:219–28.

114. Cardoso VF, Francesko A, Ribeiro C, Bañobre-López M, Martins P, Lanceros-Mendez S. 2018. Advances in magnetic nanoparticles for biomedical applications. *Adv Healthc Mater* 7:1–35.

115. El-sherbiny IM, Elbaz NM. 2017. Magnetic nanoparticles-based drug and gene delivery systems for the treatment of pulmonary diseases. *Nanomedicine* 12:387–402.

116. Lu J, Wang J, Ling D. 2017. Surface engineering of nanoparticles for targeted delivery to hepatocellular carcinoma. *Small* 1702037:1702037.

117. Deng J, Gao C. Recent advances in interactions of designed nanoparticles and cells with respect to cellular uptake, intracellular fate, degradation and cytotoxicity. *Nanotechnology* IOP Publishing; 27:1–10.

118. Kang T, Li F, Baik S, Shao W, Ling D, Hyeon T. 2017. Surface design of magnetic nanoparticles for stimuli-responsive cancer imaging and therapy. *Biomaterials* Elsevier Ltd; 136:98–114.

119. Montiel Schneider MG, Lassalle VL. 2017. Magnetic iron oxide nanoparticles as novel and efficient tools for atherosclerosis diagnosis. *Biomed Pharmacother* Elsevier Masson SAS; 93:1098–115.

120. Vuong QL, Gillis P, Roch A, Gossuin Y. 2017. Magnetic resonance relaxation induced by superparamagnetic particles used as contrast agents in magnetic resonance imaging: A theoretical review. *Wiley Interdiscip Rev Nanomed Nanobiotech* 9:1–22.

121. Nedyalkova M, Donkova B, Romanova J, Tzvetkov G, Madurga S, Simeonov V. 2017. Iron oxide nanoparticles – In vivo/in vitro biomedical applications and in silico studies. *Adv Colloid Interf Sci* Elsevier; 249:192–212.

122. Iv M, Telischak N, Feng D, Holdsworth S., Yeom K., Daldrup-Link H. 2015. Clinical applications of iron oxide nanoparticles for magnetic resonance imaging of brain tumors. *Nanomedicine (Lond)* 10:993–1018.

123. Biederer S, Knopp T, Sattel TF, Lüdtke-Buzug K, Gleich B, Weizenecker J, et al. 2009. Magnetization response spectroscopy of superparamagnetic nanoparticles for magnetic particle imaging. *J Phys D Appl Phys* 42:205007.

124. Ferguson RM, Minard KR, Krishnan KM. 2009. Optimization of nanoparticle core size for magnetic particle imaging. *J Magn Magn Mater* 321:1548–51.

125. Arami H, Krishnan KM. 2014. Intracellular performance of tailored nanoparticle tracers in magnetic particle imaging. *J Appl Phys* 115:1–4.

126. Witalison E, Thompson P, Hofseth L. 2015. HHS public access. *Curr Drug Targets* 16:700–10.

127. Arami H, Teeman E, Troska A, Bradshaw H, Saatchi K, Tomitaka A, et al. 2017. Tomographic magnetic particle imaging of cancer targeted nanoparticles. *Nanoscale* 9:18723-30.

128. Cullity BD, Graham CD. 2008. *Introduction to Magnetic Materials [Internet]. B. IEEE*, ISBN 978-0-471-47741-9. Hoboken, NJ: John Wiley & Sons, Inc.

129. Gao Y. 2005. Nanotechnologies for the life sciences. Kumar, C, Ed; New York: Wiley-VCH Verlag GmbH & Co. KGaA. ISBN 9783527610419.

130. Fan J, Lu J, Xu R, Jiang R, Gao Y. 2003. Use of water-dispersible Fe_2O_3 nanoparticles with narrow size distributions in isolating avidin. *J Colloid Interface Sci* 266:215–8.

131. Chen DH, Liao MH. 2002. Preparation and characterization of YADH-bound magnetic nanoparticles. *J Mol Catal - B Enzym* 16:283–91.

132. Portet D, Denizot B, Rump E, Lejeune JJ, Jallet P. 2001. Nonpolymeric coatings of iron oxide colloids for biological use as magnetic resonance imaging contrast agents. *J Colloid Interf Sci* 238:37–42.

133. Stöber W, Fink A, Bohn E. 1968. Controlled growth of monodisperse silica spheres in the micron size range. *J Colloid Interf Sci* 26:62–9.

134. Gao X, Yu KMK, Tam KY, Tsang SC. 2003. Colloidal stable silica encapsulated nano-magnetic composite as a novel bio-catalyst carrier. *Chem Commun (Camb)* :2998–9.

135. Kempe H, Kates SA, Kempe M. 2011. Nanomedicine's promising therapy: Magnetic drug targeting. *Expert Rev Med Devices* 8:291–4.

136. Huang Z, Pei N, Wang Y, Xie X, Sun A, Shen L, et al. 2010. Deep magnetic capture of magnetically loaded cells for spatially targeted therapeutics. *Biomaterials* Elsevier Ltd; 31:2130–40.

137. Knight L, Romano J, Krynska B. 2010. Binding and internalization of iron oxide nanoparticles targeted to nuclear oncoprotein. *J Mol* 1:1–15.

138. Gallo JM, Varkonyi P, Hassan EE, Groothius DR. 1993. Targeting anticancer drugs to the brain: II. Physiological pharmacokinetic model of oxantrazole following intraarterial administration to rat glioma-2 (RG-2) bearing rats. *J Pharmacokinet Biopharm* 21:575–92.

139. Geynisman DM, Chien CR, Smieliauskas F, Shen C, Shih YC. 2014. Economic evaluation of therapeutic cancer vaccines and immunotherapy: A systematic review. *Hum Vaccin Immunother* 10:3415–24.

140. Dunn GP, Old LJ, Schreiber RD. 2004. The immunobiology of cancer immunosurveillance and immunoediting. *Immunity* 21:137–48.

141. Lübbe AS, Bergemann C, Riess H, Lãbbe AS, Schriever F, Reichardt P, et al. 1996. Clinical experiences with magnetic drug targeting: A phase I study with 4′-epidoxorubicin in 14 patients with advanced solid tumors. *Cancer Res* 56:4686–93.

142. Bear JC, Yu B, Blanco-andujar C, Mcnaughter PD, Southern P, Ma M. 2014. A low cost synthesis method for functionalised iron oxide nanoparticles for magnetic hyperthermia from readily available materials. *Faraday Discuss* 175:83–95.

143. Gilchrist RK, Medal R, Shorey WD, Hanselman RC, Parrott JC, Taylor CB. 1957. Selective inductive heating of lymph nodes. *Ann Surg* 146:596–606.

144. Gordon RT, Hines JR, Gordon D. 1979. Intracellular hyperthermia a biophysical approach to cancer treatment via intracellular temperature and biophysical alterations. *Med Hypoth* 5:83–102.

145. Jordan A, Wust P, Fählin H, John W, Hinz A, Felix R. 1993. Inductive heating of ferrimagnetic particles and magnetic fluids: Physical evaluation of their potential for hyperthermia. *Int J Hyperth* 9:51–68.

146. Hergt R, Dutz S, Zeisberger M. 2010. Validity limits of the Néel relaxation model of magnetic nanoparticles for hyperthermia. *Nanotechnology* 21:015706.

147. Guardia P, Di Corato R, Lartigue L, Wilhelm C, Espinosa A, Garcia-Hernandez M, et al. 2012. Water-soluble iron oxide nanocubes with high values of specific absorption rate for cancer cell hyperthermia treatment. *ACS Nano* 6:3080–91.

148. Gonzales-Weimuller M, Zeisberger M, Krishnan KM. 2009. Size-dependant heating rates of iron oxide nanoparticles for magnetic fluid hyperthermia. *J Magn Magn Mater* 321:1947–50.

149. Xu Y, Qin Y, Palchoudhury S, Bao Y. 2011. Water-soluble iron oxide nanoparticles with high stability and selective surface functionality. *Langmuir* 27:8990–7.

6 Magnesium-Based Nanocomposites for Biomedical Applications

Bhaskar Thakur, Shivprakash Barve, and Pralhad Pesode
MIT World Peace University Pune

CONTENTS

6.1 INTRODUCTION

Nowadays, metallic biopolymers are profoundly utilized in clinical applications. In biomedical applications, biopolymers are utilized for the manufacturing of surgical embeds just as in load-bearing medical usages. Magnesium alloys and metal-based

DOI: 10.1201/9781003286806-6

nanocomposites are utilized broadly in biomedical applications [1]. Most of the metals are not biofunctional; however, they can be coated with biomaterials to make them biocompatible or bioactive. Nowadays, metals are having very few implementations in dentistry, hip inserts, stent joints and bone fixation [2]. The most well-known biomedical composites are developed from cobalt, iron, magnesium, titanium and their alloys. Numerous examinations are accomplished to research the mechanical behavior of magnesium-based biomedical alloys [3–6]. Fabrication is the method of constructing compounds by combining standardized components using one or more individual processes. Different methods used for the fabrication of magnesium alloys are equal channel angular extrusion, powder metallurgy, spark plasma-assisted powder metallurgy sintering, dual-stage sintering-assisted powder metallurgy, microwave-assisted powder metallurgy, additive manufacturing, friction stir process (FSP), accumulative roll bonding process, stir-casting process and disintegrated melt deposition [7]. Characterization is an important step in the commercialization of new materials. For material commercialization, makers should approve their manufacturing cycle. This guarantees that the manufacturing cycle provides a quality item so that the patient is not in danger. Different methods used for the characterization of Mg alloys are surface free energy analysis, MAF (microarc fluorination) treatment, surface characterization, immersion corrosion tests and electrochemical corrosion tests [8].

Since 1878, magnesium-based materials have been utilized in biomedical applications [9]. After clinical use, magnesium degrades in the human body as it is a biodegradable substance. Patients experiencing bone injuries, dental issues and coronary vein-related issues need backing and degradation during the healing process as far as biocompatibility, bioactivity, mechanical integrity and biodegradability are concerned. The specific design and choice of Mg alloys depend on specific applications. Magnesium-based materials are utilized to create cardiovascular stents, which should accomplish the required angiographic result in 4 months period by complete and secure desorption [10–12]. For the most part, composites that are of nanometer scale in any of their dimensional stages are named nanocomposites. Magnesium alloys are emerging materials for bio-clinical applications and are furthermore projected as proper replacements for existing materials. A nanocomposite has more extensive application in the biomedical field that incorporates drug delivery, medical implants, tissue engineering and so on. These nanocomposites have come into focus as a proper substitute to overcome the limits of solid and miniature composites while presenting readiness challenges associated with the control arrangement of components and stoichiometry in the nanocluster stage. Nanocomposites have concerned responsiveness in both industrial and research areas because of their adequacy in creating multifunctional materials with predominant properties. These nanocomposites are the rising materials in the field of bio-clinical application and due to their design attribute and exceptional properties that incorporate better healing over broken bone surfaces, they are light in weight with a high strength to weight ratio. Nanocomposites comprise a natural lattice stage in which inorganic nanomaterials are consistently scattered. For this, the support might be nanotubes, nanorods, nanoclays, nanowires and so forth like microcomposites; these nanocomposite materials can be grouped into three significant types depending on the nature of the matrix material: metallic-related nanocomposites, ceramic-related nanocomposites and polymer-related nanocomposites [13]. One of the disadvantages of magnesium alloys is their low corrosion resistance. For better corrosion resistance in vivo like aqueous environment having chlorine ions, for example, extracellular fluid needs protective coating on the substrate surface. To get better corrosion resistance of magnesium alloys, a variety of surface adjustment methods are available [14]. Among all methods, the plasma electrolytic oxidation (PEO) method gives excellent corrosion resistance to magnesium alloys used for biomedical applications. Plasma electrolytic oxidation is an electrochemical surface treatment method to provide corrosion resistance coating on magnesium and other similar light metals. The required coating property can be obtained by the PEO method for variables like electrolyte composition, applied voltage, current density, duty cycles, etc. [15]. It has been observed that coating produced by PEO techniques showed excellent adhesion to the substrate surface [16].

6.2 MAGNESIUM ALLOYS USED IN BIOMEDICAL APPLICATIONS

The most frequently utilized metals in biomedical applications are stainless steel, titanium alloys, magnesium alloys and cobalt–chromium alloys. Recent studies have stated that stainless steel can cause toxicity in the body and it is also heavy. Titanium alloys have high ductility, but as compared to natural bone, they have a high elastic modulus. Cobalt alloys have a high elastic modulus compared to natural bone and also their wear resistance is inadequate. Nowadays, the popularity of magnesium alloys is increasing as they have good corrosion rates, appropriate mechanical properties and the capacity for precipitation of a bone-like apatite layer on their outer surface.

6.2.1 MAGNESIUM ZINC (Mg–Zn) ALLOY

Zinc is abundantly available in all the cells of the body and is perhaps the most plentiful fundamental component in humans [17]. Zinc is a typical alloying component in Mg alloy and has a solubility of 6.1% and can adequately improvise mechanical behavior of Mg [18]. Different sorts of Mg–Zn composites were discussed in the past literature. Mg6Zn alloy comprises a single phase after fine solution treatment and hot working, so here corrosion can be neglected. Here the mechanical behavior of the Mg6Zn combination is accepted to be reasonable for biomedical applications. The in-vitro cytotoxicity of the Mg6Zn cells was discovered to be of grade 1 and the hemolysis rate is 3.4% showing that the Mg6Zn compound displays great biocompatibility in vitro. The Mg6Zn composite poles were inserted into the bones of the rabbits and slowly sucked in vivo at a demolition speed of 2.320 mm/year with recently framed bone encompassing the insert. The entrails histology assessment and the biomedical estimations were demonstrated, in which demolition of the Mg–Zn alloy did not harm the important organs [19].

6.2.2 MAGNESIUM CALCIUM (Mg–Ca) ALLOY

Ca is a significant part of the human body structure and is fundamental in chemical reactions with tissues. Additionally, magnesium is fundamental for inserting calcium into the bone, which may be required to be important for the healing of bone with the emission of Mg and Ca ions [20]. Calcium is likewise important to the grain processing of Mg alloys. In Mg–Ca alloy, the dissolvability limit of calcium in magnesium is 1.340 wt. % [18]. The Mg–Ca alloys are chiefly made out of the α-Mg stage and Mg–2Ca stage. With expanding Ca substance, more and coarser Mg–2Ca stage encourages along with grain limits, debilitating both the corrosion resistance and mechanical behavior of as-cast Mg–Ca alloys. After the hot extrusion or hot rolling process, the coarse Mg_2Ca stage transforms into more modest parts and then the grain size is processed, adding to the enhanced mechanical behavior and resistance to corrosion [21]. The strength of expelled double Mg–Ca composites increments with the Ca content, yet the malleability will get decreased. It is tracked down that the solid Mg3Ca amalgam strips show a much smaller grain structure, good resistance to corrosion and improved tissue cell response than the projected Mg3Ca compound ingot [22]. An in-vitro cytotoxicity test showed that Mg1Ca alloy does not initiate harmfulness to L929 cells. Mg1Ca alloy sticks to step-by-step degradation in vivo within 3 months and new bone tissue is shaped [21]. The extruded Mg–0.8Ca combination kept up the greater part of their underlying volume in the come round and is inserted into rabbit tibiae for a half year [23].

6.2.3   Magnesium Strontium (Mg–Sr) Alloy

Sr alongside calcium and magnesium has a place with set II-A of the ancient periodic chart and offers the same chemical, mechanical and metallurgical properties. One hundred and forty milligrams of strontium is available in human beings and 99% of the strontium is situated in the body structure [24]. In reality, in view of the bone development incitement impact of strontium, oral organization of strontium salts is utilized for treating osteoporotic patients for the expansion of bone mass and lessens the rate of cracks. From the scientific perspective, appropriate expansion of strontium can refine the particle size of magnesium alloys and improve the corrosion resistance [25]. The hot moved Mg–Sr binary alloy with the Sr value going from 1 to 4 wt. % and discovered Mg_2Sr composite displayed the most elevated potency and the slowest corrosion rate. The in-vivo results show the degradation as rolled Mg–2Sr compound advanced bone formation and pre-implant new bone formation without prompting any particular unfriendly effect [26]. MgZnSr and MgCaSr are the ternary alloys that recommend that the existence of a superior measure of derivative inter metallic stages prompts poor corrosion resistance.

6.2.4   Magnesium Silicon (Mg–Si) Alloys

Normally, regular consumption of Si goes from around 25 to 50 mg/day with fewer values for a non-vegetarian diet and high values for a vegetarian diet. A follow measure of silicon is accounted for to be the most important in human beings and might be significant for the development and advancement of bone tissue. Mg–Si combination has low ductility because of the presence of fine Mg–2Si since there is no solubility for silicon in magnesium, calcium and zinc components being refined and the state of Mg2Si is changed to develop the mechanical behavior and resistance to corrosion [27]. In Mg–Si alloys, the mixing of calcium can develop the consumption of

Mg–Si alloys; however, no changes were seen in the potency and stretching and the expansion of 1.60 wt.% zinc into Mg-0.6Si can change the state of the Mg–2Si stage from the course of eutectic design to a little dab or tiny rectangular shape so that the rigidity, elongation and resistance to corrosion are enhanced [28].

6.2.5 MAGNESIUM RARE-EARTH ALLOYS

RE metals in Mg alloys are transcendently utilized for reinforcing and to develop the resistance to corrosion [29]. There are 17 components, for example scandium, yttrium, lanthanum, cerium, praseodymium, neodymium, europium, gadolinium, terbium, dysprosium, holmium, erbium, thulium, ytterbium, lutetium and promethium. They are brought into magnesium alloys by ace composites, which contain fundamentally one or two rare-earth metals and practically any remaining RE components in more modest sums. In the ASTM terminology of Mg alloys, RE components are on the whole addressed by E but yttrium is exceptionally addressed by W. Refined human muscle cells with chlorides of sixteen rare-earth components and tracked down RE metals at small fixation show no major unfavorable consequences for the expansion of vascular smooth muscle cells but lead to the up-regulation of inflammatory qualities at high accumulation [30]. This compound for biomedical utilization incorporates MgY, MgGd, WE43, etc. The mentioned WE43 alloy is generally seriously examined for its amazing mechanical behavior and resistance to corrosion. The MgNdZnZr composite beats WE43 on mechanical behavior and resistance to corrosion [31]. Although Mg-based composites in muscular applications are as yet in the preliminaries stage, Mg-based cardiovascular stents have efficiently entered clinical preliminaries in humans with secondary blood vessel blocks and coronary artery illness. Mg compounds researched for cardiovascular application are mostly MgRE-dependent alloys as referenced in the literature. Nonetheless, the biosafety of RE components is still not fully discovered [7] (Table 6.1).

6.3 FABRICATION TECHNIQUES OF Mg USED IN BIOMEDICAL APPLICATIONS

Different methods used for the fabrication of magnesium alloys are equal channel angular extrusion, powder metallurgy, spark plasma-assisted powder metallurgy sintering,

TABLE 6.1
Comparison of Different Magnesium Alloys Used

Composition	Rate of Corrosion (mm/Year)	Viability of Cell (%)	Tensile Strength (MPa)	Solubility (wt.%)
Mg–6Zn	1.671	100	228	6.1
Mg–2Ca	0.34	55	200	1.34
Mg–Sr	0.1	84	56	1.4
Mg–2Si	–	88.3	179	1.6
Mg–Re	–	–	280	–

dual-stage sintering-assisted powder metallurgy, microwave-assisted powder metallurgy, additive manufacturing, FSP, accumulative roll bonding process, stir-casting process and disintegrated melt deposition.

6.3.1 EQUAL CHANNEL ANGULAR EXTRUSION

Mg and its nanocomposites show similar mechanical strength to human bones (Figure 6.1). These biocompatible materials are created by ordinary material techniques, for example, powder metallurgy, stir casting and so on, through agglomeration and unreliable performance. To ensure the widespread utilization of Mg-based hydroxyapatite (HA) composites, broad exploration has been required in the initial stage. Extreme plastic deformity measures, viz., the accumulative roll bonding process, equal channel angular extrusion process, high shear solidification and so on, are considered one of the processing methods to accomplish fine-grained nanocomposites [33]. In this shear dissolve-based treatment, the rotor–stator instrument helps in diminishing the agglomeration tendency and starts the uniform dispersion of composite materials. In certain investigations, consolidated extreme plastic deformity, i.e. equal channel angular extrusion process and high shear hardening, was utilized to achieve nanocomposites with better functional properties. Thus, the base material (Mg–Zn–Zr) was created by dissolving pure Mg ingot under protective climate and then the measure of an alloying component was added to liquid Mg for up to 1 hour to create a base matrix material. At first, the base composite was dissolved totally

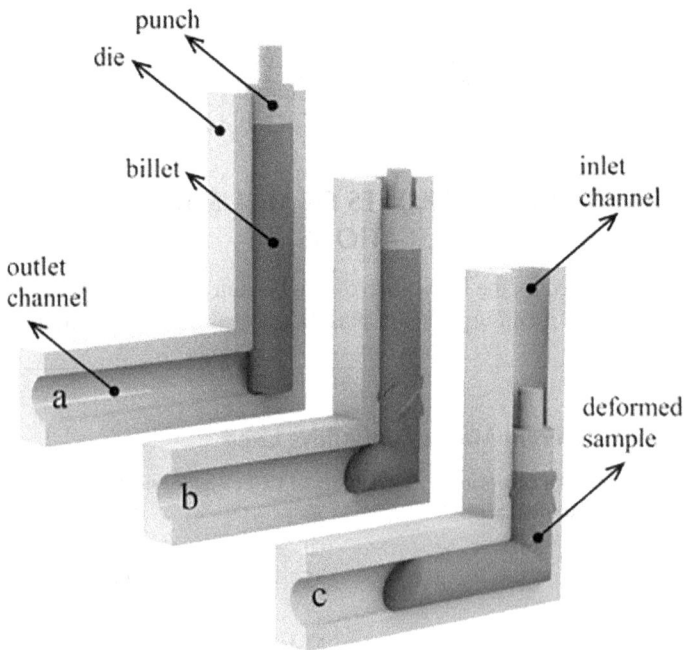

FIGURE 6.1 Representation of equal channel angular extrusion [32].

and preheated nano-HA particles are raced into the matrix material by the collaborators of a drill-driven propeller. The liquid composite materials were adjusted through shearing with the collaborators of the rotor–stator component with a speed of up to 10,000 rpm for around 20 minutes. During blending measure, rapid revolution helps in starting a high shear rate over the composite liquefied. At that point, the dissolve was poured into a steel shape with accurate measurement. After the composite turn of events, the projected composite materials are seized into a square billet for the equal channel angular extrusion process [34]. This technique comprises two equivalent channels that meet at a pre-set point. At first, the created composite square billet was squeezed throughout the main outlet and pulled out from other outlets that start the events of cut-off plastic deformation through the shear component (Figure 6.1). This aids in accomplishing a high grain refined composite material. In certain investigations, cyclic expulsion and compression combined equivalent channel angular extrusion-based forward extrusion process (C-ECAP-FE) was carried out to grow high-strength Mg–HA composites for bio-clinical applications. In this, high-virtue Mg and HA nanoparticles are preheated up to 50°C. The fundamental benefit of the joined interaction was to solidify the composite powders without the help of outer backpressure. At first, the C-ECAP-FE pass on was preheated up to 400°C; the composite powders are forced into the die at a constant speed of 0.2 mm/min [35].

6.3.2 POWDER METALLURGY

The powder metallurgy measure includes three significant steps: (i) mechanical alloying, (ii) compaction and (iii) sintering [36]. At first, the determined weight or volume level of reinforcement particles and base matrix materials are taken as a powder. The acquired composite blenders are mixed with the help of planetary ball processing. During the powder mixing process, stearic acid is added to the composite powder to accomplish homogeneous blending. During mechanical alloying, the composite materials are turned into a barrel-shaped chamber containing a circular width ball comprising hard ceramic materials like TiC or WC. Thus, the ceramic balls are chosen depending on the hardness of the base metric material. The powder mixing measure is constrained by two principal measure boundaries specifically powder to ball proportion and revolution speed. For lessening the size of particles from full scale to miniature size, the ball having a greater diameter is utilized with a lower rotational speed [37]. Moreover, the greatest chamber speed and more modest diameter balls are utilized for downsizing the smaller molecule to the nanoscale. For scale bringing down to nano-size, the composite powders are mixed with natural solvents to keep away from the possibility of agglomeration. Further, the composite blends are dried for 30 minutes and afterward permitted to ball mill [38]. Titanium-based alloys are widely utilized in creating biomedical inserts that incorporate dental prostheses and so on because they have good mechanical strength and biocompatibility. Silicon carbide-based Ti–Cu intermetallic composites can be delivered with a powder metallurgy course, which is hard to create in projecting-based techniques. The introductory phase of powder metallurgy starts with ball processing measure in this cold welding, and the collision of metal powder, plastic deformation and fracture of the composite powder occur frequently. This event produces disengagements of composite powders.

The processing cycle was performed with the powder to ball weight proportion of 1:10 under argon assurance at 300 rpm for 30 hours. The tempered steel balls with various widths could be utilized for achieving appropriate scattering of composites. Stearic acid-based controlling catalysts can be utilized to accelerate the processing interaction. The ball-processed powders were compacted under tube-shaped steel molds under the pressure of 1 GPa and afterward sintered at 900°C for 1 hour to achieve silicon carbide-based Ti–Cu [39] (Figure 6.2).

6.3.3 Microwave-Assisted Powder Metallurgy

HA-based Mg nanocomposites are typically prepared by solid-state processing, for example, powder metallurgy, where sintering of composite materials is performed in an electrical heater, which results in a high time and energy-consuming method [41]. To keep away from this reality, microwave-assisted heating was utilized to guarantee uniform heating and low energy utilization. At first, the Mg and HA nanopowder was ball milled for up to 4 hours. The accomplished composite blenders are cold compacted in tube-shaped kick the bucket. The accomplished green compact is sintered

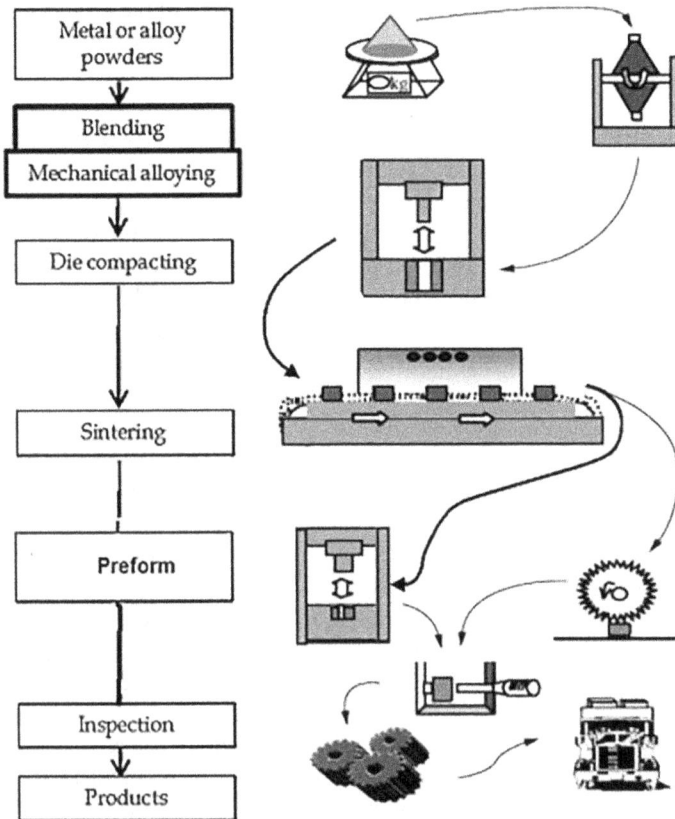

FIGURE 6.2   Representation of the powder metallurgy process [40].

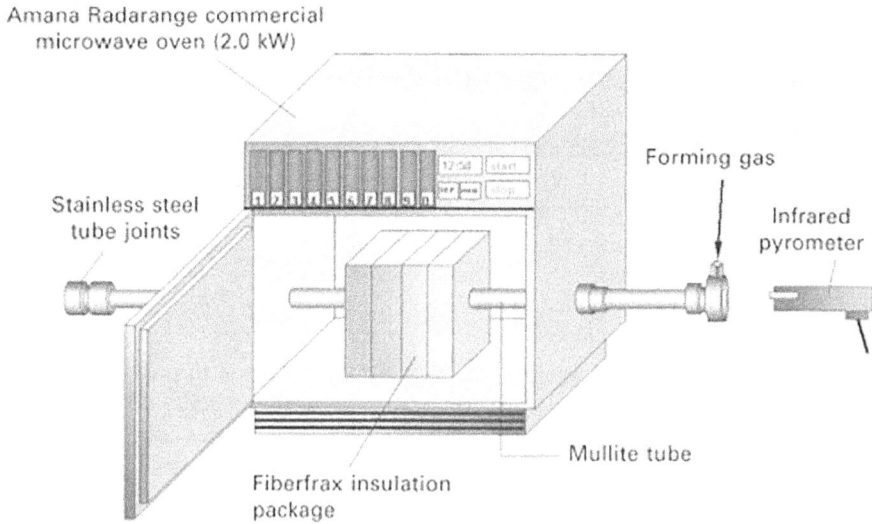

FIGURE 6.3 Representation of microwave-assisted powder metallurgy [43].

under a microwave heater at 500°C for 10 minutes under an inert gas atmosphere to achieve the Mg–HA composite [42] (Figure 6.3).

6.3.4 DUAL-STAGE SINTERING-ASSISTED POWDER METALLURGY

For bone tissue designing applications, HA–titanium dioxide-based composite materials are utilized because of their better biocompatibility [44]. Powder metallurgy-based methodologies are utilized for building up these sorts of biomaterials. For preparing ceramic-based materials, the sintering process acts as vital for composite strength. Inappropriate segment of sintering temperature brings about dehydroxylation, coarse grain arrangement and disintegration of HA-based ceramic materials. To stay away from these imperfections, double stage sintering approaches are utilized. Like old solid-state processing, the composite powder is first cold-welded by a ball mill. The composite powders are solidified and cold compacted at a pressing factor of 150 MPa to get green compacted pellets. In the double stage sintering approach, the samples are at first sintered at 900°C for 1–5 minutes to stay away from dehydroxylation and to accomplish the mass thickness of the created composite. The subsequent stage was trailed by fast cooling from 900°C to 800°C and then the temperature was kept at 800°C for 5–10 hours to achieve dense and homogeneous nanostructures with high strength to avoid decomposition [7].

6.3.5 ADDITIVE MANUFACTURING

Cobalt–chromium–molybdenum (Co–Cr–Mo) alloys are widely utilized in a few load-bearing implants, viz., hip, spinal and knee applications because of their good wear resistance. Alternately, these alloys show poor biocompatibility during vivo corrosion resistance, which could be improved by adding reasonable reinforcement particles. In certain examinations, calcium phosphate has been utilized as a support to improve the essential and effective conduct of Co–Cr–Mo alloys [45]. These nano-composites could be manufactured by a laser-designed net molding approach. The Co–Cr–Mo composite powder and calcium phosphate nanopowder were heat treated. The feedstock powder was set up with a various mix of reinforcement and afterward handled with a laser-designed net forming approach. In this, a laser power wellspring of 400 W and an output speed of 45–60 cm/min were accustomed to storing the Co–Cr–Mo–Ca–P composites alongside a powder feed pace of 60 g/min. The laser surface dissolving tests were led in an argon climate with an oxygen content of less than 10 parts per million [46].

The powder bed framework comprises two powder beds with position changes in Z bearing with the help of a piston (placed underneath the bed) [47]. The nano-composite powders are kept at the feeding bed. At first, a slender layer of compos-ite powders is spread on the feeding bed. Then, the part pushes ahead to inject the fastener over the building bed dependent on the CAD design. The feeding chamber piston pushes the feeding bed up to restricted layer thickness after the injection of the fluid binder. Next, the compartment advances toward a reverse direction to spread the powder to the next layer with the assistance of a rotating roller. The spread layers of composite powders are set up to inject the binder for another layer as shown in Figure 6.4. A similar method was repeated to accomplish a permeable design, and afterwards, the sample was dried to remove the binders [48].

6.3.6 Friction Stir Process

FSP is a plastic distortion strategy that helps in achieving better surface properties and furthermore adjusts the microstructure of the materials [42]. These strategies enjoy a few benefits like the uniform scattering of support particles and change over surface properties and so. Titanium-based materials find applications in dental and muscu-lar implants and have less wear resistance that restricts the more extensive scope of

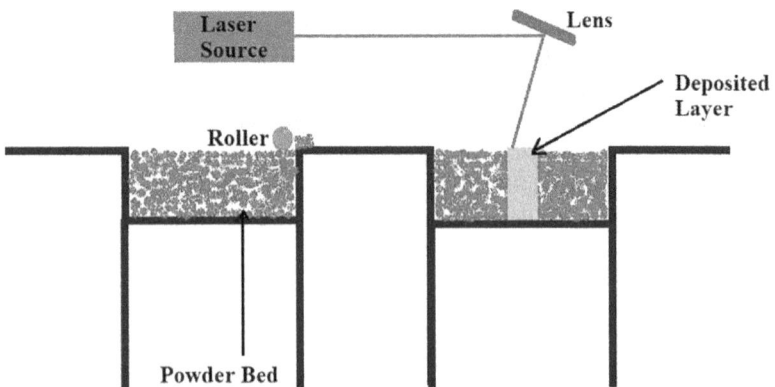

FIGURE 6.4 Representation of powder bed additive manufacturing.

their application. In certain examinations, Si–C-based nanoceramic materials were utilized as a support to improve the wear resistance of Ti-based matrix materials. For growing a Si–C supported Ti composite, at first the outside of the Ti plate is polished and cleaned using acetone to remove the impurities [49]. Openings are made over the outside of the cleaned Ti plate's surface with 1 and 2-mm diameters. At that point, the nano Si–C particles are stacked in the openings at a steady speed of 50.0 mm/min and the rotational speed of the tungsten steel apparatus was adjusted to 500 rpm. The FSP was completed in an idle gas environment to avoid oxidation owing to high temperatures close to FSP zones. The test was 10 mm in diameter with the inward shoulder; pin height was 2 mm skewed by 2.5°. The probe was embedded into the workpiece for microstructural alteration to coat the FSP region. Several passes of FSP with 100% total cover after three passes were initiated for additional structure modifications [7] (Figure 6.5).

6.3.7 SPARK PLASMA-ASSISTED POWDER METALLURGY SINTERING

Biocompatible composite materials, for example, MgZnMnSiHA composites, can be synthesized by the spark plasma sintering process, which is assisted by solid-state processing as shown in Figure 6.6. The commercially pure metal powders, viz., Mg, Mn, Si, Zn and HA, are ball milled with a calculated weight level of support particles utilizing planetary ball milling with SS balls with 5 mm diameter for mechanical alloying [51]. For the most part, the powder to ball proportion is maintained at 1:10 with a speed of 300 rpm for 12 hours. During mechanical alloying, reagents like stearic acid are added to avoid agglomeration that is formed due to cold welding. The accomplished composite powder was then preheated in an argon climate to kill the wetness of mechanically alloyed powder. Recently, composite blenders are

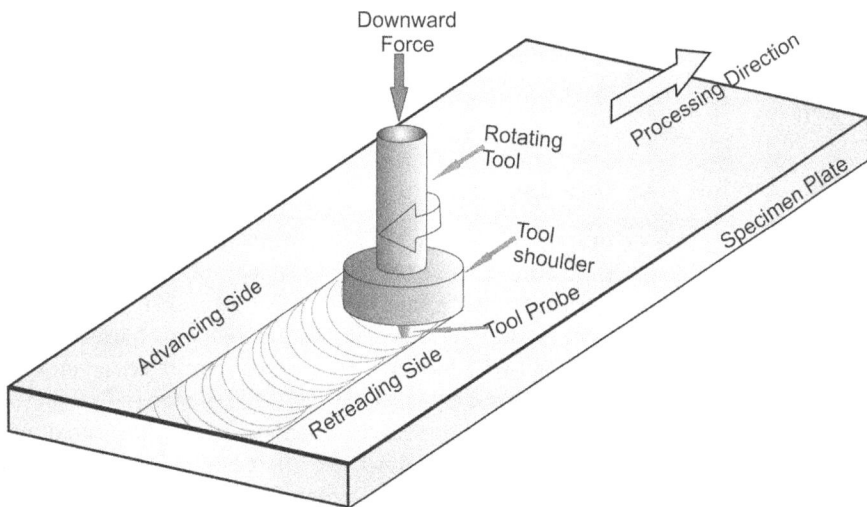

FIGURE 6.5   Representation of the friction stir process.

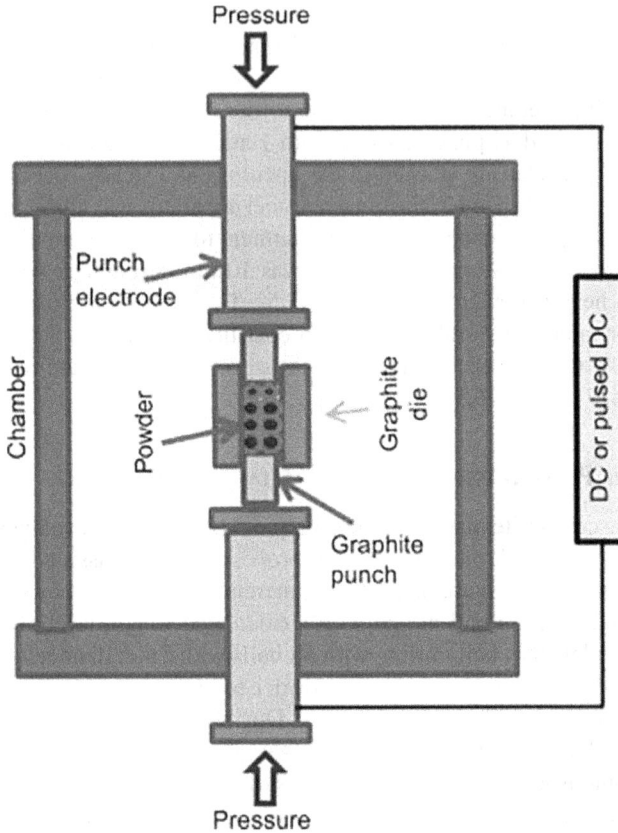

FIGURE 6.6   Representation of spark plasma-assisted sintering [50].

sintered by spark plasma sintering measure. The sintering cycle is carried out at a heat flow of 50°C/min under a vacuum climate with fluctuating applied pressure and temperature [7].

6.3.8 Accumulative Roll Bonding Process

This method depends on the principle of severe plastic degradation enforced by rolling rolls on metallic pieces to accomplish materials with fine-grain refinement [53]. Metal matrix nanocomposites are manufactured by Al/CNT, Mg/CNT and so forth. At first, the base network metal examples are cut into the required measurement. At that point, the lattice plates are wire bushed all together to eliminate the impurities and oxide layer that shaped over the outside of the network material as shown in Figure 6.7. After that, weight or volume level of nanoparticles is measured and sprayed on the matrix metal surface. After this cycle, the metal sheets are stacked into two sheets on top. At that point, the thicknesses of stacked composite sheets are reduced to 50% thickness with the help of roll bonding. After that, roll bonded samples are separated into bits and a similar cycle can be repeated for several passes,

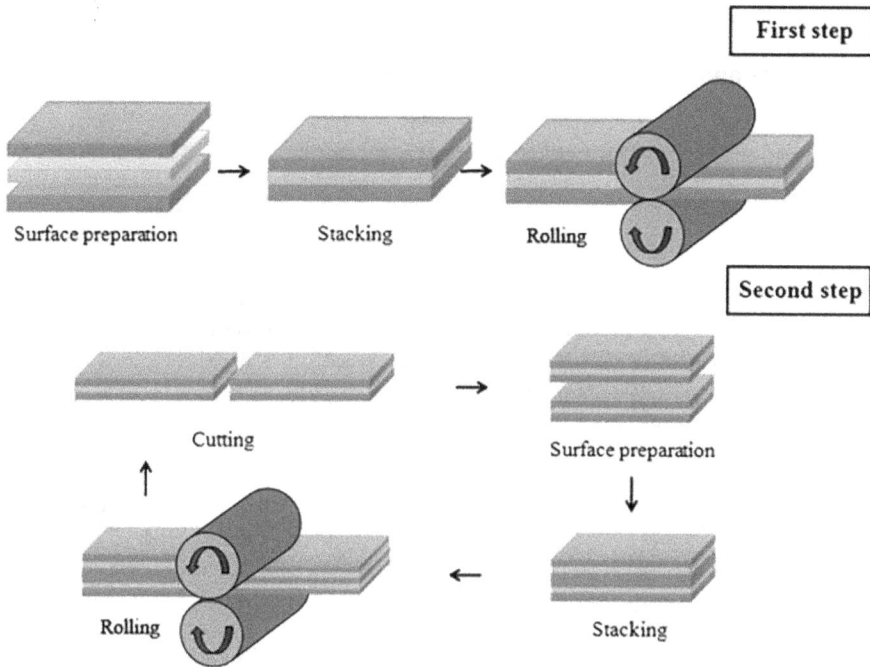

FIGURE 6.7   Representation of the accumulative roll bonding process [52].

which depend on our necessity to achieve composite materials with fine-grain refinements [7] (Table 6.2).

6.4   CHARACTERIZATION OF Mg ALLOYS

Different methods used for characterization of Mg alloys are surface free energy analysis, MAF treatment, surface characterization, immersion corrosion tests and electrochemical corrosion tests.

6.4.1   SURFACE CHARACTERIZATION

Surface state and basic components of tests were noticed by FESEM and EDS. Surface composition tests were performed by XRD [54]. At 40 kV and 30 mA, the scan speed was 1°/min utilizing a CuKα stripe. Surface scars were estimated by three-dimensional optical profilometry. The scattering point was fixed at a value less than 1. According to a single diffuse scattering scan a single diffuse dispersal check Ra, Rp, Rq, Rt and Rv esteem were calculated dependent on the ISO-4287 norm. The testing region vicinity is $0.170 \times 0.20 \text{mm}^2$ [8].

6.4.2   MAF TREATMENT

In 100 mL of the electrolyte, AZ-31 magnesium alloy in HCl was utilized as an anode and a graphite bar was utilized as a cathode in the MAF treatment process as shown

TABLE 6.2
Advantages and Disadvantages of Different Methods Used for Fabrication

Method	Advantages	Disadvantages
Equal channel angular extrusion	• Selective heating process and rapid heating	• Material strength depends on the characteristics of the powder used
Powder metallurgy	• Manufacturing near net-shaped products • Produced component will have controlled porosity	• Difficulty in choosing optimal process parameters, viz., sintering and pressing • Powder materials are costly
Microwave-assisted powder metallurgy	• Selective heating process and rapid heating	• Expensive process
Dual-stage sintering-assisted powder metallurgy	• High production rate and flexible low cost	• Attaining uniform dispersion and lower porosity is quite difficult due to the agglomeration tendency of nanomaterials
Additive manufacturing	• Fabrication of complex component shapes • Combine manufacturing and assembly into a single process	• Material strength depends on the characteristics of the powder used • Not efficient in producing a high volume of parts
Friction stir processing	• Fine-grain refinement in microstructure	• Only surface composite can be developed • Developed material will have poor resistance to intergranular corrosion
Spark plasma-assisted powder metallurgy sintering	• Efficient energy-saving process	• Only symmetrical parts can be developed
Accumulative roll bonding	• Bulky sheet materials with improved strength can be developed	• Not advisable for developing complex parts

in Figure 6.8. After various tests, it was tracked down that a lot of hydro fluoric corrosive gas was delivered at a brutal response of HCl at a high current, contaminating the climate and hurting the wellbeing. Thusly, 100, 150, 200, 250 and 300 V were picked as test voltages in the examination. Five arrangements of different voltages are applied at a voltage with a most extreme current of 2 A for 30 seconds. MAF treated AZ-31 magnesium combination was then arranged and washed with deionized water three times and blow-dried. An outline of the MAF cycle is shown in Figure 6.8 [55].

6.4.3 ELECTROCHEMICAL CORROSION TEST

The corrosion resistance of AZ-31 and MAF treated AZ31 magnesium alloys is checked with the open circuit potential and potential dynamic polarization test. An Ag–K–Cl

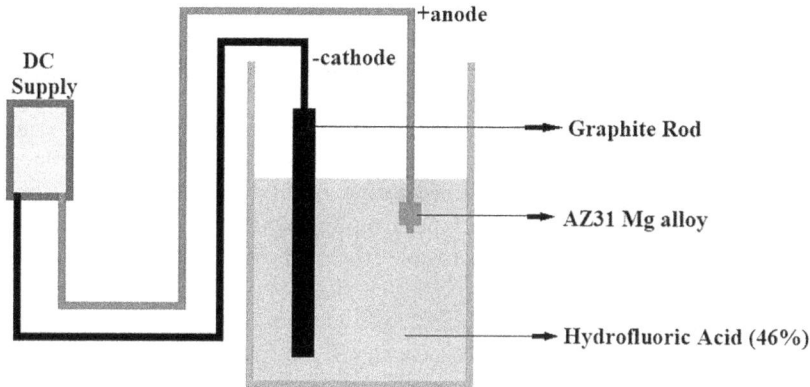

FIGURE 6.8 Representation of the MAF treatment process of AZ31 magnesium alloy.

cathode was utilized as a source of perspective terminal [56]. A fine graphite pole was utilized as a response cathode. The sample was exposed 1 cm² as a functioning electrode and 1000 mL of HBSS was utilized as an electrolyte. The heat of the electrolyte was kept up at 37°C. In this process, to balance out the capability of the process, the sample was first submerged in PBS for 1 hour to play out its open circuit potential mode. At that point, a potential dynamic polarization (PDP) test was conducted. An electrochemical test was conducted utilizing a Versa STAT3 potentiostat combined with a Versa Studio 2.43.3 programming for electrochemical control and data analysis [8].

6.4.4 IMMERSION CORROSION TEST

AZ-31 and MAF treated AZ-31 magnesium alloy was upward drenched in HBSS at 37° for 8 and 30 days. Each gathering had three equal samples. The proportion of the HBSS volume to the solution region was 20 mL/cm². HBSS was changed week after week. After submersion for 8 and 30 days, samples were ultrasonically cleaned neatly with a chromium trioxide (Cr-O₃) liquid for 3–4 minutes, flushed with deionized water three times and dried. The level of mass loss was determined [57]:

$$\text{Mass loss percent} = \eth M_0 - M_1 / M_0 \text{þ} \times 100\%.$$

Here,

M_0 is the weight of the test prior to the immersion.
M_1 is the weight of the test after the immersion.

Examples in every group should be tested and weight loss should be shown as mean standard deviation (SD).

6.5 CONCLUSION

In this chapter, a detailed review of different magnesium alloys used for biomedical applications is carried out. Magnesium is a biodegradable matter that degrades totally in the human body after clinical use and because of this property, demand for magnesium alloys is increasing day by day. Magnesium also has flexible corrosion rates, appropriate mechanical properties, and the capacity for the formation of precipitation of a bone-like apatite layer on its outer layer. Among the different magnesium alloys used in biomedical applications, Mg–6Zn is the most suitable for biomedical applications, as it shows 100% cell viability.

Different fabrication and characterization techniques of magnesium used for biomedical applications are studied in this chapter. It was observed that for bone tissue designing applications, the dual-stage sintering-assisted powder metallurgy method is mostly preferred to stay away from the imperfections. A comparative study of different fabrication techniques of magnesium nanocomposites is carried out, which will help the researcher to understand the different techniques used for processing nanocomposites for biomedical applications. Surface state and basic components of tests were noticed utilizing FESEM and EDS. The corrosion resistance of AZ31 MAF treated AZ31 magnesium alloys was measured with the open circuit potential and PDP test.

REFERENCES

1. N.R. Patel, P.P. Gohil, "A review on biomaterials: Scope, applications & human anatomy significance", *Int. J. Emerg. Technol. Adv. Eng.* 2(4) 91e101, 2012.
2. M.A. Hussein, A.S. Mohammed, N. Al-Aqeeli, "Wear characteristics of metallic biomaterials: A review", *Materials (Basel)* 8(5) 2749e2768, 2015.
3. S. Agarwal, J. Curtin, B. Duffy, S. Jaiswal, "Biodegradable magnesium alloys for orthopaedic applications: A review on corrosion, biocompatibility and surface modifications", *Mater. Sci. Eng. C* 68 948e963, 2016.
4. Y. Xin, T. Hu, P.K. Chu, "In vitro studies of biomedical magnesium alloys in a simulated physiological environment: A review", *Acta Biomater.* 7(4) 1452e1459, 2011.
5. R.C. Zeng, J. Zhang, W.J. Huang, W. Dietzel, K.U. Kainer, C. Blawert, K.E. Wei, "Review of studies on corrosion of magnesium alloys", *Trans. Nonferrous Metals Soc. China* 16 s763es771, 2006.
6. J. Liu, H. Yu, C. Chen, F. Weng, J. Dai, "Research and development status of laser cladding on magnesium alloys: A review", *Optic Laser. Eng.* 93 195e210, 2017.
7. V. Kavimani, P.M. Gopal, "Processing of nanocomposites for biomedical applications", *Proceedings of the 5th NA International Conference on Industrial Engineering and Operations* Management Detroit, MI, August 10–14, 2020.
8. L. Sun, B.C. Zhao, T. Wang, J.Y. Cui, S.X. Zhang, "Surface characterization and corrosion resistance of biomedical AZ31 Mg alloy treated by microarc fluorination", *Hindawi Scan* 2020, Article ID 5936789, 2020.
9. N.T. Kirkland, N. Birbilis, M.P. Staiger, "Assessing the corrosion of biodegradable magnesium implants: A critical review of current methodologies and their limitations", *Acta Biomater.* 8(3) 925e936, 2012.
10. R. Erbel, C. Di Mario, J. Bartunek, J. Bonnier, B. de Bruyne, F.R. Eberli, P. Erne, M. Haude, B. Heublein, M. Horrigan, C. Ilsley, D. Bose, J. Koolen, T.F. Lüscher, N. Weissman, R. Waksman, "Temporary scaffolding of coronary arteries with bioabsorbable magnesium stents: A prospective, non-randomised multicentre trial", *Lancet* 369(-9576) 1869e1875, 2007.

11. P. Peeters, M. Bosiers, J. Verbist, K. Deloose, B. Heublein, "Preliminary results after application of absorbable metal stents in patients with critical limb ischemia", *J. Endovasc. Ther.* 12(1) 1e5, 2005.

12. C. Di Mario, H.U.W. Griffiths, O. Goktekin, N. Peeters, J.A.N. Verbist, M. Bosiers, K. Deloose, B. Heublein, R. Rohde, V. Kasese, C. Ilsley, "Drug-eluting bioabsorbable magnesium stent", *J. Interv. Cardiol.* 17(6) 391e395, 2004.

13. V. Kavimani, K. Soorya Prakash. "Tribological behaviour predictions of R-GO reinforced Mg composite using ANN coupled Taguchi approach", *J. Phys. Chem. Solids* 110 2017, 409–19. Doi: 10.1016/j.jpcs.2017.06.028, 2017.

14. R.B. Heimann, "Magnesium alloys for biomedical application: Advanced corrosion control through surface coating", *Surf. Coat. Technol.* 2018, Doi: 10.1016/j.surfcoat.2020.126521.

15. P. Pesode, S. Barve, "Surface modification of titanium and titanium alloy by plasma electrolytic oxidation process for biomedical applications: A review", *Mater. Today: Proceed.* 2020, Doi: 10.1016/j.matpr.2020.11.294.

16. P.A. Pesode, S.B. Barve, "Recent advances on the antibacterial coating on titanium implant by micro-arc oxidation process", *Mater. Today: Proceed.* 2021, Doi: 10.1016/j.matpr.2021.03.702.

17. H. Tapiero, K.D. Tew, "Trace elements in human physiology and pathology: Zinc and metallothioneins", *Biomed. Pharmacot.* 57(9) 2003, 399–411. doi:10.1016/s0753-3322(03)00081-7.

18. M. Avedesian, H. Baker, *ASM Specialty Handbook: Magnesium and Magnesium Alloys,* , ASM International, 1999.

19. S.X. Zhang, X.N. Zhang, C.L. Zhao, J.A. Li, Y. Song, C.Y. Xie, H.R. Tao, Y. Zhang, Y.H. He, Y. Jiang, "Research on an Mg-Zn alloy as a degradable biomaterial", *Bian, Acta Biomater.* 6 626e640, 2010.

20. C.M. Serre, M. Papillard, P. Chavassieux, J.C. Voegel, G. Boivin, "Influence of magnesium substitution on a collagen-apatite biomaterial on the production of a calcifying matrix by human osteoblasts", *J. Biomed. Mater. Res.* 42 626e633, 1998.

21. Z. Li, X. Gu, S. Lou, Y. Zheng, "The development of binary Mg–Ca alloys for use as biodegradable materials within bone", *Biomaterials*, 29(10) 1329–1344, 2008. doi:10.1016/j.biomaterials.2007.12.021.

22. X.N. Gu, X.L. Li, W.R. Zhou, Y. Cheng, Y.F. Zheng, "Microstructure, biocorrosion and cytotoxicity evaluations of rapid solidified Mg-3Ca alloy ribbons as a biodegradable material", *Biomed. Mater.* 5 035013, 2010.

23. A. Krause, N. von der Hoh, D. Bormann, C. Krause, F.W. Bach, H. Windhagen, A. Meyer-Lindenberg, "Degradation behaviour and mechanical properties of magnesium implants in rabbit tibiae", *J. Mater. Sci.* 45 624e632, 2010.

24. H.G. Seiler, H. Sigel, A. Sigel, *Handbook on Toxicity of Inorganic Compounds*, Marcel Dekker, New York, 1988.

25. Y.C. Lee, A.K. Dahle, D.H. StJohn, "Metallurgical and materials transactions", *Metal. Mater. Trans.* 31A 2895e2906, 2000.

26. H.S. Brar, J. Wong, M.V. Manuel, "Investigation of the mechanical and degradation properties of Mg–sr and Mg–zn–sr alloys for use as potential biodegradable implant material", *J. Mech. Behav. Biomed. Mater.* 7 87e95, 2012.

27. X. Gu, Y. Zheng, Y. Cheng, S. Zhong, T. Xi. "In vitro corrosion and biocompatibility of binary magnesium alloys", *Biomaterials* 30(4) 484–498. doi:10.1016/j.biomaterials.2008.10.021, 2009.

28. D.M. Reffit, N. Ogston, R. Jugdaohsingh, H.F.J. Cheungb, B.A.J. Evansc, R.P.H. Thompsona et al., "Hampson Orthosilicic acid stimulates collagen type I synthesis and osteoblastic differentiation in human osteoblast-like cells in vitro", *Bone* 32 127–35, 2003.

29. L.L. Rokhlin, *Magnesium Alloys Containing Rare Earth Metals: Structure and Properties*, CRC Press, 2003.
30. A. Drynda, N. Deinet, N. Braun, "Rare earth metals used in biodegradable magnesium-based stents do not interfere with proliferation of smooth muscle cells but do induce the upregulation of inflammatory genes", *J. Biomed. Mater. Res. Part A.* 91A(2) 360–369, 2009. doi:10.1002/jbm.a.32235.
31. X. Zhang, G. Yuan, L. Mao, J. Niu, W. Ding, "Enhanced biocorrosion resistance and biocompatibility of degradable Mg-Nd-Zn-Zr alloy by brushite coating", *Mater. Lett.* 66 209e211, 2012.
32. Fadaei, A., Farahafshan, F., & Sepahi-Boroujeni, S. (2017). Spiral equal channel angular extrusion (Sp-ECAE) as a modified ECAE process. Materials & Design, 113, 361-368.
33. S.R. Agnew, P. Mehrotra, T.M. Lillo, G.M. Stoica, P.K. Liaw, "Texture evolution of five wrought magnesium alloys during route a equal channel angular extrusion: Experiments and simulations", *Acta Materialia* 53(11) 3135–46, 2005.
34. R.Z. Valiev, T.G. Langdon. "Principles of equal-channel angular pressing as a processing tool for grain refinement", *Progress Mater. Sci.* 51(7) 881–981, 2006.
35. Y. Huang, J. Li, L. Zhou. "Mg–3Zn–0.5 Zr/HA nanocomposites fabricated by high shear solidification and equal channel angular extrusion", *Mater. Sci. Technol.* 34(15) 1868–79, 2018.
36. G. Singh, N. Sharma, D. Kumar, H. Hegab. "Design, development and tribological characterization of Ti-6Al-4V/hydroxyapatite composite for bio-implant applications", *Mater. Chem. Phys.*, 243, 122662, 2020.
37. V. Kavimani, K. Soorya Prakash, M. S. Starvin, B. Kalidas, V. Viswamithran, S. R. Arun. "Tribo-surface characteristics and wear behaviour of SiC@r-GO/Mg composite worn under varying control factor", *Silicon* 12(1) 29–39, 2020. doi:10.1007/s12633-019-0095-2.
38. V. Kavimani, K. Soorya Prakash, T. Thankachan "Investigation of graphene-reinforced magnesium metal matrix composites processed through a solvent-based powder metallurgy route", *Bullet. Mater. Sci.* 42(1) 39, 2019. doi:10.1007/s12034-018-1720-1.
39. S.M. Javadhesari, S. Alipour, M.R. Akbarpour "Microstructural characterization and enhanced hardness, wear and antibacterial properties of a powder metallurgy SiC/Ti-Cu nanocomposite as a potential material for biomedical applications", *Ceramics Inter.* 45(8) 10603–11, 2019.
40. P. Radha, G. Chandrasekaran, N. Selvakumar, "Simplifying the powder metallurgy manufacturing process using soft computing tools", *Appl. Soft Comput.* 27, February 2015.
41. G. Xiong, Y. Nie, D. Ji, J. Li, C. Li, W. Li, Y. Zhu, H. Luo, Y. Wan. "Characterization of biomedical hydroxyapatite/magnesium composites prepared by powder metallurgy assisted with microwave sintering", *Curr. Appl. Phys.* 16(8) 830–36, 2016.
42. G. Radha, S. Balakumar, B. Venkatesan, E. Vellaichamy. "Evaluation of hemocompatibility and in vitro immersion on microwave-assisted hydroxyapatite–alumina nano-composites", *Mater. Sci. Eng.: C* 50 143–50, 2015.
43. D. Agrawal, "Microwave sintering of metal powders", Editor(s): Isaac Chang, Yuyuan Zhao, In Woodhead Publishing Series in Metals and Surface Engineering, Advances in Powder Metallurgy, Woodhead Publishing Sawston United Kingdom, 2013, Pages 361–379. doi.org/10.1533/9780857098900.3.361.
44. C. Marinescu, A. Sofronia, E.M Anghel, R. Baies, D. Constantin, A.-M. Seciu, O. Gingu, and S. Tanasescu. "Microstructure, stability and biocompatibility of hydroxyapatite–titania nanocomposites formed by two step sintering process", *Arab. J. Chem.*, 12(6) 857–867, 2017.

45. H. Li, M. Wang, D. Lou, W. Xia, and X. Fang. "Microstructural features of biomedical cobalt–chromium–molybdenum (CoCrMo) alloy from powder bed fusion to aging heat treatment", *J. Mater. Sci. Technol.* 45 146–56, 2020.

46. A. Bandyopadhyay, A. Shivaram, M. Isik, J.D Avila, W.S Dernell, and S. Bose. "Additively manufactured calcium phosphate reinforced CoCrMo alloy: Bio-tribological and biocompatibility evaluation for load-bearing implants", *Additive Manufact.* 28. Elsevier: 312–24, 2019.

47. A. Azhari, E. Toyserkani, C. Villain "Additive manufacturing of graphene–hydroxyapatite nanocomposite structures", *Int. J. Appl. Ceramic Technol.* 12(1) 8–17, 2015.

48. X. Yao, S.K. Moon, B.Y. Lee, and G. Bi. "Effects of heat treatment on microstructures and tensile properties of IN718/TiC nanocomposite fabricated by selective laser melting", *Int. J. Precision Eng. Manufact.* 18(12) 1693–1701, 2017.

49. C. Zhu, Y. Lv, C. Qian, H. Qian, T. Jiao, L. Wang, F. Zhang. "Proliferation and osteogenic differentiation of rat BMSCs on a novel Ti/SiC metal matrix nanocomposite modified by friction stir processing", *Sci. Rep.* 6(1) 1–15, 2016.

50. R. Madugundo, N. V. R. Rao, A. M. Schönhöbel, D.Salazar, A. A. El-Gendy. Recent Developments in Nanostructured Permanent Magnet Materials and Their Processing Methods. Editor(s): Ahmed A. El-Gendy, José M. Barandiarán, Ravi L. Hadimani, In *Micro and Nano Technologies, Magnetic Nanostructured Materials*, Elsevier, 2018, Pages 157–198. doi.org/10.1016/B978-0-12-813904-2.00006-1.

51. C. Prakash, S. Singh, M. Gupta, M. Mia, G. Królczyk, N. Khanna. "Synthesis, characterization, corrosion resistance and in-vitro bioactivity behaviour of biodegradable Mg–Zn–Mn–(Si–HA) composite for orthopaedic applications", *Materials* 11(9) 1602, 2018.

52. V.Y. Mehr, A. Rezaeian, M.R. Toroghinejad. Application of accumulative roll bonding and anodizing process to produce Al–Cu–Al2O3 composite. *Materials & Design* 70 53–59, 2015.

53. A. Bhardwaj, A.K. Gupta, S.K. Padisala, and K. Poluri. "Characterization of mechanical and microstructural properties of constrained groove pressed nitinol shape memory alloy for biomedical applications", *Mater. Sci. Eng.: C* 102 730–42, 2019.

54. P.R. Hall, "Introduction to surface roughness and scattering", *Precision Eng.* 13(1) 62, 1991.

55. C.Y. Zhang, J.C. Gao, and C.L. Liu, "Effect of fluoride treatment on corrosion property of AZ31 magnesium alloy in Hank's solution", *Adv. Mater. Res.* 239–242 186–190, 2011.

56. J. Zhang, S. Hiromoto, T. Yamazaki et al., "Macrophage phagocytosis of biomedical Mg alloy degradation products prepared by electrochemical method", *Mater. Sci. Eng.: C* 75 1178–1183, 2017.

57. L. Yang and E. Zhang, "Biocorrosion behaviour of magnesium alloy in different simulated fluids for biomedical application", *Mater. Sci. Eng.: C* 29(5) 1691–1696, 2009.

7 Magnesium Alloy for Biomedical Applications

Pralhad Pesode, Shivprakash Barve,
and Dr. Vishwanath Karad
MIT-World Peace University Pune

CONTENTS

7.1 INTRODUCTION

Since the last few decades, interest in Mg alloys as biodegradable alloys has been growing. Magnesium alloys are getting attention due to their outstanding biocompatibility, moderate corrosion rate and excellent mechanical properties, when proper alloying elements and processes are utilized. Likely, magnesium alloys are used as materials for temporary cardiovascular devices and orthopedic applications. Body absorbs these implants after they complete their functions such as bonding to tissue, scaffolding and mechanical support. While developing a magnesium alloy, the focus is mainly on the design, fatigue, corrosion resistance, deformability and uniform corrosion morphology. Researchers working on magnesium alloys mainly focus on in vitro and in vivo properties, which will help to minimize animal testing and support

DOI: 10.1201/9781003286806-7

simulation to select a proper alloy [1]. The natural inspiration for picking biodegradable implant materials instead of nondegradable implants is because of many issues, such as stress shielding, secondary infection, particle release and so forth. Because of nondegradability and the longer healing time span of an implant, many times, another surgery (secondary surgery) is required to replace or eliminate an implant once the healing process is completed [2–4].

Because of their excellent properties, magnesium alloys have displayed greater potential and arisen as solid competitors for use in creating biodegradable types of implants [5,6]. Magnesium has a lower density (1.8 g/cm^3). The amazing compressive yield strength, higher strength-to-weight ratio and elastic modulus of Mg are nearly similar to those of natural human bone, making it a favored choice over generally utilized metallic implant materials [7]. But, the widespread use of magnesium alloys is limited due to some of the unfortunate properties [8], including production of a higher amount of hydrogen gas, faster corrosion rate, increase in local pH of the body fluid and gathering of the hydrogen bubbles near to the implant (hindering the healing of wound). However, magnesium tends to be a perfect biodegradable implant material whenever alloying it with some bioactive elements. A few elements like Ca, Zn and Sr are found to be excellent alloying elements for magnesium-based materials for the biomedical field [9].

There are primarily two main possibilities to delay the degradation of Mg alloys: (i) coating or surface treatment and (ii) alloying. To improve the corrosion resistance of Mg alloys, alloying with suitable elements is an effective way. Alloyed magnesium offers the extraordinary potential for developing new magnesium alloys with excellent physical and mechanical properties by changing the structure and phase distribution [10,11], which influences the corrosion rate of magnesium alloy altogether. The important alloying elements of magnesium alloys are Ca, Al, Zn, Fe, Mn, Li, etc. Al has been accounted to be cytotoxic and hence, it will make adverse impacts on body tissues [12]. A high percentage of Ca and Zr in magnesium alloy can increase the corrosion rate [13]; however, a limited quantity of Zr could give finer grain and improve properties [14]. Due to the implantation of these artificial materials in the human body, safety should be considered while picking alloying elements. Although it has been realized that alloying is advantageous to corrosion resistance, the impact is not as expected.

Zn is discovered mostly in bones and muscles, and it improves the yield strength of an implant material, lessens H$_2$ gas release during biocorrosion because of Mg and furthermore keeps away from the antagonistic impact of nickel and iron impurities that may be present in magnesium [9]. Sr improves corrosion resistance and strength by grain size refinement of magnesium alloys. Sr gives an inactive layer on magnesium alloys, which results in human osteoblast development and bone mass. Ca is an indispensable bone component and possibly fundamental for keeping up bone health [15–17]. Magnesium alloys have set another standard in orthopedic implant materials because of their higher corrosion resistance, particularly in vitro [14]. A biodegradable implant material needs to remain in the human body for sensibly longer spans and it should dissolve entirely after satisfying the proposed purposes. However, it should keep up its mechanical strength for at least 12–18 weeks during the process of bone tissue healing. Biodegradable magnesium-based alloys offer additional benefits over Sr-based, Ca-based, Zn-based and Fe-based alloys [18,19]. During the bone tissue healing time, biodegradable materials are unpredictable because of the nonstop degradation process with changeable degradation rates in the complicated physiological environment. Biodegradable types of implants might lose their strength very early on account of localized corrosion, which is reliant upon pitting, corrosion fatigue and so forth. A perfect biodegradable material should have a lower rate of degradation.

Another reasonable and attractive alternative to prevent degradation of magnesium against corrosion is surface treatment. Many surface modification techniques are available for magnesium and its alloys, including sol–gel technique, anodization, electrochemical deposition and micro-arc oxidation (MAO). Among available techniques, MAO has got extensive consideration. MAO, also called plasma electrolytic oxidation (PEO), is based on a conversional anodic oxidization technique, generally utilized for the surface modifications on magnesium alloys and other light metals such as Ti and Al [20]. The MAO process produces coatings with fantastic properties, for example, higher hardness [21], great wear resistance [22], great corrosion performance [23], good thermal stability [24] and excellent thermal emissivity [24].

7.1.1 Need of Coating on Magnesium Alloys

Mg and its alloys are interesting light-weight metals for aviation, transportation, biomedical usage and hydrogen storage [25,26]. One of the limitations of a magnesium alloy is its poor resistance toward corrosion [27] and faster rate of degradation [28]. Mg gets corroded faster in chlorine-containing solutions, i.e., human body fluid [29,30]. Consequently, due to the faster rate of degradation, it causes the following issues: (i) hydrogen evolution happens at cavities close to the injury parts after implantation treatment [2]. Luckily, the developed hydrogen air pockets will vanish within half a month and are not a significant worry in clinical cases [31,32]. (ii) Alkalization near the surface of a magnesium-based implant, due to Mg degradation, prompts the high hemolysis of red platelets [33]. A higher value of pH attaining up to highly alkaline micro-environments is unsafe to the living organism [2]. (iii) Osmotic pressure of human body liquid will be raised with increasing Mg^{2+}. Thus, keeping up the ionic concentration of the local area under a specific value is the most important [33]. (iv) The structural defects of magnesium and its alloys lead to a fast decrease in the mechanical strength of implants due to long-term degradation in vivo [34], which can bring mechanical pre-failure. In the course of the most recent 20 years, one of the researchers [35] investigated the degradation phenomenon of Mg alloys in vitro and in vivo. Recent studies show a lot of progress in surface modification methods for Mg alloys utilized for biomedical applications [36], with respect to biodegradability [37], bioactivity [37], biocompatibility [38] and improvement in corrosion behavior [27]. This paper focuses on surface treatments of magnesium alloys by the MAO process utilized in the biomedical field.

7.1.2 Coating Techniques

Generally, there are two basic kinds of surface treatment strategies: wet and dry coating techniques. The dry technique includes different vapor deposition processes, and wet coating techniques include different anodizing processes.

7.1.2.1 Dry Coating Methods

Both CVD and PVD come under the vapor deposition category, which incorporates atomic layer deposition (ALD) and a sputtering method. PVD comes under a dry treatment process where a high vacuum is required. Solid precursors move in the vapor stage after that they get condensed to frame a stronger and thicker film. Sputtering is the most widely recognized PVD method in which the object is targeted by nitrogen and argon plasma emitted and ultimately deposited on the specimen, creating a thinner layer. The layer thickness might come to ~0.05 mm created through interlocking. Then again, CVD using vaporous materials, rather than solid precursors, occurs in the vapor stage framing a thin layer. The parameters include gas flow rate, precursor composition and temperature. Nonetheless, CVD might experience effects of nonconsistency because of a quick reaction associated deposition process. ALD gives a more uniform coating with superb adaptability and controllability. ALD is similar to the CVD; but it varies in the depositing process, where ALD does not occur in the vaporous stage; however, it is presented in a reactor successively by means of cleansing by N_2 or Ar in the middle. There are two fundamental types of precursors present in CVD. On account of elemental precursors, a depositing layer will not have any sort of contamination; notwithstanding, the decision is restricted for the materials having a higher vapor pressure. Metal halides, then again, are extremely receptive so the deposition will be sped up notwithstanding a wide temperature range, albeit antagonistic responses may bring about lesser purity of depositing layer. The total clarification of CVD and PVD strategies is not the scope of this chapter, along these lines, further information needs to be found somewhere else.

In the past studies, several researchers have reported the deposition of ceramics on lighter metals like Al, Mg and Ti. For example, hydroxyapatite (HA) deposition through PVD has essentially modified the bioactivity of the substrate surface. When TiN was deposited on Al by means of PVD, which has changed the physicochemical performance of Al, it gives excellent adhesive strength to the Al-to-Al joint. Considering magnesium, due to the deposition of SiOx on magnesium by the CVD technique, a thin film is formed without any microdefects. Even though different methodologies previously mentioned are accessible to deposit different ceramics and oxides of metal, the majority of processes needed higher temperatures; however, such techniques are less reasonable for Mg and Al because of their lower melting temperatures. What is more, lower coating thickness and poorer coating attachment are the principal disadvantages of the above techniques. From a modern viewpoint, confounded preparation, tediousness and significant expense are the primary limitation of the deposition technique mentioned above. Hence, a different technique that will wipe out the above-mentioned limitation will be ideal.

7.1.2.2 Wet Coating Techniques

Different dry coating strategies were set up to deposit metal oxides on metallic implants and were carried out under vacuum conditions and at a higher temperature, which made these methods somewhat unsuitable for different light metals including Mg, Al and Ti. In addition, dry coating methods can create conformal and thinner films having lesser evident of microdefects. For modern industrial applications including biomedical applications, those strategies are not effective, concerning a few significant limitations previously mentioned. Several wet coating strategies, including chemical conversion coating, sol–gel technique, anodizing process and metal plating, turned into a viable choice to create the thicker protective coating on the light metals mentioned above. Out of these, anodizing is the straightforward electrochemical technique that started approximately in the 1930s, which was utilized effectively in industrial applications for surface coating of light metals particularly Ti, Mg and Al in electrolytes such as chromic acid, sulfuric acid, phosphoric, oxalic acid and so on. Traditional anodizing is normally done at a lower voltage such as 20–80 V; on the other hand, hard anodizing is carried out at high voltages such as 120 V approximately, which can give a higher thickness of the coating and better hardness value. However, both yet experience a few limitations emerging from the utilization of electrolyte which is environmentally nonfriendly, with a slower depositing rate as well as critical pre-treatment requirements. In this manner, a large number of investigations have been carried out to manufacture inorganic oxide layers on light metal surfaces in environmentally viable electrolytes through the modern strategy created from the anodizing technique, in particular, MAO. Developed from anodizing, MAO is carried out at a higher voltage, where the previously deposited coating will probably not be going to survive the stronger electrical field; hence, dielectric breakdown happened with sparking starting over the entire substrate. Development of coating in anodizing is determined exclusively by electrochemical reactions, whereas in the MAO technique, the electrochemical reaction occurs along with plasma discharges that happened at the same time in the electrolyte–metal interface. Plasma releases are essential for the development of the coating layer. Such release discharges give a higher energy for the melting of a specimen and an already deposited layer of coating.

There are different surface modification and coating methods available for Mg and other light metal alloys such as physical, mechanical, chemical, biomimetic, biological, etc. [39,40]. Various surface modification techniques are shown in Figure 7.1. Among available techniques, MAO has got extensive consideration. MAO is a high-voltage plasma-assisted oxidation method, based on a conversional anodic oxidization technique, generally utilized for the surface modifications on magnesium alloys and other light metals such as Ti and Al [41].

7.2 METHODOLOGY

The MAO process was utilized to develop hard, abrasion resistance, electronic insulator, shock resistance and thermal barrier coating. Coating created by the MAO technique has excellent adhesion to implant surfaces by using a potential above the dielectric breakdown potential [42,43]. Even though the MAO process may look similar to the traditional anodizing process, it is essentially different [44,45]. MAO required a higher potential than the breakdown potential value of primary oxide films (150–800 V), whereas anodizing is done at very low voltages (10–80 V) [46]. During an MAO process, discrete discharge is seen at random spots over the whole surface, when the provided voltage surpasses the breakdown voltage [47,48]. Such discrete discharges appear because of the loss of dielectric stability, during which gas development and visible light emission can be seen clearly [49]. Two fundamental characteristics of coatings are the occurrence of micropores and microcracks which

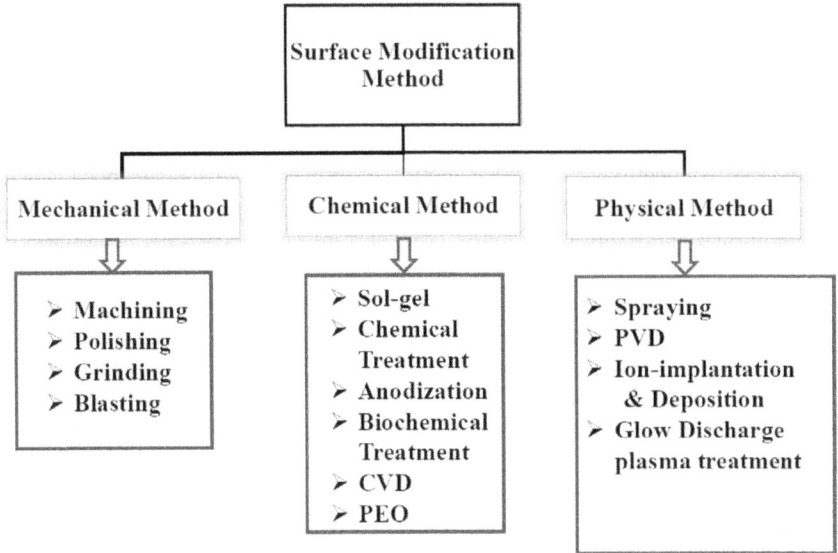

FIGURE 7.1   Different surface modification techniques [41].

are distributed randomly all over the surface of the coating. The development of these microcracks on the surface of coating can be credited to the thermally induced stresses that are developed at the time of coating. The underlying reason for such thermal stresses is that the ceramic experiences quick melting and solidification in stronger discharge channels [50–52]. On the other hand, micropores development was due to the removal of melt products from the micro-discharge channel to electrolyte solution and successive quick solidification of melted regions [53]. These pores developed in a variety of forms such as through or closed and also have a variety of shapes such as channel, point or porosity, which also changes significantly in size [54]. The performance of the MAO coating is straightforwardly impacted by the size and number of such micropores and microcracks [55].

The properties of MAO coatings are controlled by the type of electrolyte, alloying element and furthermore by the processing parameters, such as duty cycle, pulse frequency [56], voltage applied and time of reaction [44]. Electrical discharges started because of the flow of electric current locally through the developing layer; as a result, the typical holes are created on the surface of the coating [57]. Porous coatings give substantial corrosion protection to the substrate and improve the binding force of a coating. In one of the study, corrosion behaviors of MAO-coated Mg–Zn–Ca at constant compressive stress near that of the human tibia were explored in vitro [58]. Results demonstrated that the applied compressive stress could change the degradation style of the coated sample and speed up corrosion rate. As referred above, other than the constrained chemical compositions and higher energy utilization, the various micropores are the fundamental disadvantages of MAO coatings to accomplish long-term security or functional surfaces [59]. Due to the porous nature of MAO coating, it allows solution and caustic ions to pass into, contact and react with the specimen. Sealing pores can essentially help to solve these problems for magnesium alloys. The basic pore-sealing strategies are self-sealing or in-situ [60] and ex-situ sealing, for example, phosphate and silicate [61], sol–gel technique [62], polymeric coating [63] and alkaline treatment [64]. In one of the studies [65], attempt has been made to get a compact MAO coating, where pores are sealed through in-situ sealing of carbon sphere. Post-treatment is carried out by submerging the coated specimen in an alkaline electrolyte solution [66]. Subsequently, the development of $Mg(OH)_2$ prompts the pore sealing. MAO coating is not just biocompatible but also biodegradable, showing that it is an excellent coating technique for orthopedic application. It was observed that MAO coating on Mg–Ca alloys shows a very good impact on cell adhesion, differentiation, proliferation and corrosion resistance [66]. Presently, a researcher focuses on improving biocompatibility, cytocompatibility and corrosion resistance of MAO coating [67].

In one of the studies [68], it has been claimed that the porous silicon-containing micro-arc coating on pure magnesium provides excellent corrosion resistance and also supported antibacterial activity, because of the direct contact of microorganisms and released Mg^{2+} particles. Fundamentally, three kinds of defects are found in coating prepared by the MAO technique. They are open micropores on a superficial level, segregated pores in the center and through-cracks [69]. These pores can convert into one another, for example, isolated pores and close pores can be converted into open pores and through-crack, respectively, with degradation of the coating. Subsequently, for MAO coating, there are two degradation mechanisms that exist on magnesium alloy [69]. One is electrochemical corrosion, developed by through-crack, by which water molecules enter into the interface of a coating substrate, which prompts better dissolution of the magnesium matrix and electron release. The other is chemical dissolution, due to open pores. Electrons are accepted by water molecules, resulting in the formation of hydroxide ions and hydrogen gas. The significant benefits of MAO coating are improved wear and corrosion resistance, biodegradability, biocompatibility, etc. The porous surface morphology plays double role. On the one hand, the pores affect top-coat positively for adhesion strength. On the other hand, the pores have a negative impact, such as development of fatigue crack and creating path for access of aggressive medium.

7.2.1 Mechanism of the MAO Process

A significant amount of knowledge of the MAO coating mechanism will be needed to achieve the characteristics of the phenomenal coating to the extent electrochemical, bioactive and mechanical properties are concerned. Generally, a stable micro-discharge with gas delivery would occur on the substrate surface on utilization of an exceptionally high voltage, subsequently, a coating film would be developed on the substrate surface [70]. MAO started from the conventional anodization technique, in which the workpiece is kept in an electrolyte solution and 10–80 V voltage is given to the workpiece and cathode. The MAO technique permits creation of a metal oxide coating as per the required morphology and thickness by changing the process parameters [71]. The MAO technique required high voltages (~250–800 V) with AC supply, to facilitate continuous dielectric breakdown all over the surface of a substrate. During the process, a large number of micro-discharges are produced, which are randomly spread on the entire substrate surface. This mechanism promotes the formation of a thicker layer of oxide, which brings crystalline and a harder coating structure, basically plasma discharges dissipated large quantity of heat, tending to propel crystallization in the enveloping oxide layer. Essentially, MAO coatings have very high porosity with intricate geometry, yet have overall excellent wear resistance than coatings developed by the anodizing process; similarly, MAO coating can be made thicker [72].

During the MAO process, gaseous oxygen is released and specimen oxidation occurs on the anode; on the other hand, gaseous hydrogen is released on the cathode [73,74]. One of the important parts of the technique is the development of micro-discharges on an anode surface in an electrolyte by utilizing a high voltage [75,76]. The anodic process occurs in three different phases and can be seen easily from the V-t chart as shown in Figure 7.2. In the initial stage, because of the electrolysis of water, vaporous oxygen discharges at the anode and voltage straightforwardly increases as per time. In this stage, no significant sparks are found on the substrate surface and total current is characterized by the ionic current because of the diffusion process of electrolyte ions. The ionic current plays a significant role in current in forming the oxide layer [77,78].

During the second stage, the V–t graph starts deviating from the previously detected linearity, also the slope is decreased. In the subsequent second stage, the dielectric breakdown happens on account of a higher electric field, and a large number of tiny sparks reliably spread over the whole surface of a substrate. At the point when the sparking starts, the current density is calculated by the sum of the electron current

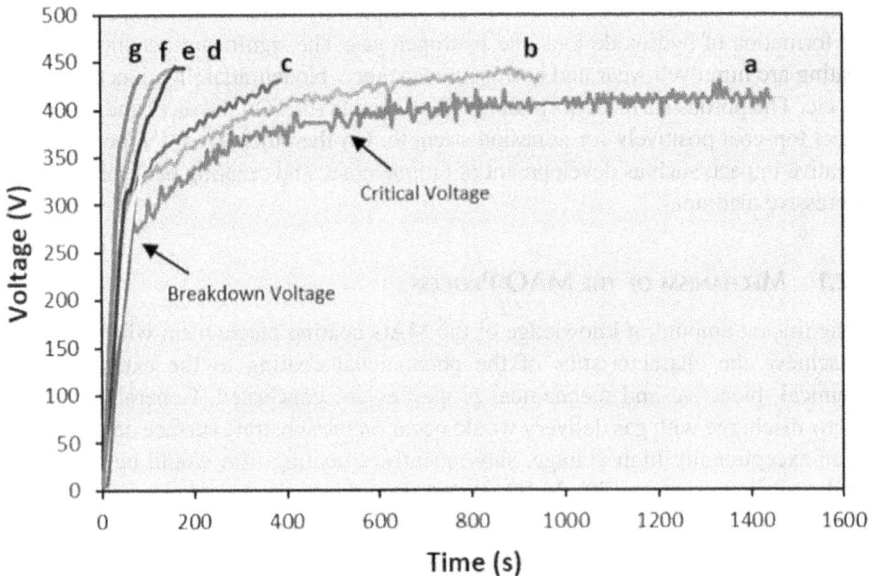

FIGURE 7.2 MAO voltage–time graph at (a) 30, (b) 40, (c) 50, (d) 60, (e) 80, (f) 100 and (g) 120 mA/cm^2 current densities [73].

caused due to sparking at the surface of the substrate and ionic current. During the second stage, commonly voltage increases according to current, contrasted with the starting stage on the grounds that the current density is basically because of sparking and independent of the coating resistance. In the last third stage, the voltage reaches to steady-state value, indicating that coating reached a constant resistance state and no noteworthy increase in the anodic voltage is required to maintain the constant current as demonstrated in Figure 7.2 [73].

7.3 RESULTS AND DISCUSSION

Microstructure, phase composition, corrosion resistance and different other properties of MAO-coated implants can be affected by different variables [79]. Important process parameters of the MAO technique are electrolyte composition, current density, processing time, electrolyte temperature, applied voltage and frequency [80]. It was seen that the MAO is a multi-variable controlled technique, which is affected by various extrinsic or intrinsic parameters. The workpiece material and electrolyte are seen as intrinsic variables, which play a vital role in the construction and microstructure of MAO coatings, while electric parameters, processing time and processing temperature are the extrinsic parameters. It has been seen that the working variable of MAO, which exceptionally affects the properties of the coating, can be classified into three types, related to the composition of the electrolyte, workpiece material and electric parameters [81].

7.3.1 ELECTROLYTE

The composition of electrolytes incredibly affects plasma discharge and coating developed by the MAO technique. In the past, different types of electrolyte composition were utilized for MAO coating. Electrolyte's composition used for MAO was created by blending zinc, manganese, silicon, magnesium, calcium and prosperous particles into NaF, $NaAlO_2$, KOH, $NA_2P_4O_7$ and Na_2SiO_3 [82]. Most of the time, alkaline electrolyte with a pH of around 13 was used for the MAO process. Why a higher pH is perfect for the MAO technique is not clear yet [72]. An electrolyte conductivity is also important since it impacts current, and voltage drops across electrolyte segments in little pores inside the coating, and would affect the beginning of plasma discharge [82,83]. An electrolyte conductivity is by and large in the range of 5–100 ms/cm for the MAO technique [72]. Furthermore, it has been seen that the aging of an electrolyte can affect the performance of the MAO technique and coating developed by it [84].

7.3.2 FREQUENCY

From past investigates, it was seen that frequency has a significant impact on the properties of MAO coating. The coating created at a lower frequency has a greater pore size and higher roughness value than a high-frequency value coating [85]. It was observed from past research [86] that coatings created using AC conditions are by and large of superb quality than DC. It has furthermore been shown that the quality of the coating is improved if the cathodic voltage is increased [87]. It is obviously the circumstances that, in most of the conditions discharges for the most part occur in an anodic half-cycle, even though the current is flowing during both the cycles. However, under some conditions, discharge was found in the cathodic half-cycle, particularly in alkaline electrolytes [88,89], and for discreetly thick coatings. It is furthermore significant that in the MAO technique, the coating was made under the conditions in which the cathodic discharge is dominant. It undeniably gives off an impression that the workpiece material can be oxidized quickly inside the cathodic discharge than an anodic one. For MAO of Ti or other light metal nowadays, the pulsed bipolar type of power source is broadly utilized, due to its magnificent coating properties [41]. It was detected that the thickness of the coating decreases when a smaller cathode pulse was used in comparison to an anodic single polar pulse. However, the coating thickness increases as the cathodic pulse value increases [90]. It has been observed that the coating prepared by the MAO technique has higher hardness and surface roughness. Higher roughness is attributed to the higher energy density per pulse. At lower frequencies, high energy density causes intense melting and subsequently produces oxide coating on the workpiece surface. It was observed that coating properties will be better at low energy per pulse. The micro-crack is limited at a lower energy per pulse, also it significantly affects the surface roughness of coating [91].

Types of current waveform impact the MAO coating on an Mg alloy. During one of the past studies, researchers developed 37 μm thick MAO coating under three different conditions, constant, stepped and decaying current conditions. It has been observed that the energy required to achieve the expected thickness was much higher in decaying and stepped conditions, indicating that the constant current density provides higher energy for a faster development rate of coating [91–93]. Under higher growth rate conditions, high surface roughness was observed for MAO coating. It was observed that high energy per pulse was created because of high pulse on time under low-frequency conditions and subsequently this had supported a high growth rate of coating as shown in Figure 7.3 [91]. With an increase in frequency from 100 to 800 Hz, the growth of coating decreases considerably during coating on an Mg alloy in a phosphate-containing electrolyte solution. At a high-frequency value, a greater number of tiny pores were seen [94,95].

7.3.3 Temperature of Electrolyte

The MAO coating is developed at high voltages when micro-discharges occur on a specimen surface. Microspark discharge helps the crystalline phase formation, which is generally formed at high temperatures [96] and includes the particles from the electrolyte [97–99]. During the process, specimens are regularly kept at low temperatures to avoid degradation of the mechanical properties [100]. It was observed that the initial discharge (15s) is uniform at all temperature values. Highly intensive discharges are created at 278 K temperature and the number of discharges increases with time. At 278 K temperature, the discharge is uniformly distributed over the complete surface of workpiece. At a temperature of 293 K, same performance was observed like that at 278; however, the quantity of discharges is decreased. Also, a rise in the electrolyte temperature gives a smaller number of discharges and occurs

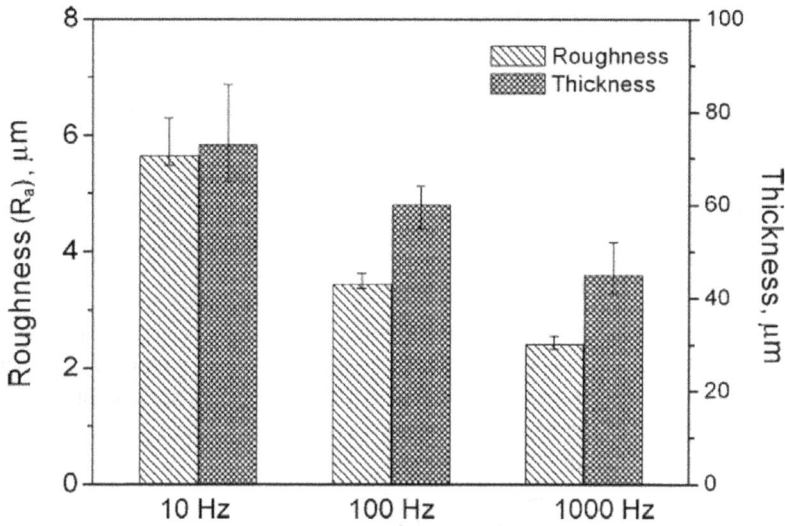

FIGURE 7.3 Processing frequencies' effect on surface roughness and coating thickness during the MAO process [91].

TABLE 7.1

Effect of Electrolyte Temperature on Coating Thickness during the MAO Process [100]

Parameters	Temperature and Thickness Values			
Electrolyte temperature (K)	278	293	303	313
Thickness (μm)	13–18	13–17	13–48	19–49

at local area than the entire area of a specimen, particularly at 313 K temperature. The micro-discharge region moves slowly and start concentrating at a limited area. Nonuniform coating was developed because of the discharge concentration at higher temperatures of electrolyte, particularly at higher temperatures of 303 and 313 K as shown in Table 7.1. So, it was concluded that, a lower electrolyte temperature is more sensible for making a uniform coating [100].

The morphology of the coating surface not only depends on the electrolyte temperature but depends on other factors as well. During the MAO process, a large number of discharge pores of tiny diameter (~2 μm) are produced on the coating surfaces. It has been observed that coating developed at a higher temperature has high porosity than coating developed at 278 K temperature. It has been seen that for the most part, bigger size void and high density of pores are responsible for the improper adhesion of coating on substrate [101]. It was observed that coating thickness variation is less at temperatures of 278 and 293 K, getting significantly greater at 303 and 313 K temperatures [100].

It has been observed that coatings created at higher temperatures show the indication of wear and excellent wear resistance was observed for coatings developed at low electrolyte temperature. The coating made at 278 K temperature was denser, uniform and exhibits phenomenal wear resistance when contrasted with coating made at higher than 293 K temperature [100]. For excellent properties and uniform coating thickness, the temperature needs to be maintained around 20°C by utilizing a cooling system [102].

7.3.4 CURRENT DENSITY

The current density is one of the main variables, which influences the microstructure and other properties of the MAO coating [103]. In addition, voltage is an essential factor in the MAO technique since it fundamentally impacts some coating properties, like crystal structure and surface morphology [104]. Different electrical conditions, for example, AC and DC, can be used in MAO. Under AC power conditions, the coatings are of superb quality due to the efficient running of the process. First, set the current at the desired level and change voltage as required to get that current. Regardless, there are various other options, like controlling capacitance or applied voltage [72]. In the MAO process, qualities of discharge can be adjusted by varying the current amplitude, duty cycle, waveform shape and frequency of the applied current. Among the three key current modes used in MAO, for instance, pulse current, AC and DC, AC gives the greatest process control flexibility [105]. In one of the studies [73], it was observed that the complete current in the MAO process comprises electronic current because of sparking and ionic current because of an electrolyte ion diffusion into the oxide. Ionic current has very little contribution to total current at lower charge densities like $30–40 \, mA/cm^2$. The electronic current contribution is still higher at moderate current densities, such as $50–100 \, mA/cm^2$; there is higher incorporation rate of ionic charge but there are generally a very few numbers of particles available for oxide formation. Equal amounts of ionic and electronic charges were observed when coating was made at current densities of 120 and $140 \, mA/cm^2$. This case gives a higher coating development rate. From the literature, it has been observed that, at equal contributions of ionic and electronic charges, the development rate of coating is high. It was also noticed that reducing current density values gives higher average roughness and high porosity. As a result of the higher contribution by electronic current at a lower current density value, large quantity of micro-discharges are created, which increases porosity and roughness of coating. Table 7.2 indicates

TABLE 7.2
Effect of Current Densities on Various Parameters [73]

Current density (mA/cm^2)	30	40	50	60	80	100	120
Average roughness (μm)	2	1.6	1.5	1.4	1.4	1.3	1.5
Porosity (%)	20.1	15.2	13.3	12.8	11.9	8.2	7.9
Thickness (μm)	2.3	1.7	2.4	1.9	2.2	2.6	2.7
Growth rate (nm/s)	1.6	1.8	6.1	7.6	11.9	17.1	30

the effects of current density on various parameters. It was fascinating to observe that as the current density value increases, the porosity reduces due to a higher rate of ionic current and subsequently sealing of pores [73].

7.3.5 DUTY CYCLE

In the MAO process, voltage increases within a very short period of time, nearly about 15 seconds, and after that, there is a decline in the slope of the voltage–time chart. The sparking or breakdown voltage is shown by a point where the voltage–time chart changes its slope [106]. In the MAO process because of dielectric breakdown, an enormous number of micro-discharges [76,107], contact glow discharge [108], gas discharge [76] or any of their mixes are happening, which are an outstanding component of the MAO process in relation to common anodization [107]. During the MAO process, the color, intensity and density of micro-discharge continuously change. The intensity of micro-discharges increases as the micro-discharge density decreases, with the shade of micro-discharge changing from pale blue white to yellowish and finally to orange [41]. At lower duty cycles, it was observed that the micro-discharge has high spatial density and low intensity. Smaller size craters were observed on the surface of the coating due to these soft micro-discharges. In the MAO process when a high duty cycles value was used, micro-discharges get stronger yet their number decreases, especially during a long processing time. However, at a lower value of duty cycles, the substrate surface was entirely occupied by discharges even at final stages. Because of the increase in duty cycles, a high quantity of energy is delivered to the process of oxidation, delivering extremely energetic channels, producing molten oxides as well as gas bubbles on the substrate surface, resulting in the porous morphology [109]. The MAO power supply provides more energy per cycle because of which current travels a more profound way through the coating to make an extra-oxidized coating material. This can be achieved when discharges are produced in the lower resistance region of coating and due to that, the discharge channel diameter increases accordingly [110]. It has been observed that a lower number of tiny pores are yet present on the coating, even though with an increase in the duty cycle value. The presence of tiny pores was due to microplasma burst during starting periods of the interaction because of dielectric discharge [111]. Due to an increase in the breaking stress value, various size pores are developed. This is a direct result of an increase in discharge diameter as shown in Figure 7.4, when the MAO power supply unit provides a higher energy per pulse [112].

7.3.6 MG ALLOYS CORROSION PERFORMANCE

Due to the poor corrosion resistance of Mg and its alloys, it has limited application in the biomedical and industrial areas [113]. MAO has been perceived as a viable strategy to deal with this issue. The effectiveness of MAO-based coatings on corrosion performance was examined in many reports. From the literature, it was seen that the corrosion performance of an uncoated specimen was found to be multiple times [114] less than that of the coated specimen. Impacts of different variables including the composition of electrolyte solution, electrical parameters, for example, intensity and

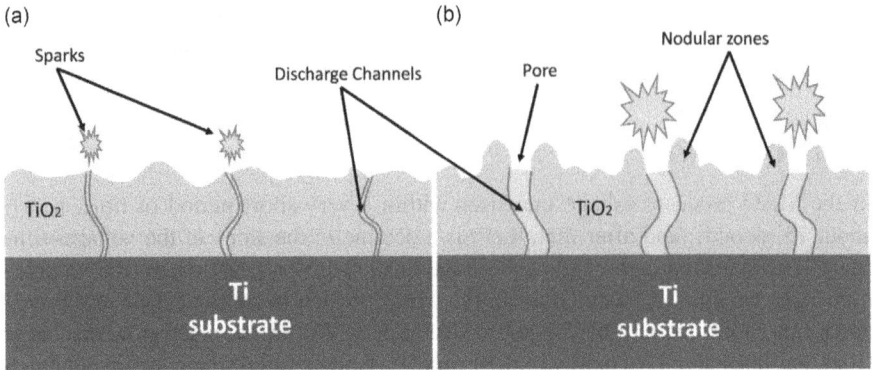

FIGURE 7.4 MAO coating formation at different duty cycles, (a) low duty cycle and (b) high duty cycle [112].

current type, time of processing, the composition of alloys and pre-treatment used on the magnesium alloys are deliberated in this chapter. Corrosion of MAO-based coating on Mg alloys increases in chloride-containing electrolyte with an increase in the chloride percentage. Corrosion tests on AZ91D Mg alloy prepared by MAO using AC in a silicate-based solution of electrolyte show that pitting happened at higher concentrations of NaCl (1%, 3.5% and 5%); however, the corrosion rate of coatings was uniform at lower concentrations (0.1% and 0.5%). MAO of AZ91D gives a superior corrosion performance in dilute NaCl solution [107]. When MAO coating was created on AZ31 alloy in a sodium sulfate-based electrolyte solution, then it was observed that, increase in the concentration of chloride results in an increasing rate of corrosion and the electrochemical impedance decreases. Coatings were created on AM50 utilizing phosphate-based electrolyte solution and mainly having MgO. In the case of a neutral NaCl electrolyte, this event gets delayed and damage due to corrosion becomes local. However, MgO undergoes degradation in alkaline NaCl solution (pH = 11) [109]. Due to the accumulation of corrosion products, charge transfer gets disrupted after 48 hours. As the corrosion product gets accumulated, stress starts to build up, with an additional duration of testing of up to 120 hours, prompting the production of newer types of microcracks in the coating, which further provokes corrosion [115]. The following section explains the effects of different parameters on corrosion performance coating.

7.3.6.1 Electrolyte

For MAO treatment of Mg alloys, generally alkaline electrolytes are used to get stable coating and fast dissolution of the anode can be avoided, due to the higher chemical activity of Mg in acidic media [116]. NaOH and KOH are commonly used to change the pH of the MAO electrolyte [117]. Along with adjusting pH, these metal hydroxides improve electrolyte conductivity utilized in the MAO process [116]. Some of the researchers used acidic electrolytes, comprising fluoro zirconate and a similar kind of inorganic salt for the MAO process; however, the first treatment is carried out in alkaline electrolyte to get stable coating and restrict the anodic dissolution of Mg [109,118]. The properties of MAO coating can be varied by adding different compounds in the electrolyte solution [119]. It was seen that KF-bearing electrolyte was giving better corrosion resistance than one without KF-containing electrolyte. Even though larger pores are there on the surface of the coating, the layer of oxide had a very compact passive coating with fluoride particles. It has been observed that the presence of MgO and MgF_2 could give better corrosion resistance. It has been observed that bringing potassium fluoride in the solution of electrolyte will reduce the size of pores and surface roughness value, also coating becomes more compact. Due to the presence of KF at the time of coating, it changes the compositions of coating [4,120]. It was observed that the thickness of coating increased by adding KF in an aluminate-based electrolyte. Moreover, the corrosion performance of coating was increased due to the creation of an internal dense film with $MgAl_2O_4$ crystalline and fluorine ions [52].

In one of the studies [121], it was announced that the existence of KF in MAO electrolyte bath for AM50 might be vital in the event of in-situ closing of pores, due to the low solidifying point of MgF_2 in comparison to other constituents of coating [121]. The coating produced was more compact when potassium ions are present in the form of phosphate, hydroxide or combined as compared to those having sodium compounds. However, small size pores were found on the outer surface of coatings when developed in Na-containing electrolytes [122]. Under longer anodizing and current density conditions, the corrosion performance of coating developed in 3M KOH electrolyte solution was better than that of 1.5M KOH. This was observed, because of a decrease in porosity of coating [123]. It was additionally revealed that there was significant variation in the coating morphology due to variation in the concentration of KOH [124]. As per a report, the MgO content increased in the coating due to an increase in the concentration of KOH. MAO coatings developed by using silicate-based electrolyte solution were thinner and has a smooth surface compared to coating obtained from phosphate-based electrolytes. It was noticed that the corrosion resistance of Si-MAO coating was excellent in both long-term and short-term testing. The excellent corrosion resistance of Si-MAO-based coating in the long-duration corrosion test was due to dense inner layer, lesser porosity and excellent adhesion at the interface with better chemical stability of Mg_2SiO_4 [125]. In another investigation on Mg alloy utilizing AC, it was observed that coating developed in a phosphate electrolyte has high porosity and thickness as compared to the silicate-based electrolyte under the same current densities condition. This was due to the loss of dielectric stability and the use of a low current value. The coating performance might be related to its compact and uniform structure, which will block the movement of corrosive ions from the electrolyte solution into an oxide coating [37]. One researcher [95] examined the optimized proportion of the two anions in an electrolyte having both phosphate and silicate. They understood that microcanals and micropores become small at lower concentrations of phosphate and provide additional corrosion resistance. But, pitting type of corrosion was reported in these coatings.

7.3.6.2 Electrical Parameters

Due to the electrochemical nature of the MAO process, current, frequency, voltage, duty cycle, etc. of power supply greatly influence the coating characteristics. Generally, bipolar and unipolar power supplies are utilized for the MAO process. More concentration was given on bipolar current in accomplishing expected corrosion performance. When bipolar and unipolar current types were utilized for AJ62 MAO coating in aluminate-based electrolytes, both were observed to be effective in increasing the corrosion performance of coated specimens. But it was observed that as compared to the unipolar type, the bipolar current type was more effective [52]. This might be because of defects and pores created by entangled gas inside the coating during processing with unipolar types of current [52]. Bipolar current improves the thermal condition of plasma. It was observed that with exact control of positive and negative pulses proportion, it was possible to avoid extremely strong discharge and therefore abruptly extreme high temperatures. Therefore, coating quality would be improved. Coating created by the bipolar current is normally thicker than those developed by means of unipolar current. The utilization of cathodic current during the MAO technique is very effective in accomplishing a more thick and uniform coating. It was reported that bipolar pulse coating provides excellent corrosion protection [126].

Conversely, in one of the studies [127], it was observed that unipolar MAO coating on pure Mg showed superior in vitro corrosion properties. It was observed that bipolar coatings showed lesser porosity with a thick interior film, but large-scale imperfection was observed on the coating. However, unipolar coating showed high stability, which results in excellent coating performance. Because of the transient passivity state, MAO coating cannot be developed by an increase in cathodic density beyond a certain value [127]. Corrosion performance and morphology of coating are greatly influenced by cathodic current density. During corrosion testing, EIS results show that the polarization resistance of a specimen, in which the anodic/cathodic proportion is 2:3, was practically 44% higher in comparison to a similar proportion of 2:1. This means, by increasing the cathodic current density, there is improvement in corrosion performance, which can be credited to more compactness and lower porosity of coating developed at higher current densities [121]. Duty cycle is another important parameter that affects the properties of the coating. Water electrolysis and anodic reaction were intensified by an increase in duty cycle at a constant frequency and voltage, which gives higher porosity and thickness of the coating. Coatings could not give an efficient corrosion performance under 40% or over 60% duty cycle [122]. But, in the last stage, voltage drop down under 480 V, which makes the duty cycle immaterial [123]. Frequency is another factor that influences corrosion resistance and morphology of MAO coating on Mg alloys. Apparently, corrosion resistance, morphology and chemical composition can be significantly improved by taking precise frequency control [124].

During MAO treatment, it was observed that the size of the pores decreases by an increase in alternating current (AC) frequency. High intensity of micro-discharge during the process is liable for an increase in the size of pores at a lower value of frequencies [128]. The corrosion performance of MAO coating is better when the process is carried out at a higher frequency [124,128]. As indicated by EIS results, corrosion resistance of MAO coating created at 1000 Hz was roughly multiple times higher compared to 100 Hz frequency, as at a high frequency, coating is more compact and porous [125]. With an increase in applied frequency, accordingly quantity of discharge channels increases but their size decreases. Subsequently, there were decreases in porosity, finally resulting in too thick coating [124,125,128]. It was additionally seen that the MgO percentage increases at a higher frequency [128]. It was observed that with an increase in frequency value, residual stresses decreases. At a higher frequency, micro-discharge present for a very short period of time in each cycle; consequently few numbers of micro-discharge happen at a particular location and sparks are very weak. Therefore, the coatings appear to be smooth with fewer defects. In one of the studies, it was reported that coating created at 100 Hz frequency has more surface roughness and poor corrosion resistance as compared to 800 Hz frequency. In any case, long discharge results in high temperature, which increases the molten material into discharge channels, which results in a higher growth rate [128].

Current density is an important variable of the MAO technique that influences the performance of the coating. At current densities of 15, 75 and 150 mA/cm², the growth rates of coating recorded are 1, 2 and 3 mm/min, respectively. Coatings created at lower current densities are usually dense and have limited imperfections. As indicated by electrochemical testing, these coatings show excellent corrosion performance [129]. The coating thickness was increased linearly according to the current density value [129,130]. It was noticed that corrosion performance was improved with an increase in the oxidation time or current density up to their optimized value. However, further increment unfavorably affected corrosion performance [131]. The coating growth rate increases with an increase in current density, but it results in a nonuniform coating. One of the researchers [132] performed the coating process in two distinct methods of current applications, in which current value was reduced at the end of the process by two methods, one decreasing current density and the other was decreasing stepped current density. Researchers observed that optimizing current waveforms might improve the microstructure of coating as compared to the constant current condition, because of the change in the sparking condition. It was observed that decaying freely current density condition can give optimum sparking, in which a homogeneous and most intact microstructure was accomplished. It was reported that the corrosion resistance of this coating was roughly 56% higher as compared to coating produced by utilizing constant current density [93].

7.3.6.3 Oxidation Time

It was observed that current density and oxidation time have the same influence on the corrosion resistance of MAO coating [131]. But, the impact of oxidation time was less in comparison to current density [133]. It was seen that the coating had excellent corrosion resistance during a longer oxidation time and lower current densities [123]. At the beginning, the corrosion performance of the coating is enhanced by a longer oxidation time; however, corrosion resistance is reduced after the oxidation time surpasses an optimum value [131,134]. Under extreme long durations, it might be possible that the coating is destroyed completely due to dissolution of the coating, which results in a significant decrease in corrosion resistance [135].

7.4 CONCLUSIONS

Magnesium alloys are widely used as biodegradable materials for implants in recent years due to their good biocompatibility, biodegradability and reasonable mechanical properties. Nonetheless, their lower corrosion resistance and quick degradation in the physiological environment remain challenges for their wide application. Surface modifications to change surface attributes have been demonstrated powerful in improving the corrosion resistance of the materials. Many surface modifications and coating methods were inspected in recent times to improve the cell–implant interaction and enhance the surface properties of magnesium alloys. Contrasted with other surface modification methods, MAO can give great adhesion, hard, wear-resistant and corrosion-resistant coating on magnesium and its alloys. Following are important observations noted from the literature.

Generally, an alkaline electrolyte is used for the MAO process. The electrolyte concentration is one of the most significant parameters that impact the growth mechanism of the coating. Higher concentration of electrolyte gives the fast deposition rate of electrolyte compounds on the implant surface.

MAO coating carried out at a lower electrolyte temperature gives homogeneous and better wear resistance coating in comparison to high-temperature electrolyte coatings. The electrolyte temperature should be maintained at around 20°C during the MAO process for excellent coating properties.

Utilization of cathodic current during the MAO technique is very effective in accomplishing a more thick and uniform coating. It is seen that a bipolar pulse coating provides excellent corrosion protection.

The pore size decreases by an increase in AC frequency, also the corrosion performance of a coating is excellent at a higher frequency. EIS results show that the corrosion resistance of MAO coating created at 1000 Hz was multiple times higher as compared to 100 Hz frequency.

Current density is also one of the significant variables of the MAO technique that influences the properties of coatings. Coatings created at lower current densities are usually dense, have limited imperfections and have excellent corrosion resistance. Corrosion performance can be improved with an increase in the time of oxidation or current density up to the optimized value; however, beyond a certain limit, it unfavorably affected corrosion performance. The coating growth rate increases with an increase in current density, but it results in a nonuniform coating. Current density and oxidation time have the same influence on the corrosion resistance of coatings.

REFERENCES

1. Maier, P., & Hort, N. (2020). Magnesium alloys for biomedical applications. Metals, 10(10), 1328.
2. Guo, Y., Sealy, M. P., & Guo, C. (2012). Significant improvement of corrosion resistance of biodegradable metallic implants processed by laser shock peening. *CIRP Annals*, 61(1), 583–586.
3. Nagels, J., Stokdijk, M., & Rozing, P. M. (2003). Stress shielding and bone resorption in shoulder arthroplasty. *Journal of Shoulder and Elbow Surgery*, 12(1), 35–39.
4. Zheng, Y. F., Gu, X. N., & Witte, F. (2014). Biodegradable metals. *Materials Science and Engineering: R: Reports*, 77, 1–34.
5. Xin, Y., Liu, C., Huo, K., Tang, G., Tian, X., & Chu, P. K. (2009). Corrosion behavior of ZrN/Zr coated biomedical AZ91 magnesium alloy. *Surface and Coatings Technology*, 203(17–18), 2554–2557.

6. Xu, L., Pan, F., Yu, G., Yang, L., Zhang, E., & Yang, K. (2009). In vitro and in vivo evaluation of the surface bioactivity of a calcium phosphate coated magnesium alloy. *Biomaterials*, 30(8), 1512–1523.

7. Poinern, G. E. J., Brundavanam, S., & Fawcett, D. (2012). Biomedical magnesium alloys: A review of material properties, surface modifications and potential as a bio-degradable orthopaedic implant. *American Journal of Biomedical Engineering*, 2(6), 218–240.

8. Gray, J., & Luan, B. (2002). Protective coatings on magnesium and its alloys—a critical review. *Journal of Alloys and Compounds*, 336(1–2), 88–113.

9. Venezuela, J., & Dargusch, M. S. (2019). The influence of alloying and fabrication techniques on the mechanical properties, biodegradability and biocompatibility of zinc: A comprehensive review. *Acta Biomaterialia*, 87, 1–40.

10. Zhang, W., Li, M., Chen, Q., Hu, W., Zhang, W., & Xin, W. (2012). Effects of Sr and Sn on microstructure and corrosion resistance of Mg–Zr–Ca magnesium alloy for biomedical applications. *Materials & Design*, 39, 379–383.

11. Baril, G., Blanc, C., & Pébère, N. (2001). AC impedance spectroscopy in characterizing time-dependent corrosion of AZ91 and AM50 magnesium alloys characterization with respect to their microstructures. *Journal of the Electrochemical Society*, 148(12), B489.

12. Verstraeten, S. V., Aimo, L., & Oteiza, P. I. (2008). Aluminium and lead: Molecular mechanisms of brain toxicity. *Archives of Toxicology*, 82(11), 789–802.

13. Li, Y., Wen, C., Mushahary, D., Sravanthi, R., Harishankar, N., Pande, G., & Hodgson, P. (2012). Mg–Zr–Sr alloys as biodegradable implant materials. *Acta Biomaterialia*, 8(8), 3177–3188.

14. Staiger, M. P., Pietak, A. M., Huadmai, J., & Dias, G. (2006). Magnesium and its alloys as orthopedic biomaterials: A review. *Biomaterials*, 27(9), 1728–1734.

15. Han, H. S., Minghui, Y., Seok, H. K., Byun, J. Y., Cha, P. R., Yang, S. J., & Kim, Y. C. (2013). The modification of microstructure to improve the biodegradation and mechanical properties of a biodegradable Mg alloy. *Journal of the Mechanical Behavior of Biomedical Materials*, 20, 54–60.

16. Cipriano, A. F., Sallee, A., Tayoba, M., Alcaraz, M. C. C., Lin, A., Guan, R. G., … Liu, H. (2017). Cytocompatibility and early inflammatory response of human endothelial cells in direct culture with Mg-Zn-Sr alloys. *Acta Biomaterialia*, 48, 499–520.

17. Cheng, M., Chen, J., Yan, H., Su, B., Yu, Z., Xia, W., & Gong, X. (2017). Effects of minor Sr addition on microstructure, mechanical and bio-corrosion properties of the Mg-5Zn based alloy system. *Journal of Alloys and Compounds*, 691, 95–102.

18. Moravej, M., & Mantovani, D. (2011). Biodegradable metals for cardiovascular stent application: Interests and new opportunities. *International Journal of Molecular Sciences*, 12(7), 4250–4270.

19. Yun, Y., Dong, Z., Lee, N., Liu, Y., Xue, D., Guo, X., … Fox, C. (2009). Revolutionizing biodegradable metals. *Materials Today*, 12(10), 22–32.

20. Dou, Q., Li, W., Zhang, G., & Wan, X. (2015). Preparation and characterisation of black ceramic coating on AZ91D magnesium alloy by plasma electrolytic oxidation with reduced energy consumption. *Materials Research Innovations*, 19(sup2), S2–23.

21. Nie, X., Leyland, A., Song, H. W., Yerokhin, A. L., Dowey, S. J., & Matthews, A. (1999). Thickness effects on the mechanical properties of micro-arc discharge oxide coatings on aluminium alloys. *Surface and Coatings Technology*, 116, 1055–1060.

22. Voevodin, A. A., Yerokhin, A. L., Lyubimov, V. V., Donley, M. S., & Zabinski, J. S. (1996). Characterization of wear protective Al–Si–O coatings formed on Al-based alloys by micro-arc discharge treatment. *Surface and Coatings Technology*, 86, 516–521.

23. Shahri, Z., Allahkaram, S. R., Soltani, R., & Jafari, H. (2020). Optimization of plasma electrolyte oxidation process parameters for corrosion resistance of Mg alloy. *Journal of Magnesium and Alloys*, 8(2), 431–440.

24. Curran J. A., & T. W. Clyne. (2005). The thermal conductivity of plasma electrolytic oxide coatings on aluminium and magnesium. *Surface and Coatings Technology* 199(2–3), 177–183.

25. Luo, Q., Li, J., Li, B., Liu, B., Shao, H., & Li, Q. (2019). Kinetics in Mg-based hydrogen storage materials: Enhancement and mechanism. *Journal of Magnesium and Alloys,* 7(1), 58–71.

26. Song, M. S., Zeng, R. C., Ding, Y. F., Li, R. W., Easton, M., Cole, I., & Chen, X. B. (2019). Recent advances in biodegradation controls over Mg alloys for bone fracture management: A review. *Journal of Materials Science & Technology,* 35(4), 535–544.

27. Atrens, A., Song, G. L., Liu, M., Shi, Z., Cao, F., & Dargusch, M. S. (2015). Review of recent developments in the field of magnesium corrosion. *Advanced Engineering Materials,* 17(4), 400–453.

28. Ding, Z. Y., Cui, L. Y., Zeng, R. C., Zhao, Y. B., Guan, S. K., Xu, D. K., & Lin, C. G. (2018). Exfoliation corrosion of extruded Mg-Li-Ca alloy. *Journal of Materials Science & Technology,* 34(9), 1550–1557.

29. Esmaily, M., Svensson, J. E., Fajardo, S., Birbilis, N., Frankel, G. S., Virtanen, S., ... Johansson, L. G. (2017). Fundamentals and advances in magnesium alloy corrosion. *Progress in Materials Science,* 89, 92–193.

30. Wang, Y., Ding, B. H., Gao, S. Y., Chen, X. B., Zeng, R. C., Cui, L. Y., ... Liu, Q. Y. (2019). In vitro corrosion of pure Mg in phosphate buffer solution—Influences of isoelectric point and molecular structure of amino acids. *Materials Science and Engineering: C,* 105, 110042.

31. Witte, F. (2010). The history of biodegradable magnesium implants: A review. *Acta Biomaterialia,* 6(5), 1680–1692.

32. Witte, F., Kaese, V., Haferkamp, H., Switzer, E., Meyer-Lindenberg, A., Wirth, C. J., & Windhagen, H. (2005). In vivo corrosion of four magnesium alloys and the associated bone response. *Biomaterials,* 26(17), 3557–3563.

33. Zhen, Z., Liu, X., Huang, T., Xi, T., & Zheng, Y. (2015). Hemolysis and cytotoxicity mechanisms of biodegradable magnesium and its alloys. *Materials Science and Engineering: C,* 46, 202–206.

34. Hofstetter, J., Martinelli, E., Weinberg, A. M., Becker, M., Mingler, B., Uggowitzer, P. J., & Löffler, J. F. (2015). Assessing the degradation performance of ultrahigh-purity magnesium in vitro and in vivo. *Corrosion Science,* 91, 29–36.

35. Witte, F., Fischer, J., Nellesen, J., Crostack, H. A., Kaese, V., Pisch, A., ... Windhagen, H. (2006). In vitro and in vivo corrosion measurements of magnesium alloys. *Biomaterials,* 27(7), 1013–1018.

36. Wang, Y., Chen, M., & Zhao, Y. (2019). Preparation and corrosion resistance of micro-arc oxidation-coated biomedical Mg–Zn–Ca alloy in the silicon–phosphorus- mixed electrolyte. *ACS Omega,* 4(25), 20937–20947.

37. Li, Z., Gu, X., Lou, S., & Zheng, Y. (2008). The development of binary Mg–Ca alloys for use as biodegradable materials within bone. *Biomaterials,* 29(10), 1329–1344.

38. Willbold, E., Gu, X., Albert, D., Kalla, K., Bobe, K., Brauneis, M., ... Witte, F. (2015). Effect of the addition of low rare earth elements (lanthanum, neodymium, cerium) on the biodegradation and biocompatibility of magnesium. *Acta Biomaterialia,* 11, 554–562.

39. Rahman, M., Li, Y., & Wen, C. (2020). HA coating on Mg alloys for biomedical applications: A review. *Journal of Magnesium and Alloys,* 8(3), 929–943.

40. Kurup, A., Dhatrak, P., & Khasnis, N. (2021). Surface modification techniques of titanium and titanium alloys for biomedical dental applications: A review. *Materials Today: Proceedings,* 39, 84–90.

41. Pesode, P., & Barve, S. (2020). Surface modification of titanium and titanium alloy by plasma electrolytic oxidation process for biomedical applications: A review. *Materials Today: Proceedings.*

42. Pesode, P. A., & Barve, S. B. (2021). Recent advances on the antibacterial coating on titanium implant by micro-arc oxidation process. *Materials Today: Proceedings.*

43. Molaei, M., Fattah-Alhosseini, A., & Keshavarz, M. K. (2019). Influence of different sodium-based additives on corrosion resistance of PEO coatings on pure Ti. *Journal of Asian Ceramic Societies*, 7(2), 247–255.

44. Narayanan, T. S., Park, I. S., & Lee, M. H. (2014). Strategies to improve the corrosion resistance of microarc oxidation (MAO) coated magnesium alloys for degradable implants: Prospects and challenges. *Progress in Materials Science*, 60, 1–71.

45. Chu, H. J., Liang, C. J., Chen, C. H., & He, J. L. (2017). Optical emission spectroscopic determination of the optimum regions for micro-arc oxidation of titanium. *Surface and Coatings Technology*, 325, 166–173.

46. Shao, L., Li, H., Jiang, B., Liu, C., Gu, X., & Chen, D. (2018). A comparative study of corrosion behavior of hard anodized and micro-arc oxidation coatings on 7050 aluminum alloy. *Metals*, 8(3), 165.

47. Yang, W., Xu, D., Guo, Q., Chen, T., & Chen, J. (2018). Influence of electrolyte composition on microstructure and properties of coatings formed on pure Ti substrate by micro arc oxidation. *Surface and Coatings Technology*, 349, 522–528.

48. Martin, J., Melhem, A., Shchedrina, I., Duchanoy, T., Nomine, A., Henrion, G., ... Belmonte, T. (2013). Effects of electrical parameters on plasma electrolytic oxidation of aluminium. *Surface and Coatings Technology*, 221, 70–76.

49. Wang, Y., Yu, H., Chen, C., & Zhao, Z. (2015). Review of the biocompatibility of micro-arc oxidation coated titanium alloys. *Materials & Design*, 85, 640–652.

50. Hussein, R. O., Northwood, D. O., & Nie, X. (2013). The effect of processing parameters and substrate composition on the corrosion resistance of plasma electrolytic oxidation (PEO) coated magnesium alloys. *Surface and Coatings Technology*, 237, 357–368.

51. Zhang, Y., Wu, Y., Chen, D., Wang, R., Li, D., Guo, C., ... Nash, P. (2017). Micro- structures and growth mechanisms of plasma electrolytic oxidation coatings on aluminium at different current densities. *Surface and Coatings Technology*, 321, 236–246.

52. Hussein, R. O., Zhang, P., Nie, X., Xia, Y., & Northwood, D. O. (2011). The effect of current mode and discharge type on the corrosion resistance of plasma electrolytic oxidation (PEO) coated magnesium alloy AJ62. *Surface and Coatings Technology*, 206(7), 1990–1997.

53. Chaharmahali, R., Fattah-Alhosseini, A., & Esfahani, H. (2020). Increasing the in-vitro corrosion resistance of AZ31B-Mg alloy via coating with hydroxyapatite using plasma electrolytic oxidation. *Journal of Asian Ceramic Societies* 8(1), 39–49.

54. Markov, M. A., Gerashchenkov, D. A., Krasikov, A. V., Ulin, I. V., Bykova, A. D., Shishkova, M. L., & Yakovleva, N. V. (2018). Porous functional coatings by microarc oxidation. *Glass and Ceramics*, 75(7), 258–263.

55. Vakili-Azghandi, M., Fattah-alhosseini, A., & Keshavarz, M. K. (2016). Effects of Al_2O_3 nano-particles on corrosion performance of plasma electrolytic oxidation coatings formed on 6061 aluminum alloy. *Journal of Materials Engineering and Performance*, 25(12), 5302–5313.

56. Gu, Y., Chen, C. F., Bandopadhyay, S., Ning, C., Zhang, Y., & Guo, Y. (2012). Corrosion mechanism and model of pulsed DC microarc oxidation treated AZ31 alloy in simulated body fluid. *Applied Surface Science*, 258(16), 6116–6126.

57. Hornberger, H., Virtanen, S., & Boccaccini, A. R. (2012). Biomedical coatings on magnesium alloys–a review. *Acta Biomaterialia*, 8(7), 2442–2455.

58. Wang, B., Gao, J., Wang, L., Zhu, S., & Guan, S. (2012). Biocorrosion of coated Mg–Zn–Ca alloy under constant compressive stress close to that of human tibia. *Materials Letters*, 70, 174–176.

59. Lu, X., Mohedano, M., Blawert, C., Matykina, E., Arrabal, R., Kainer, K. U., & Zheludkevich, M. L. (2016). Plasma electrolytic oxidation coatings with particle additions–A review. *Surface and Coatings Technology*, 307, 1165–1182.

60. Dong, K., Song, Y., Shan, D., & Han, E. H. (2015). Corrosion behavior of a self-sealing pore micro-arc oxidation film on AM60 magnesium alloy. *Corrosion Science*, 100, 275–283.

61. Malayoglu, U., Tekin, K. C., & Shrestha, S. (2010). Influence of post-treatment on the corrosion resistance of PEO coated AM50B and AM60B Mg alloys. *Surface and Coatings Technology*, 205(6), 1793–1798.

62. Gao, J. H., Shi, X. Y., Yang, B., Hou, S. S., Meng, E. C., Guan, F. X., & Guan, S. K. (2011). Fabrication and characterization of bioactive composite coatings on Mg–Zn–Ca alloy by MAO/sol–gel. *Journal of Materials Science: Materials in Medicine*, 22(7), 1681–1687.

63. Narayanan, T. S., & Lee, M. H. (2016). A simple strategy to modify the porous structure of plasma electrolytic oxidation coatings on magnesium. *RSC Advances*, 6(19), 16100–16114.

64. Cui, L. Y., Gao, S. D., Li, P. P., Zeng, R. C., Zhang, F., Li, S. Q., & Han, E. H. (2017). Corrosion resistance of a self-healing micro-arc oxidation/polymethyltrimethoxysilane composite coating on magnesium alloy AZ31. *Corrosion Science*, 118, 84–95.

65. Li, C. Y., Feng, X. L., Fan, X. L., Yu, X. T., Yin, Z. Z., Kannan, M. B., ... Zeng, R. C. (2019). Corrosion and wear resistance of micro-arc oxidation composite coatings on magnesium alloy AZ31—the influence of inclusions of carbon spheres. *Advanced Engineering Materials*, 21(9), 1900446.

66. Gu, X. N., Li, N., Zhou, W. R., Zheng, Y. F., Zhao, X., Cai, Q. Z., & Ruan, L. (2011). Corrosion resistance and surface biocompatibility of a microarc oxidation coating on a Mg–Ca alloy. *Acta Biomaterialia*, 7(4), 1880–1889.

67. Zhang, L., Zhang, J., Chen, C. F., & Gu, Y. (2015). Advances in microarc oxidation coated AZ31 Mg alloys for biomedical applications. *Corrosion Science*, 91, 7–28.

68. Ren, L., Lin, X., Tan, L., & Yang, K. (2011). Effect of surface coating on antibacterial behavior of magnesium based metals. *Materials Letters*, 65(23–24), 3509–3511.

69. Cui, L. Y., Zeng, R. C., Guan, S. K., Qi, W. C., Zhang, F., Li, S. Q., & Han, E. H. (2017). Degradation mechanism of micro-arc oxidation coatings on biodegradable Mg-Ca alloys: The influence of porosity. *Journal of Alloys and Compounds*, 695, 2464–2476.

70. Kaseem, M., Fatimah, S., Nashrah, N., & Ko, Y. G. (2020). Recent progress in surface modification of metals coated by plasma electrolytic oxidation: Principle, structure, and performance. *Progress in Materials Science*, 100735.

71. Wong, Y. H., Affendy, M. G., Lau, S. K., Teh, P. C., Lee, H. J., Tan, C. Y., & Ramesh, S. (2017). Effects of anodisation parameters on thin film properties: A review. *Materials Science and Technology*, 33(6), 699–711.

72. Clyne, T. W., & Troughton, S. C. (2019). A review of recent work on discharge characteristics during plasma electrolytic oxidation of various metals. *International Materials Reviews*, 64(3), 127–162.

73. Mortazavi, G., Jiang, J., & Meletis, E. I. (2019). Investigation of the plasma electrolytic oxidation mechanism of titanium. *Applied Surface Science*, 488, 370–382.

74. Meletis, E. I., Nie, X., Wang, F. L., & Jiang, J. C. (2002). Electrolytic plasma processing for cleaning and metal-coating of steel surfaces. *Surface and Coatings Technology*, 150(2–3), 246–256.

75. Yerokhin, A. L., Nie, X., Leyland, A., Matthews, A., & Dowey, S. J. (1999). Plasma electrolysis for surface engineering. *Surface and Coatings Technology*, 122(2–3), 73–93.

76. Hussein, R. O., Nie, X., Northwood, D. O., Yerokhin, A., & Matthews, A. (2010). Spectroscopic study of electrolytic plasma and discharging behaviour during the plasma electrolytic oxidation (PEO) process. *Journal of Physics D: Applied Physics*, 43(10), 105203.

77. Chang, L. (2009). Growth regularity of ceramic coating on magnesium alloy by plasma electrolytic oxidation. *Journal of Alloys and Compounds*, 468(1–2), 462–465.

78. Matykina, E., Arrabal, R., Monfort, F., Skeldon, P., & Thompson, G. E. (2008). Incorporation of zirconia into coatings formed by DC plasma electrolytic oxidation of aluminium in nanoparticle suspensions. *Applied Surface Science*, 255(5), 2830–2839.

79. Fattah-alhosseini, A., Molaei, M., & Babaei, K. (2020). The effects of nano-and micro-particles on properties of plasma electrolytic oxidation (PEO) coatings applied on titanium substrates: A review. *Surfaces and Interfaces*, 21, 100659.

80. Li, J. F., Wan, L., & Feng, J. Y. (2006). Study on the preparation of titania films for photocatalytic application by micro-arc oxidation. *Solar Energy Materials and Solar Cells*, 90(15), 2449–2455.

81. Laveissière, M., Cerda, H., Roche, J., Cassayre, L., & Arurault, L. (2019). In-depth study of the influence of electrolyte composition on coatings prepared by plasma electrolytic oxidation of TA6V alloy. *Surface and Coatings Technology*, 361, 50–62.

82. Simchen, F., Sieber, M., & Lampke, T. (2017). Electrolyte influence on ignition of plasma electrolytic oxidation processes on light metals. *Surface and Coatings Technology*, 315, 205–213.

83. Venkateswarlu, K., Rameshbabu, N., Sreekanth, D., Sandhyarani, M., Bose, A. C., Muthupandi, V., & Subramanian, S. (2013). Role of electrolyte chemistry on electronic and in vitro electrochemical properties of micro-arc oxidized titania films on Cp Ti. *Electrochimica Acta*, 105, 468–480.

84. Martin, J., Leone, P., Nomine, A., Veys-Renaux, D., Henrion, G., & Belmonte, T. (2015). Influence of electrolyte ageing on the plasma electrolytic oxidation of aluminium. *Surface and Coatings Technology*, 269, 36–46.

85. Wang, Y., Wang, L., Zheng, H., Du, C., Shi, Z., & Xu, C. (2010). Effect of frequency on the structure and cell response of Ca-and P-containing MAO films. *Applied Surface Science*, 256(7), 2018–2024.

86. Xin, S., Song, L., Zhao, R., & Hu, X. (2006). Influence of cathodic current on composition, structure and properties of Al2O3 coatings on aluminum alloy prepared by micro-arc oxidation process. *Thin Solid Films*, 515(1), 326–332.

87. Li, Q., Liang, J., Liu, B., Peng, Z., & Wang, Q. (2014). Effects of cathodic voltages on structure and wear resistance of plasma electrolytic oxidation coatings formed on aluminium alloy. *Applied Surface Science*, 297, 176–181.

88. Rakoch, A. G., Gladkova, A. A., Linn, Z., & Strekalina, D. M. (2015). The evidence of cathodic micro-discharges during plasma electrolytic oxidation of light metallic alloys and micro-discharge intensity depending on pH of the electrolyte. *Surface and Coatings Technology*, 269, 138–144.

89. Sah, S. P., Tsuji, E., Aoki, Y., & Habazaki, H. (2012). Cathodic pulse breakdown of anodic films on aluminium in alkaline silicate electrolyte–understanding the role of cathodic half-cycle in AC plasma electrolytic oxidation. *Corrosion Science*, 55, 90–96.

90. Yao, Z., Liu, Y., Xu, Y., Jiang, Z., & Wang, F. (2011). Effects of cathode pulse at high frequency on structure and composition of Al2TiO5 ceramic coatings on Ti alloy by plasma electrolytic oxidation. *Materials Chemistry and Physics*, 126(1–2), 227–231.

91. Srinivasan, P. B., Liang, J., Balajeee, R. G., Blawert, C., Störmer, M., & Dietzel, W. (2010). Effect of pulse frequency on the microstructure, phase composition and corrosion performance of a phosphate-based plasma electrolytic oxidation coated AM50 magnesium alloy. *Applied Surface Science*, 256(12), 3928–3935.

92. Fattah-alhosseini, A., Molaei, M., Attarzadeh, N., Babaei, K., & Attarzadeh, F. (2020). On the enhanced antibacterial activity of plasma electrolytic oxidation (PEO) coatings that incorporate particles: A review. *Ceramics International*, 46(13), 20587–20607.

93. Liang, J., Hu, L., & Hao, J. (2007). Improvement of corrosion properties of micro-arc oxidation coating on magnesium alloy by optimizing current density parameters. *Applied Surface Science*, 253(16), 6939–6945.

94. Nominé, A., Nominé, A. V., Braithwaite, N. S. J., Belmonte, T., & Henrion, G. (2017). High-frequency-induced cathodic breakdown during plasma electrolytic oxidation. *Physical Review Applied*, 8(3), 031001.

95. Lv, G. H., Chen, H., Gu, W. C., Li, L., Niu, E. W., Zhang, X. H., & Yang, S. Z. (2008). Effects of current frequency on the structural characteristics and corrosion property of ceramic coatings formed on magnesium alloy by PEO technology. *Journal of Materials Processing Technology*, 208(1–3), 9–13.

96. Yerokhin, A. L., Lyubimov, V. V., & Ashitkov, R. V. (1998). Phase formation in ceramic coatings during plasma electrolytic oxidation of aluminium alloys. *Ceramics International*, 24(1), 1–6.

97. Xue, W., Deng, Z., Ma, H., Chen, R., & Zhang, T. (2001). Microstructure and phase composition of microarc oxidation coatings formed on Ti–6Al–4V alloy in aluminate solution. *Surface Engineering*, 17(4), 323–326.

98. Sah, S. P., Aoki, Y., & Habazaki, H. (2010). Influence of phosphate concentration on plasma electrolytic oxidation of AZ80 magnesium alloy in alkaline aluminate solution. *Materials Transactions*, 51(1), 94–102.

99. Luo, H., Cai, Q., Wei, B., Yu, B., He, J., & Li, D. (2009). Study on the microstructure and corrosion resistance of ZrO2-containing ceramic coatings formed on magnesium alloy by plasma electrolytic oxidation. *Journal of Alloys and Compounds*, 474(1–2), 551–556.

100. Habazaki, H., Tsunekawa, S., Tsuji, E., & Nakayama, T. (2012). Formation and characterization of wear-resistant PEO coatings formed on β-titanium alloy at different electrolyte temperatures. *Applied Surface Science*, 259, 711–718.

101. Nakajima, M., Miura, Y., Fushimi, K., & Habazaki, H. (2009). Spark anodizing behaviour of titanium and its alloys in alkaline aluminate electrolyte. *Corrosion Science*, 51(7), 1534–1539.

102. O'Hara, M., Troughton, S. C., Francis, R., & Clyne, T. W. (2020). The incorporation of particles suspended in the electrolyte into plasma electrolytic oxidation coatings on Ti and Al substrates. *Surface and Coatings Technology*, 385, 125354.

103. Li, J., Wan, L., & Feng, J. (2009). Micro arc oxidation of S-containing TiO_2 films by sulfur bearing electrolytes. *Journal of Materials Processing Technology*, 209(2), 762–766.

104. Yangi, Y., & Wu, H. (2012). Effects of current density on microstructure of titania coatings by micro-arc oxidation. *Journal of Materials Science & Technology*, 28(4), 321–324.

105. Khan, R. H., Yerokhin, A. L., & Matthews, A. (2008). Structural characteristics and residual stresses in oxide films produced on Ti by pulsed unipolar plasma electrolytic oxidation. *Philosophical Magazine*, 88(6), 795–807.

106. Dehnavi, V., Luan, B. L., Shoesmith, D. W., Liu, X. Y., & Rohani, S. (2013). Effect of duty cycle and applied current frequency on plasma electrolytic oxidation (PEO) coating growth behavior. *Surface and Coatings Technology*, 226, 100–107.

107. Wu, H., Wang, J., Long, B., Long, B., Jin, Z., Naidan, W., ... Bi, D. (2005). Ultra-hard ceramic coatings fabricated through microarc oxidation on aluminium alloy. *Applied Surface Science*, 252(5), 1545–1552.

108. Yerokhin, A. L., Snizhko, L. O., Gurevina, N. L., Leyland, A., Pilkington, A., & Matthews, A. (2003). Discharge characterization in plasma electrolytic oxidation of aluminium. *Journal of Physics D: Applied Physics*, 36(17), 2110.

109. Matykina, E., Arrabal, R., Skeldon, P., & Thompson, G. E. (2009). Investigation of the growth processes of coatings formed by AC plasma electrolytic oxidation of aluminium. *Electrochimica acta*, 54(27), 6767–6778.

110. Stojadinovic, S., Vasilic, R., Belca, I., Petkovic, M., Kasalica, B., Nedic, Z., & Zekovic, L. (2010). Characterization of the plasma electrolytic oxidation of aluminium in sodium tungstate. *Corrosion Science*, 52(10), 3258–3265.

111. Rakoch, A. G., Khokhlov, V. V., Bautin, V. A., Lebedeva, N. A., Magurova, Y. V., & Bardin, I. V. (2006). Model concepts on the mechanism of microarc oxidation of metal materials and the control over this process. *Protection of Metals*, 42(2), 158–169.

112. Torres-Ceron, D. A., Restrepo-Parra, E., Acosta-Medina, C. D., Escobar-Rincon, D., & Ospina-Ospina, R. (2019). Study of duty cycle influence on the band gap energy of TiO2/P coatings obtained by PEO process. *Surface and Coatings Technology*, 375, 221–228.

113. Schultze, J. W., & Lohrengel, M. M. (2000). Stability, reactivity and breakdown of passive films. Problems of recent and future research. *Electrochimica Acta*, 45(15–16), 2499–2513.

114. Guo, H. F., & An, M. Z. (2005). Growth of ceramic coatings on AZ91D magnesium alloys by micro-arc oxidation in aluminate–fluoride solutions and evaluation of corrosion resistance. *Applied Surface Science*, 246(1–3), 229–238.

115. Wang, Y., Huang, Z., Yan, Q., Liu, C., Liu, P., Zhang, Y., … Shen, D. (2016). Corrosion behaviors and effects of corrosion products of plasma electrolytic oxidation coated AZ31 magnesium alloy under the salt spray corrosion test. *Applied Surface Science*, 378, 435–442.

116. Zhang, R. F. (2010). Film formation in the second step of micro-arc oxidation on magnesium alloys. *Corrosion Science*, 52(4), 1285–1290.

117. Khaselev, O., Weiss, D., & Yahalom, J. (2001). Structure and composition of anodic films formed on binary Mg–Al alloys in KOH–aluminate solutions under continuous sparking. *Corrosion Science*, 43(7), 1295–1307.

118. Ghasemi, A., Raja, V. S., Blawert, C., Dietzel, W., & Kainer, K. U. (2008). Study of the structure and corrosion behavior of PEO coatings on AM50 magnesium alloy by electrochemical impedance spectroscopy. *Surface and Coatings Technology*, 202(15), 3513–3518.

119. Ko, Y. G., Namgung, S., & Shin, D. H. (2010). Correlation between KOH concentration and surface properties of AZ91 magnesium alloy coated by plasma electrolytic oxidation. *Surface and Coatings Technology*, 205(7), 2525–2531.

120. Mori, Y., Koshi, A., Liao, J., Asoh, H., & Ono, S. (2014). Characteristics and corrosion resistance of plasma electrolytic oxidation coatings on AZ31B Mg alloy formed in phosphate–silicate mixture electrolytes. *Corrosion Science*, 88, 254–262.

121. Su, P., Wu, X., Guo, Y., & Jiang, Z. (2009). Effects of cathode current density on structure and corrosion resistance of plasma electrolytic oxidation coatings formed on ZK60 Mg alloy. *Journal of Alloys and Compounds*, 475(1–2), 773–777.

122. Chang, L. R., Cao, F. H., Cai, J. S., Liu, W. J., Zhang, Z., & Zhang, J. Q. (2011). Influence of electric parameters on MAO of AZ91D magnesium alloy using alternative square-wave power source. *Transactions of Nonferrous Metals Society of China*, 21(2), 307–316.

123. Zhang, R. F., Shan, D. Y., Chen, R. S., & Han, E. H. (2008). Effects of electric parameters on properties of anodic coatings formed on magnesium alloys. *Materials Chemistry and Physics*, 107(2–3), 356–363.

124. Bin, Z. O. U., LÜ, G. H., Zhang, G. L., & Tian, Y. Y. (2015). Effect of current frequency on properties of coating formed by microarc oxidation on AZ91D magnesium alloy. *Transactions of Nonferrous Metals Society of China*, 25(5), 1500–1505.

125. Su, P., Wu, X., Jiang, Z., & Guo, Y. (2011). Effects of working frequency on the structure and corrosion resistance of plasma electrolytic oxidation coatings formed on a ZK60 Mg alloy. *International Journal of Applied Ceramic Technology*, 8(1), 112–119.

126. Wang, S., Xia, Y., Liu, L., & Si, N. (2014). Preparation and performance of MAO coatings obtained on AZ91D Mg alloy under unipolar and bipolar modes in a novel dual electrolyte. *Ceramics International*, 40(1), 93–99.

127. Gao, Y., Yerokhin, A., & Matthews, A. (2014). Effect of current mode on PEO treatment of magnesium in Ca-and P-containing electrolyte and resulting coatings. *Applied Surface Science*, 316, 558–567.
128. Hwang, I. J., Hwang, D. Y., Ko, Y. G., & Shin, D. H. (2012). Correlation between current frequency and electrochemical properties of Mg alloy coated by micro arc oxidation. *Surface and Coatings Technology*, 206(15), 3360–3365.
129. Srinivasan, P. B., Liang, J., Blawert, C., Störmer, M., & Dietzel, W. (2009). Effect of current density on the microstructure and corrosion behaviour of plasma electrolytic oxidation treated AM50 magnesium alloy. *Applied Surface Science*, 255(7), 4212–4218.
130. Durdu, S., & Usta, M. (2012). Characterization and mechanical properties of coatings on magnesium by micro arc oxidation. *Applied Surface Science*, 261, 774–782.
131. Wang, H. M., Chen, Z. H., & Li, L. L. (2010). Corrosion resistance and microstructure characteristics of plasma electrolytic oxidation coatings formed on AZ31 magnesium alloy. *Surface Engineering*, 26(5), 385–391.
132. Darband, G. B., Aliofkhazraei, M., Hamghalam, P., & Valizade, N. (2017). Plasma electrolytic oxidation of magnesium and its alloys: Mechanism, properties and applications. *Journal of Magnesium and Alloys*, 5(1), 74–132.
133. Pezzato, L., Brunelli, K., Gross, S., Magrini, M., & Dabalà, M. (2014). Effect of process parameters of plasma electrolytic oxidation on microstructure and corrosion properties of magnesium alloys. *Journal of Applied Electrochemistry*, 44(7), 867–879.
134. Ping, W. A. N. G., Liu, D. X., Li, J. P., Guo, Y. C., & Zhong, Y. A. N. G. (2010). Growth process and corrosion resistance of micro-arc oxidation coating on Mg-Zn-Gd magnesium alloys. *Transactions of Nonferrous Metals Society of China*, 20(11), 2198–2203.
135. Zhao, L., Cui, C., Wang, Q., & Bu, S. (2010). Growth characteristics and corrosion resistance of micro-arc oxidation coating on pure magnesium for biomedical applications. *Corrosion Science*, 52(7), 2228–2234.

8 Investigation of Titanium Lattice Structures for Biomedical Implants

Vijay Kumar Meena, Prashant Kumar, and Tarun Panchal
CSIR-CSIO Chandigarh

Parveen Kalra
Punjab Engineering College Chandigarh

Ravindra Kumar Sinha
Delhi Technological University New Delhi

CONTENTS

8.1 INTRODUCTION

Unlike traditional or subtractive manufacturing, additive manufacturing (AM) is a layerwise material deposition process that can produce 3D models directly from a CAD model [1–4]. Aerospace, automobile, biomedical, and other similar industries, which require complex component fabrication, have seen an upsurge in the use of AM. Among the aforementioned industries, AM is gaining attention rapidly in the biomedical industry due to its adaptability in generating low-cost, quick surgical equipment and bio-implants that can be customized or produced in low volumes [5,6]. It is used to fabricate dental implants and orthopedic implants, as well as medical, electronic, and microfluidic devices [7–10].

A mismatch between the modulus of biomedical metal implants and that of adjacent bone would cause stress shielding. This can result in the organ or partial resorption and, eventually, failure of the implant [11]. Lattices, which are a type of porous structures centered on regularity and repeatability of unit cells, in biomedical implants can guarantee precise mechanical properties as that of the replaced bone

DOI: 10.1201/9781003286806-8

and can increase biocompatibility [12–16]. Lattice structures must have specific qualities to attain these objectives. For the ingrowth of cells and the transit of nutrients, some properties like pore size, porosity, surface finishing, and interconnectivity are important. The use of lattice structures in the biomedical industry is prevalent due to their high stiffness-to-weight proportion and ability to maximize surface area characteristics [12,17–24]. According to Wang et al., the ideal pore size for bone ingrowth is a topic of debate in the literature; studies have demonstrated that cell ingrowth and vascularization can occur at pore sizes spanning from 30 to 900 μm [25–27]. In vitro investigations by Frosch et al. revealed that porous materials with pore sizes of 0.4–0.6 mm had more osteoblasts than those with pore sizes of 0.3 and 1 mm [28]. Taniguchi et al. in their in vivo experiments also found that samples with a pore size of 0.6 mm were best suited for bone-tissue ingrowth among the samples with pore sizes 0.3/0.6/0.9 mm [27]. Pores with larger diameters allow for more cell ingrowth, whereas pores with smaller diameters can cause occlusion, resulting in the prevention of tissue regeneration [29]. The porosity of the lattice structure can be a crucial characteristic and serves two main goals. First, a porous structure allows waste materials and nutrients to disseminate, and the second goal is to attain the same elastic modulus as that of the original bone [30]. However, subsequent research revealed that a very porous structure is not necessarily the best method for a well-designed lattice structure, because biomechanical properties deteriorate even when tissue regeneration is higher [31,32]. The presence of a layer of porous structure on the top surface of a biomedical implant is critical for tissue ingrowth, which reduces recovery time. Implants with the requisite modulus, biocompatibility, and porosity can be simply fabricated if there is a good understanding of the relation between the density and elastic modulus of lattice structures [33]. Biological instrumental tools, bone structure, and biomedical implants have also made use of these lattice structures [34–38]. Titanium alloys and cobalt–chromium are the most widely used materials for orthopedic implants and prostheses due to their biocompatibility.

Fabrication of a lattice structure-based design using conventional manufacturing methods is extremely complex, costly, and difficult. Recent improvements in AM have made it possible to fabricate lattices with complicated shapes in a shorter amount of time. Additively manufactured lattice structures are designed and manufactured to conserve costly functional materials, energy, and build time while providing excellent mechanical characteristics and a high strength-to-weight ratio [39–43]. The AM technology is becoming more competitive with traditional production as the cost of the technology is reducing day by day. As a result, engineers may now develop stronger and lighter lattice structures and complex geometries [44].

Two significant lattice structures with "infinitely periodic surfaces and a mean curvature of zero" have been discovered by Schwarz and Schoen [45,46]. Triply periodic minimal surface (TPMS) Diamond and TPMS Gyroid are the names given to these lattice structures. TPMS structures, unlike manually formed structures, are constructed mathematically utilizing a variety of algorithms and have no need for any post-processing to enhance or integrate the structures [47,48]. "Triply periodic" means that the structure can be packed together in a periodic 3D pattern and "minimal surface" means that it locally minimizes the surface area for a given boundary such that the mean surface curvature at each point is zero. The lack of points of curvature-discontinuity ensured by these architectures is expected to reduce the stress concentration and ultimately to enhance the fatigue strength [49].

In this work, the elastic moduli of three TPMS lattice structures, that is, Gyroid, Diamond, and Schwarz W with three pore sizes, that is, 0.4, 0.5, and 0.6 mm manufactured using the selective laser melting (SLM) manufacturing process, are investigated experimentally. These lattice structures and pore sizes can be conveniently used in a biomedical implant for better osseointegration and to match the elastic modulus of the natural human bone to that of the implant.

8.2 MATERIALS AND METHODS

CAD models of Gyroid, Diamond, and Schwarz W lattice structures with three pore sizes, that is, 0.4, 0.5, and 0.6 mm, each (total nine models) are designed using Simpleware ScanIP 2019.09 software (Figure 8.1). The dimensions of each CAD model are 10 mm × 10 mm × 20 mm. These CAD models are then transferred to Materialise Magic software for support generation in the .stl file format. The slicing of each model (with a layer height of 30 μm) is performed in the same software. The support files are saved in the .cli file format and models with support structures are then transferred to printing software EOSPRINT.

Five samples of each model (a total of 45 samples) have been fabricated using AM. An EOS M290 metal 3D printer has been used to additively manufacture these lattice structures using the SLM process and Ti6Al4V ELI metal powder. The models are placed and oriented on the base plate according to the space availability and recoater movement. A fully neutral environment (chamber filled with argon gas) is used for manufacturing the parts to avoid oxidation at high temperatures due to laser melting. The sintering process parameters used to fabricate the models are listed in Table 8.1.

Samples attached with the base plate are then removed from the printing chamber after the completion of the whole printing process and after the temperature comes to environment temperature. To remove the residual stresses of parts generated due to high temperature in printing processes, the heat treatment process is used. The parts attached with the base plate are transferred to the inert muffle furnace chamber. It is heated to 820°C for 2 hours and then the furnace cooled up to 300°C in an inert environment with a chamber filled with argon gas (Figure 8.2). It is then removed from the furnace chamber and then left to cool up to environment temperature. All the

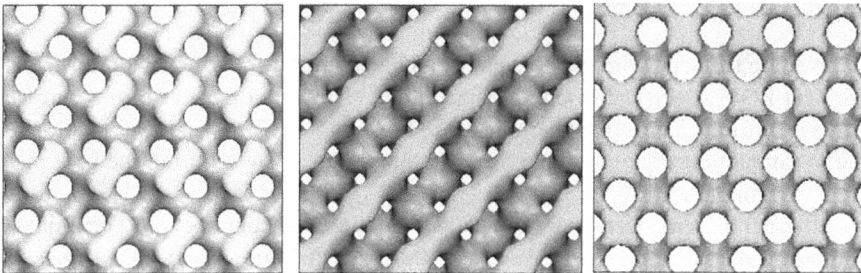

FIGURE 8.1 CAD representation of different porous structures.

TABLE 8.1
Sintering Process Parameters

Laser power	155 W
Laser type	Nd-YAG Laser
Laser beam diameter	80 µm
Layer thickness	30 µm
Scan speed	1300 mm/s
Scan strategy	EOS sorted
Particle size	27–56 µm
Base plate temperature	70°C

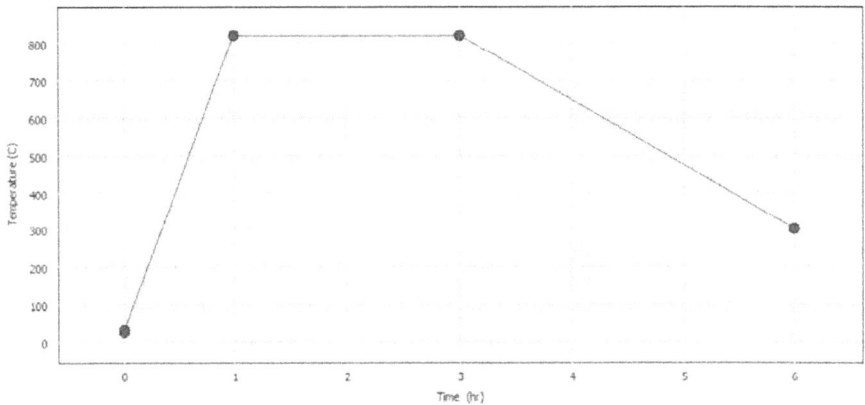

FIGURE 8.2   Heat treatment graph.

TABLE 8.2
Wire Cut EDM Parameters for the Cutting of the Samples from the Base Plate

Material	Pulse On (µs)	Pulse Off (µs)	Group On	Group Off	Current (A)	Voltage	Max Speed (µm/s)
Ti	18	10	1	0	2	Low	10

samples are then cut from the base plate and their support structures with the help of wire cut EDM (electrical discharge machining). The wire diameter of the wire cut EDM is 0.16 mm. The default parameters of the wire cut EDM machine for cutting of the Ti samples are listed in Table 8.2. The samples after cutting from the base plate are shown in Figure 8.3.

All specimens are tested mechanically under uniaxial compression. The uniaxial compression test has been performed at a strain rate of 1 mm/min on a DAK systems 7200 series universal testing machine (Figure 8.4). Each compression test resulted in elastic modulus (E) values that have been deduced by the test results.

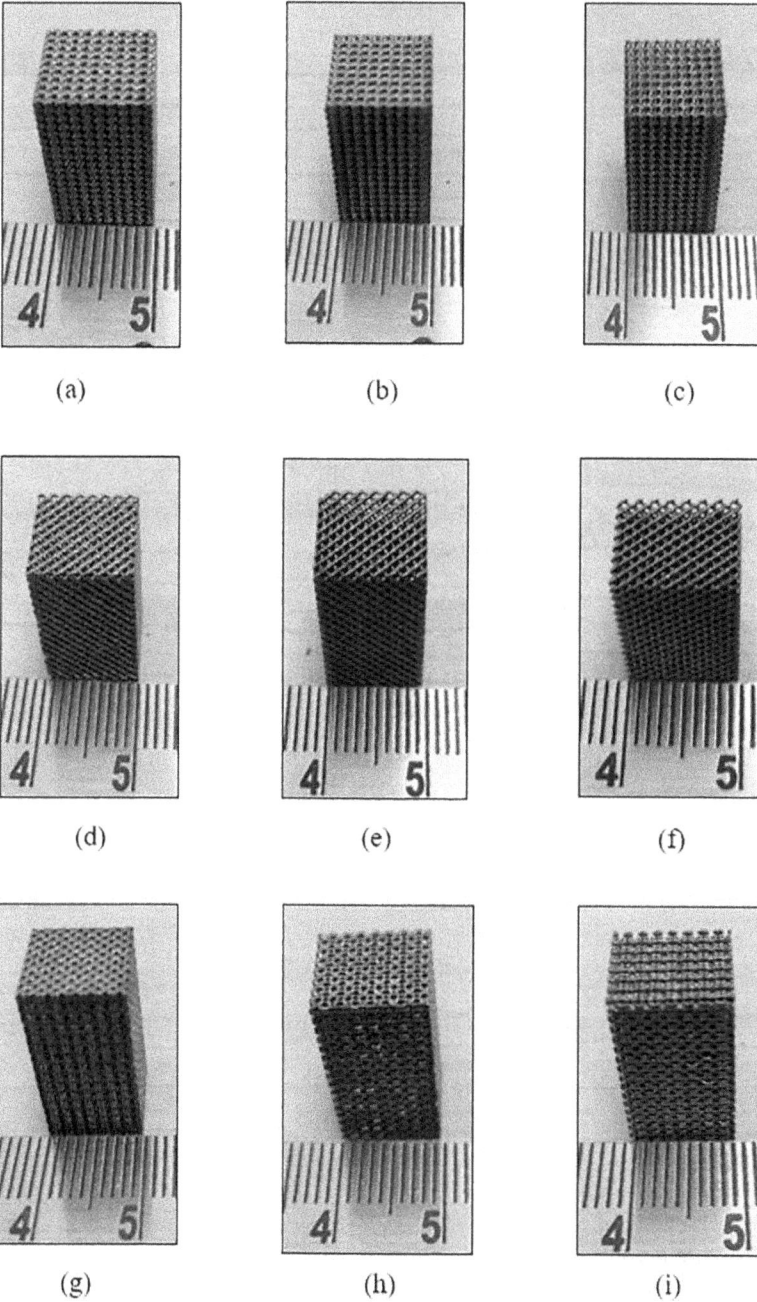

FIGURE 8.3 Fabricated samples of Gyroid porous structures with pore sizes of (a) 0.4 mm, (b) 0.5 mm, and (c) 0.6 mm. Diamond porous structures with pore sizes of (d) 0.4 mm, (e) 0.5 mm, and (f) 0.6 mm. Schwarz W porous structures with pore sizes of (g) 0.4 mm, (h) 0.5 mm, and (i) 0.6 mm.

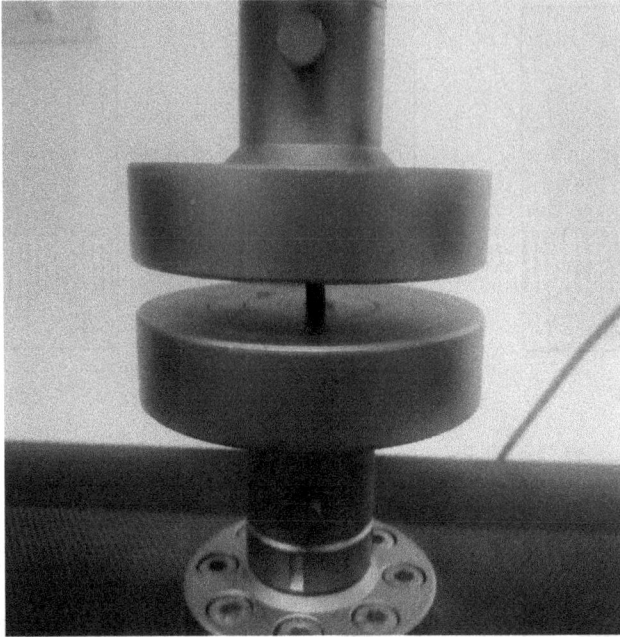

FIGURE 8.4   Tested sample between the compression anvils of UTM.

8.3   RESULTS AND DISCUSSION

All manufactured samples were tested until mechanical failure took place. No samples exhibited untypical behavior of failure, e.g., slipping or lateral buckling. So, all samples were taken into consideration for the assessment of results. The average elastic modulus (E) values for each design configuration are tabulated in Table 8.3.

The elastic modulus values varied between 2649.09 and 5941.92 MPa. The highest modulus was found for the Gyroid lattice structure having a pore size of 0.4 mm, that is, 5941.92 MPa. The lowest modulus was found for the Schwarz W lattice structure having a pore size of 0.6 mm, that is, 2649.09 MPa. A comparative graph to easily interpret the results is shown in Figure 8.5.

The results showed that lattice structures can effectively alter the elastic modulus of materials. The elastic modulus of all the studied lattice structures was found to match the elastic modulus of human cancellous bone. With the increase in pore size, the elastic modulus reduced in all the structures. The lattice structures can hence be used in biomedical implants, to lessen the stress shielding effect imparted due to the use of solid materials.

8.4   CONCLUSIONS

Titanium alloys are widely used for biomedical implants because of their high stiffness-to-weight ratio and excellent biocompatibility. However, their usage also leads to stress shielding due to their high elastic modulus when compared to human

TABLE 8.3

Average Elastic Modulus (E) Values for Each Design Configuration ($n = 5$ for Each Design)

Lattice Structure	Pore Size (mm)	Average Elastic Modulus (MPa)
Gyroid	0.4	5941.92
	0.5	4322.32
	0.6	3833.12
Diamond	0.4	5280.47
	0.5	4274.69
	0.6	3289.34
Schwarz W	0.4	4118.12
	0.5	3306.91
	0.6	2649.09

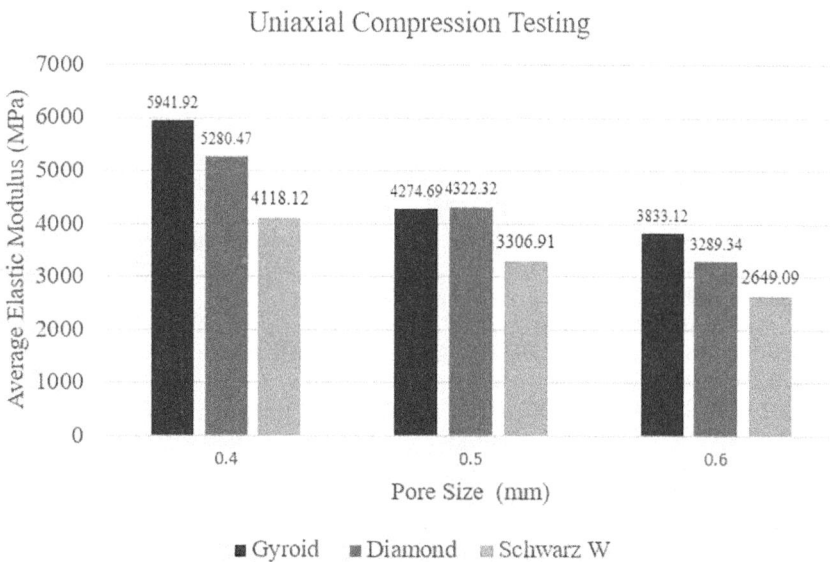

FIGURE 8.5 Comparative graphical representation of average elastic modulus values of design configurations.

cancellous bone. With AM, it is possible to alter the elastic modulus of titanium alloy (Ti6Al4V) to match the elastic modulus of human bone using lattice structures with suitable pore sizes. In the presented work Gyroid, Diamond, and Schwarz W structures with pore sizes varying from 0.4 to 0.6 mm were manufactured using SLM and tested for elastic modulus variation. The results showed a significant reduction in elastic modulus in all the structures with all porosities. Schwarz W with a pore size of 0.6 mm showed the least elastic modulus.

ACKNOWLEDGMENT

This work was supported by the SERB, New Delhi, India [Grant EEQ/2017/000154].

REFERENCES

1. J. Edgar and S. Tint. (2015). Additive manufacturing technologies: 3D printing, rapid prototyping, and direct digital manufacturing. *Johnson Matthey Technology Review*, 59(3), 193–198.
2. ASTM Committee F42 on Additive Manufacturing Technologies, & ASTM Committee F42 on Additive Manufacturing Technologies. Subcommittee F42. 91 on Terminology. (2012). *Standard Terminology for Additive Manufacturing Technologies*. ASTM International, Conshohocken, PA.
3. H.-J. Steenhuis and L. Pretorius. (2017). The additive manufacturing innovation: A range of implications. *Journal of Manufacturing Technology Management*, 28(1), 122–143.
4. T. D. Ngo, A. Kashani, G. Imbalzano, K. T. Q. Nguyen, and D. Hui. (2018). Additive manufacturing (3D printing): A review of materials, methods, applications and challenges. *Composites Part B-Engineering*, 143, 172–196. doi:10.1016/j.compositesb.2018.02.012.
5. J. Zuback and T. DebRoy. (2018). The hardness of additively manufactured alloys. *Materials*, 11(11), 2070.
6. A. Pandey, A. Awasthi, and K. K. Saxena. (2020). Metallic implants with properties and latest production techniques: A review. *Advances in Materials and Processing Technologies*, 6(2), 405–440.
7 L. Murr. (2018). Additive manufacturing of biomedical devices: An overview. *Materials Technology*, 33(1), 57–70.
8. T.-S. Jang, D. Kim, G. Han, C.-B. Yoon, and H.-D. Jung. (2020). Powder based additive manufacturing for biomedical application of titanium and its alloys: A review. *Biomedical Engineering Letters*, 10(4), 1–12.
9. T. M. Hipolito, L. R. Rodrigues, G. C. da Silva, and E. G. del Conte. (2016). Additive manufacturing of microfluidic devices. *IEEE Latin America Transactions*, 14(12), 4652–4656.
10. M. P. Francis, N. Kemper, Y. Maghdouri-White, and N. Thayer. (2018). Additive manufacturing for biofabricated medical device applications. In *Additive Manufacturing* (pp. 311–344): Elsevier, Miamisburg, OH.
11. R. Huiskes, H. Weinans, and B. Van Rietbergen. (1992). The relationship between stress shielding and bone resorption around total hip stems and the effects of flexible materials. *Clinical Orthopaedics and Related Research*, 274, 124–134.
12 D. W. Hutmacher. (2000). Scaffolds in tissue engineering bone and cartilage. *Biomaterials*, 21(24), 2529–2543.
13. C. Y. Lin, N. Kikuchi, and S. J. Hollister. (2004). A novel method for biomaterial scaffold internal architecture design to match bone elastic properties with desired porosity. *Journal of Biomechanics*, 37(5), 623–636.
14. V. S. Deshpande, N. A. Fleck, and M. F. Ashby. (2001). Effective properties of the octet-truss lattice material. *Journal of the Mechanics and Physics of Solids,* 49(8), 1747–1769.
15. A. G. Evans, J. W. Hutchinson, N. A. Fleck, M. Ashby, and H. Wadley. (2001). The topological design of multifunctional cellular metals. *Progress in Materials Science*, 46(3–4), 309–327.
16. N. A. Fleck. (2004). An overview of the mechanical properties of foams and periodic lattice materials. In *Cellular Metals and Polymers*, edited by R. F. Singer, C. Körner, and V. Altstädt, (Trans Tech Publications, Switzerland) pages 3–7. ISBN 978-0878494910.

17. V. G. Sundararajan. (2010). Topology optimization for additive manufacturing of customized meso-structures using homogenization and parametric smoothing functions. Thesis Presented to the Faculty of the Graduate School of The University of Texas, Austin. https://repositories.lib.utexas.edu/handle/2152/ETD-UT-2010-12-2302

18. A. Sutradhar, J. Park, D. Carrau, and M. J. Miller. (2014). Experimental validation of 3D printed patient-specific implants using digital image correlation and finite element analysis. *Computers in Biology and Medicine*, 52, 8–17.

19. A. Sutradhar, G. H. Paulino, M. J. Miller, and T. H. Nguyen. (2010). Topological optimization for designing patient-specific large craniofacial segmental bone replacements. *Proceedings of the National Academy of Sciences*, 107(30), 13222–13227.

20. M. T. Arafat, I. Gibson, and X. Li. (2014). State of the art and future direction of additive manufactured scaffolds-based bone tissue engineering. *Rapid Prototyping Journal*.

21. A. Armillotta and R. Pelzer. (2008). Modeling of porous structures for rapid prototyping of tissue engineering scaffolds. *The International Journal of Advanced Manufacturing Technology*, 39(5), 501–511.

22. P. Ohldin. (2010). Series production of CE-certified orthopedic implants with integrated porous structures for improved bone ingrowth. *Paper Presented at the Proceedings of the 21st International DAAAM Symposium*, Zadar.

23. M. R. Dias, J. M. Guedes, C. L. Flanagan, S. J. Hollister, and P. R. Fernandes. (2014). Optimization of scaffold design for bone tissue engineering: A computational and experimental study. *Medical Engineering & Physics*, 36(4), 448–457.

24. S. M. Giannitelli, D. Accoto, M. Trombetta, and A. Rainer. (2014). Current trends in the design of scaffolds for computer-aided tissue engineering. *Acta Biomaterialia*, 10(2), 580–594.

25. X. Wang et al. (2016). Topological design and additive manufacturing of porous metals for bone scaffolds and orthopaedic implants: A review. *Biomaterials*, 83, 127–141.

26. T. G. Van Tienen, R. G. Heijkants, P. Buma, J. H. de Groot, A. J. Pennings, and R. P. Veth. (2002). Tissue ingrowth and degradation of two biodegradable porous polymers with different porosities and pore sizes. *Biomaterials*, 23(8), 1731–1738.

27. N. Taniguchi et al. (2016). Effect of pore size on bone ingrowth into porous titanium implants fabricated by additive manufacturing: An in vivo experiment. *Materials Science and Engineering: C*, 59, 690–701.

28. K. H. Frosch et al. (2004). Growth behavior, matrix production, and gene expression of human osteoblasts in defined cylindrical titanium channels. *Journal of Biomedical Materials Research Part A: An Official Journal of The Society for Biomaterials, The Japanese Society for Biomaterials, and The Australian Society for Biomaterials and the Korean Society for Biomaterials*, 68(2), 325–334.

29. K. Leong, C. Cheah, and C. Chua. (2003). Solid freeform fabrication of three-dimensional scaffolds for engineering replacement tissues and organs. *Biomaterials*, 24(13), 2363–2378.

30. G. Savio, S. Rosso, R. Meneghello, and G. Concheri. (2018). Geometric modeling of cellular materials for additive manufacturing in biomedical field: A review. *Applied Bionics and Biomechanics*, 2018, 1654782. doi:10.1155/2018/1654782.

31. S. N. Bhatia and C. S. Chen. (1999). Tissue engineering at the micro-scale. *Biomedical Microdevices*, 2(2), 131–144.

32. S. Bruder, K. Kraus, V. Goldberg, and S. Kadiyala. (1998). Critical-sized canine segmental femoral defects are healed by autologous mesenchymal stem cell therapy. *Paper presented at the Transactions of the Annual Meeting-Orthopaedic Research Society*. Boston.

33. K. Wheeler, M. Karagianes, and K. Sump. (1983). Porous titanium alloy for prosthesis attachment. In *Titanium Alloys in Surgical Implants*, edited by H. A. Luckey and F. Kubli, 1–14, ASTM International, Conshohocken, PA.

34. B. Dabrowski, W. Swieszkowski, D. Godlinski, and K. J. Kurzydlowski. (2010). Highly porous titanium scaffolds for orthopaedic applications. *Journal of Biomedical Materials Research Part B: Applied Biomaterials*, 95(1), 53–61.

35. L. F. Cooper. (2000). A role for surface topography in creating and maintaining bone at titanium endosseous implants. *The Journal of prosthetic dentistry*, 84(5), 522–534.

36. S. Hansson and M. Norton. (1999). The relation between surface roughness and inter-facial shear strength for bone-anchored implants. A mathematical model. *Journal of Biomechanics*, 32(8), 829–836.

37. P. Colombo and H. P. Degischer. (2012). *Highly Porous Metals and Ceramics*. Wiley Online Library, Hoboken, NJ.

38. J. Banhart. (2001). Manufacture, characterisation and application of cellular metals and metal foams. *Progress in Materials Science*, 46(6), 559–632.

39. L. J. Gibson, M. F. Ashby, and B. A. Harley. (2010). *Cellular Materials in Nature and Medicine*. Cambridge University Press, Cambridge.

40. C. Chu, G. Graf, and D. W. Rosen. (2008). Design for additive manufacturing of cellular structures. *Computer-Aided Design and Applications*, 5(5), 686–696.

41. R. Lakes. (1993). Materials with structural hierarchy. *Nature*, 361(6412), 511–515.

42. M. F. Ashby, T. Evans, N. A. Fleck, J. Hutchinson, H. Wadley, and L. Gibson. (2000). *Metal Foams: A Design Guide*. Elsevier, Oxford.

43. K.-J. Kang. (2009). A wire-woven cellular metal of ultrahigh strength. *Acta Materialia*, 57(6), 1865–1874.

44. J. Hagel III, J. S. Brown, D. Kulasooriya, C. Giffi, and M. Chen. (2015). The future of Manufacturing-Making things in a changing world. *Future of the Business Landscape*, 4–18.

45. A. H. Schoen. (1970). *Infinite Periodic Minimal Surfaces without Self-Intersections*. National Aeronautics and Space Administration, Boston, MA.

46. H. A. Schwarz. (1972). *Gesammelte Mathematische Abhandlungen* (Vol. 260). American Mathematical Society, Providence, RI.

47. Y. Wang. (2007). Periodic surface modeling for computer aided nano design. *Computer-Aided Design*, 39(3), 179–189.

48. P. J. Gandy, S. Bardhan, A. L. Mackay, and J. Klinowski. (2001). Nodal surface approximations to the P, G, D and I-WP triply periodic minimal surfaces. *Chemical Physics Letters*, 336(3–4), 187–195.

49. M. Afshar, A. P. Anaraki, H. Montazerian, and J. Kadkhodapour. (2016). Additive manufacturing and mechanical characterization of graded porosity scaffolds designed based on triply periodic minimal surface architectures. *Journal of the Mechanical Behavior of Biomedical Materials*, 62, 481–494.

9 Cost Estimation of Polymer Material for Biomedical Application

Suya Prem Anand, Ashwin Sunil Kumar,
Grreshan Ramesh, and Abel Eldho Jose
Vellore Institute of Technology Vellore

CONTENTS

9.1 INTRODUCTION

Knee replacement is a surgical substitution of a knee joint where both the femoral and the tibial components meet with the assistance of an artificial implant. The knee implant consists of mainly three parts, namely femoral, liner, and tibial, as shown in Figure 9.1. Metallic materials like cobalt chromium, or titanium are used for making the femoral and tibial components due to their corrosion and wear resistance properties. The present work focuses on the liner component used in the knee implant made up of polymer materials, where the substitute material should replace the knee structures, biocompatible in nature, withstand heavy loads, possess good flexibility, and allow to move freely [1,2]. Therefore, it must be able to maintain its strength and shape for a long period after the knee implant surgery. The properties of the replacement polymer materials can be improved to exactly replace the bone behavior. Currently, material properties such as fracture toughness, compressive strength, and fatigue strength are enhanced to achieve the

DOI: 10.1201/9781003286806-9

169

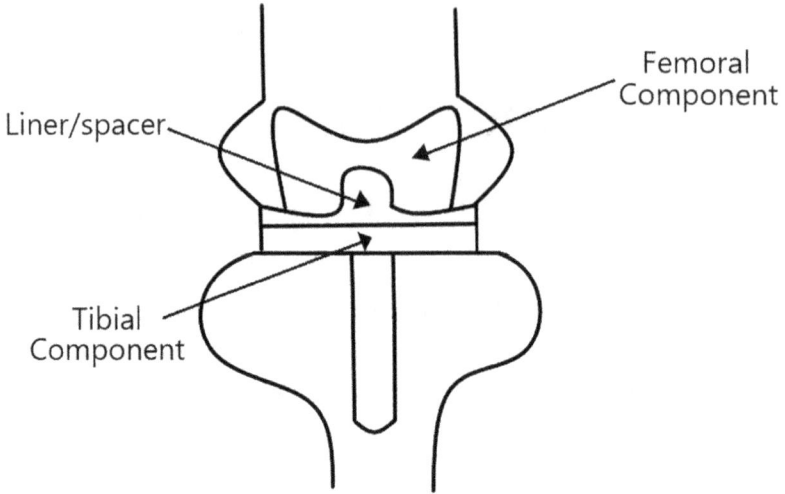

FIGURE 9.1   Schematic view of a knee implant.

appropriate mechanical properties of the human bone. However, properties like modulus of elasticity and density will be reduced but not minimized below the density of the knee bone. Additionally, important properties like osseointegration must be present to improve the quality of bone and enhance the bone growth inside the porous structure [3]. Earlier, the compression molding process was used for making the plastic liner in the knee implant but using conventional methods for fabrication tends to form more scrap and includes a higher cost. Due to this, the research work is mainly concentrated on 3D printing and the cost analysis of the plastic liner component [4].

Additive manufacturing plays a crucial role in changing the design limits to more complex products without additional expenses. This makes it easier to customize personalized parts and components sized in small batches. In comparison to different 3D printing methods, fused deposition modeling (FDM) has gained remarkable attention due to its low-cost materials, high reliability, and minimal investment [5,6]. Earlier, more studies have been pursued to pinpoint the effect of printing parameters such as raster angle, layer thickness, and nozzle temperatures on the performance of printed polymers through the FDM process. In the current situation, the most frequently used polymer materials in the FDM process are ABS, polylactic acid (PLA), and nylon. The majority of the research work focused on the high-density polyethylene material to produce the liner component, but only limited evidence is suggested for the ABS material. Recently, the research is carried out for two major materials in the FDM process such as ABS and PLA for different applications [7–9]. A thermoplastic ABS material is suitable for the FDM process where two important mechanical properties like impact resistance and toughness are excellent compared to other polymers. ABS also has a high heat resistance and chemical stability, which contribute as a promising bone repairing material to make prostheses for the human body. Overall, the ABS material is considered to have better performance compared to PLA [10]. Mathematical analyses like ANOVA and F-test were performed in the FDM process. The analysis resulted in identifying the dominant factors listed as layer thickness, number of contours, and air gap for the build cost. Meanwhile, other factors such as build orientation, raster angle, and road width will have only a marginal effect on the build cost. The main focus was to reduce build cost and build time without compromising on mechanical properties such as tensile strength, dynamic flexural modulus, and impact strength. Now, a proposed mathematical model is used to predict the amount of material consumed and build time in the FDM process. Finally, the augmentation of both the layer thickness and air gap leads to reduce the material consumption and build time [11,12]. In addition, essential process parameters such as printing temperature, filling rate, layer thickness, and printing velocity play an important role in strengthening the mechanical properties [13].

In general, the compression molding process is used to develop the liner component in conventional manufacturing, where machining is required at the final stage that consumes time and produces a lot of scrap materials. The flexibility of design and the cost of the manufacturing process are the important factors affecting the development of liner components in biomedical applications. Earlier, the traditional method used both the compression molding and machining process to produce femoral, liner, and tibial components. At present, the additive manufacturing method is proposed which consists of EBM (electron beam melting) to produce femoral and tibial components and the FDM process is considered for producing the liner component [14,15]. Therefore, there is a need to evaluate the cost of the liner component developed using the FDM process.

The present work focuses on reducing the cost of the liner component without compromising the strength and minimizing the build time. The cost estimation of polymer material ABS was performed, which was produced by both the conventional and additive manufacturing processes used in the biomedical knee implant application. The finite element analysis was also used to evaluate the stresses acting on the liner model by considering the appropriate size dimension of the implant. Finally, the cost analysis of the liner product was determined for both manufacturing processes. A comparative study was also carried out between the conventional and additive methods to produce a low-cost liner component.

9.2   MATERIALS AND METHODS

The method of approach for this paper is to make a 3D CAD model of the liner and produce the STL file. The process is subdivided into designing, printing, and post-processing during the fabrication of liner components. The prototype is designed with the assistance of ANSYS software and the printing is done using the (Prusa I3 MK3S) FDM printer. Before the printing process, the slicing is done to the 3D model to generate the tool path for the printing. The process parameters are taken into consideration and the different costs are calculated along with the build cost. At last, the prototype is printed as per the dimension in the design portion. Later, post-processing and cost estimation was done. An approximate value of the build cost for the prototype can be estimated as shown in the flowchart in Figure 9.2.

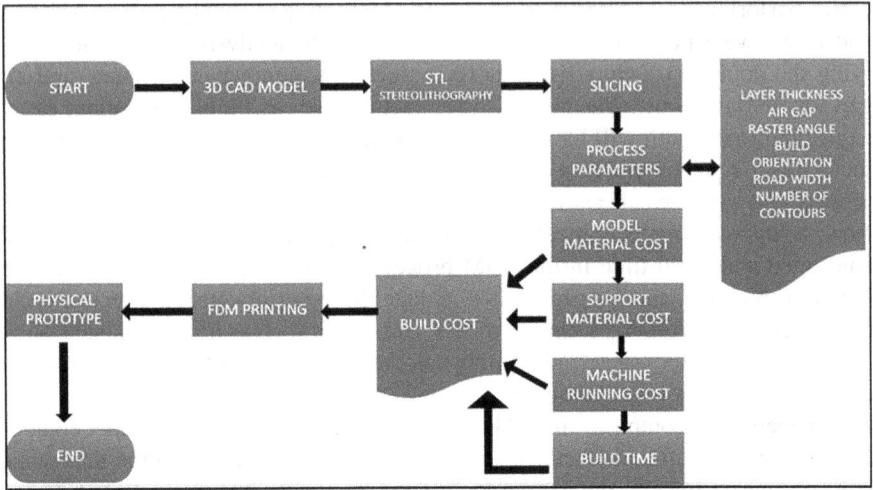

FIGURE 9.2 Flow chart for the printing of a liner component.

A systematic cost analysis is carried out, which includes processing cost, execution cost, material cost, and post-processing cost of the liner component.

9.2.1 3D CAD Model

By studying the knee prosthesis sizes in the Indian patients undergoing knee replacement, it has been found that around 53.3% population of the men have the tibial implant size three and the women have size two. The comparison chart between different tibial sizes is listed in Table 9.1. Another research work shows that shoe size is a better predictor than height size when considering tibial component sizes in the knee implant. Here, the male tibial component size varies from 3 to 4 and is considered as the most common size for male patients, and females' size varies from 2 to 3. The value of tibial size 3 was selected to be the dimension of the implant for the present work as per the literature survey [5]. The dimension of tibial component size 3 is shown in Figure 9.3.

9.2.2 Slicing and Effect of Process Parameters

Figure 9.4 shows the 3D view of the liner model with the assist of ANSYS software. The 3D prototype CAD design is converted to the .stl file format and it can be sliced into individual layers. The software then generates the tool path (gcode) that the printer will use for printing. Extensive analysis suggests that the optimal combination of printing parameters is given as a printing speed of 60 mm/s, a layer thickness of 0.3112 mm, a temperature of 260°C, and a filling ratio of 40% [7, 8]. All the factors are considered to produce the prototype with low build cost, low build time, and improved mechanical properties as listed in Table 9.2. The optimum parameters are taken for reducing the build time and feedstock material consumption while maximizing the impact strength, flexural strength, and tensile strength.

TABLE 9.1

Comparison Chart between Different Tibial Sizes

Tibial Size	A	B	C
8	54.1	88.4	60
7	51	83.4	56.5
6	48	78.7	53.2
5	45.3	74.2	50.2
4	42.7	70	47.3
3	40.6	66.5	45

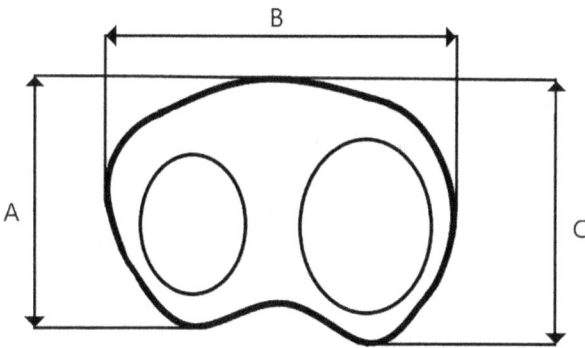

FIGURE 9.3 Model size 3 of the tibial component.

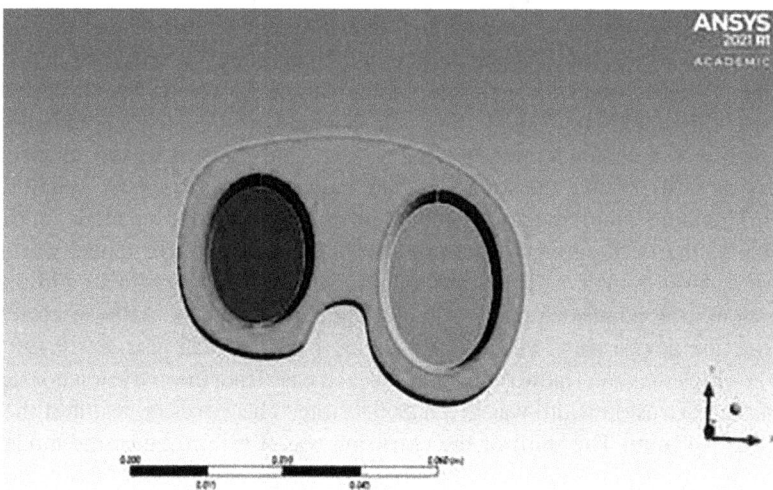

FIGURE 9.4 3D front view of the liner model.

TABLE 9.2

Factors Considered for Producing the Prototype

S. No.	Process Parameters	Specification
1	Air gap	0.499 mm
2	Build orientation	0°
3	Raster angle	45°
4	Layer thickness	0.3112 mm
5	Road width	0.484 mm
6	Printing speed	60 mm/s
7	Number of contours	5
8	Temperature of printing	260°C
9	Filling ratio	40%

9.2.3 Design of Experiments

Since the build cost of the component depends on the build time, a study was conducted to determine which process parameters influence the build time more. Therefore, a design of experiment with the Taguchi method was done to reduce the number of trials to a minimum, where 21 observations were recorded for four levels and six process parameters such as layer thickness, air gap, raster angle, build orientation, road width, and the number of contours. The design of the experiment for different parameters is listed in Table 9.3.

9.2.4 Experimental Works

The implant was designed by using Solid Works software and converted to the .stl file. The STL file was imported to PruscaSlicer 2.3.0 printer and the various parameters were adjusted. Figure 9.5 shows the experimental setup of 3D printing machine. The liner model was developed by using a 3D printer Prusca I3 MK3S. The layer thickness was made 0.3 mm and the number of contours used were five. As the number of contours increases, the process tends to increase the build time, it also assists in improving the strength of the model and increases the weight of the model. Therefore, an average of five contours were selected for the model in the 3D printing. In the infill parameter settings, the infill density of the model was made 40% to make it durable and the infill pattern selected was rectilinear and the top and bottom infill patterns were monotonic. The flow rate of the ABS material from the extrusion nozzle was 15% and the spacing between each pass was 0.499. The angle at which the material was being filled each pass from the extrusion nozzle was 45° and the extrusion width was given as 0.45 mm. The extrusion width of the first layer was 0.42 mm. The infill of the extrusion was 0.45 mm. Since the model did not require any support material, the support material infill option was neglected. In the printing speed parameters, the printing speed taken into account was 60

TABLE 9.3

Design of Experiment for Different Parameters

S. No.	Layer Thickness (mm)	Air Gap (mm)	Raster Angle (Degrees)	Build Orientation (Degrees)	Road Width (mm)	Number of Contours	Build Time (minutes)
1	0.1270	0.0	0	0	0.4572	1	87
2	0.1270	0.1	15	30	0.4814	3	89
3	0.1270	0.3	30	45	0.5056	5	94
4	0.1270	0.5	45	60	0.5298	7	93
5	0.1778	0.0	30	60	0.6000	1	56
6	0.1778	0.1	45	75	0.4572	3	73
7	0.1778	0..3	60	0	0.4814	5	76
8	0.1778	0.5	0	30	0.5056	7	75
9	0.2540	0.0	30	75	0.4814	7	63
10	0.2540	0.1	45	0	0.5056	8	61
11	0.2540	0.3	60	30	0.5298	1	51
12	0.2540	0.5	0	45	0.6000	3	49
13	0.2540	0.5	30	0	0.4572	7	61
14	0.3302	0.0	45	30	0.6000	5	44
15	0.3302	0.1	60	45	0.4572	7	56
16	0.3302	0.3	15	75	0.5056	1	45
17	0.3302	0.5	30	0	0.5298	3	46
18	0.3500	0.0	60	60	0.5056	3	47
19	0.3500	0.1	0	75	0.5298	5	48
20	0.3500	0.3	15	0	0.6000	7	45
21	0.3500	0.5	45	45	0.4814	1	48

mm/s, which proved that 60 mm of the material was pushed through the nozzle of the 3D printer per second. The acceleration of the 3D printer taken into account was 800 mm/s². The first layer was printed with an acceleration of 1000 mm/s². Once the parameters were applied, a 3D printing process was started, where the base plate (i.e. platform) and extruder temperature were heated to 115°C and 260°C. The implant was printed at an angle of 0° orientation with the *X-axis*. The build time of the product was 40 minutes and the weight of the prototype was 12.5 g, which is ideal for a knee implant. The 3D printed prototype is shown in Figure 9.6.

9.3 RESULTS AND DISCUSSION

By using the analysis of variance on each process parameter, keeping the response as build time, it was found that layer thickness plays a major role compared to other parameters. The other parameters play a marginal role in comparison to the layer thickness. To intensify the significance of the process parameters on the build time of the liner component, the Taguchi method was carried out to identify the response

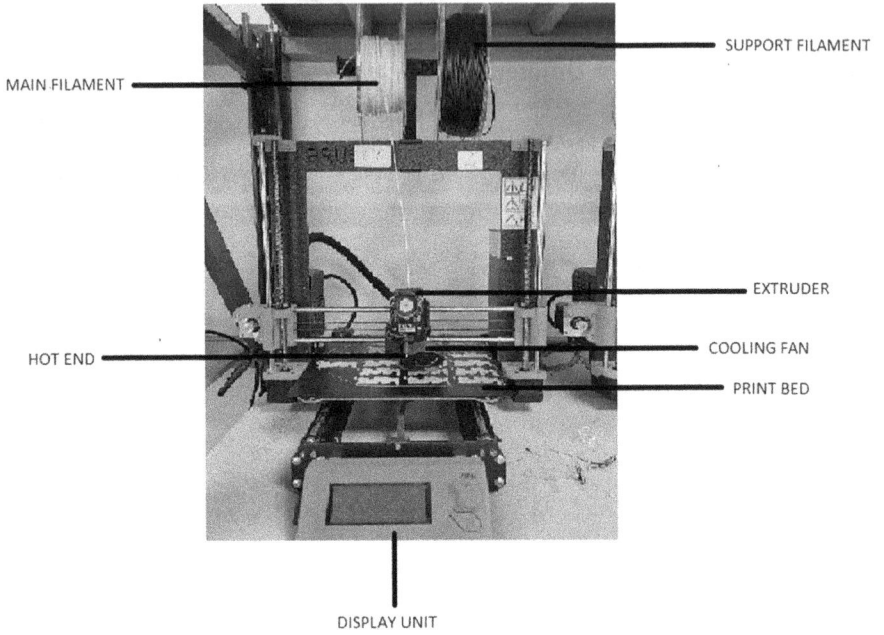

FIGURE 9.5   Experimental setup.

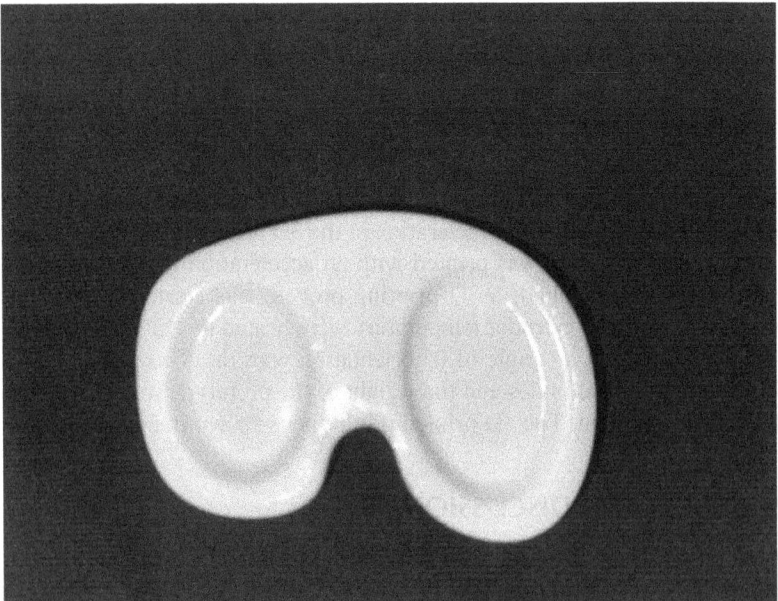

FIGURE 9.6   3D printed sample.

of the build time using Minitab software and the following regression equation was obtained as shown in Equation (9.1).

$$
\begin{aligned}
\text{Build Time} = {}& -572.9 - 1865 \text{ Layer Thickness} + 48.96 \text{ Air Gap} \\
& + 0.4698 \text{ Raster Angle} - 1.098 \text{ Build Orientation} \\
& + 3294 \text{ Road Width} - 9.589 \text{ Number of Contours} \\
& + 769.9 \text{ Layer Thickness} \times \text{Layer Thickness} + 56.90 \text{ Air Gap} \\
& \times \text{Air Gap} - 0.008438 \text{ Raster Angle} \times \text{Raster Angle} \\
& + 0.005788 \text{ Build Orientation} \times \text{Build Orientation} \\
& - 3334 \text{ Road Width} \times \text{Road Width} \\
& - 0.4074 \text{ Number of Contours} \times \text{Number of Contours} \\
& + 403.2 \text{ Layer Thickness} \times \text{Air Gap} + 2.845 \text{ Layer Thickness} \\
& \times \text{Raster Angle} + 3.796 \text{ Layer Thickness} \\
& \times \text{Build Orientation} + 1319 \text{ Layer Thickness} \times \text{Road Width} \\
& + 68.64 \text{ Layer Thickness} \times \text{Number of Contours} \\
& - 0.6950 \text{ Air Gap} \times \text{Raster Angle} + 0.6597 \text{ Air Gap} \\
& \times \text{Build Orientation} - 205.0 \text{ Air Gap} \times \text{Road Width}
\end{aligned}
\tag{9.1}
$$

Figure 9.7 shows the effect of layer thickness on the build time. An interval plot was created for the effect of layer thickness on the build time using the obtained data as listed in Table 9.4. This supports us to understand how the build time reduces with increasing layer thickness.

Figure 9.8 shows the residual plots for build time. The points in the residual plots are randomly distributed around the horizontal axis which means that the regression model obtained is appropriate. Also, the data set is approximately distributed in a normal probability plot.

The effects of different parameters on the build time are shown in Figure 9.9. The surface plot is also plotted using Minitab software to understand the effect of road width, layer thickness, and the number of contours on the build time. The most influential factors such as road width, number of contours, and layer thickness are taken for predicting the variation of the build time.

The Ansys 2021 R1 software is used for stress–strain analysis. The tibial size 3 is used for the analysis of human body weight ranging from 75 to 100 kg. Different activities such as walking and jogging are taken into consideration while selecting the load applied by the femur on the knee. The average load that is applied by a human body on the knee joint is taken as 4218 N. Different properties of the ABS polymer are given as input to the Ansys software as listed in Table 9.5. Later, the output variables like stress, strain, and total deformation solutions are generated.

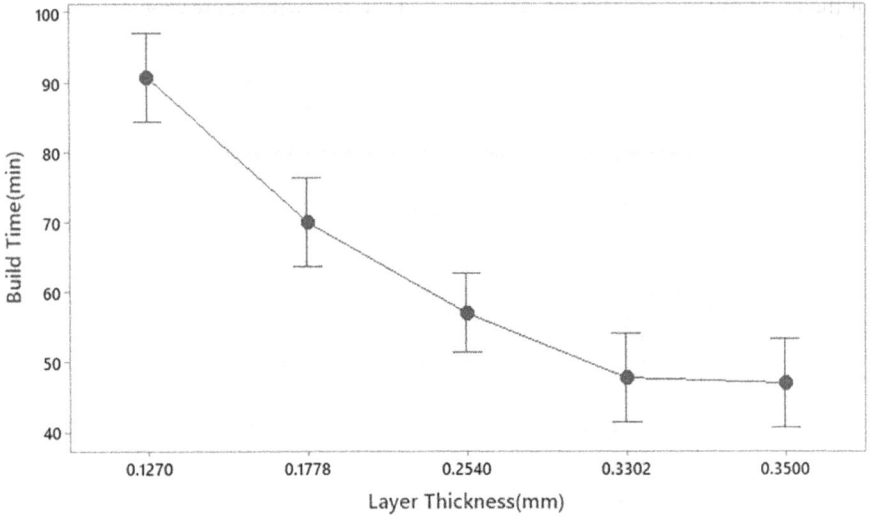

FIGURE 9.7   Effect of layer thickness on build time.

TABLE 9.4
Analysis of Variance

Source	DF	Adj SS	Adj MS	F-Value	P-Value
Layer thickness (mm)	4	5398.3	1349.58	38.18	0.000
Error	16	565.5	35.34	–	–
Total	20	5963.8	–	–	–

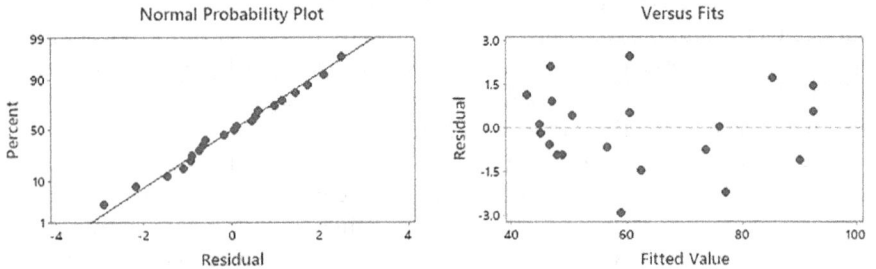

FIGURE 9.8   Residual plots for build time.

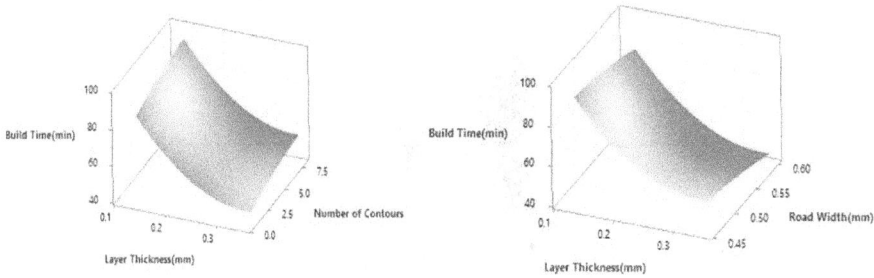

FIGURE 9.9 Effects of different parameters on the build time.

TABLE 9.5

Input Variables for the Stress–Strain Analysis

S. No.	Input Parameters	Values
1	Density	1 g/cm³
2	Melting temperature	240°C
3	Poisson's ratio	0.35
4	Young's modulus	1.5 GPa
5	Yield strength	80 MPa
6	Tangent modulus	500 MPa
7	Coefficient of thermal expansion	0.00008 /C
8	Tensile strength	28 MPa
9	Compressive strength	65 MPa
10	Tensile ultimate strength	45 MPa

9.3.1 ANALYZING THE STRESS DISTRIBUTION

The load is applied to the liner model as shown in Figure 9.10. This observation shows that the stress is minimal and does not affect the liner. The two oval-shaped pockets on the liner component, where the femoral component is placed, experience more stress than the flat surface of the liner. Figure 9.11 shows the solution for the strain analysis. Here, the strain developed was very much minimal and does not affect the liner component in the knee implant. As the stress applied was in the range of the plastic region, the deformation was not detected. The analysis shows that no deformation has taken place. The total deformation of the model is shown in Figure 9.12. It was observed that the inner middle region of the pockets was more affected than the rest of the liner due to the direct contact with the femoral component.

9.3.2 STRESS–STRAIN CURVE

To produce the stress–strain curve, the solution graphs of stress and strain were extracted and plotted. The strain values were projected along the X-axis and stress values were projected along the Y-axis.

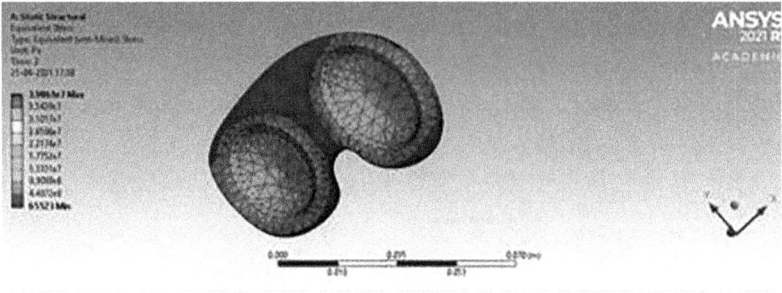

FIGURE 9.10 Stress distribution applied on the liner model.

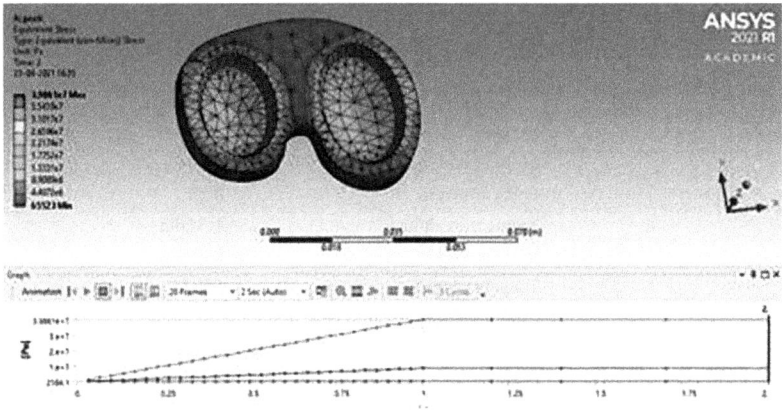

FIGURE 9.11 Strain experienced by the liner model.

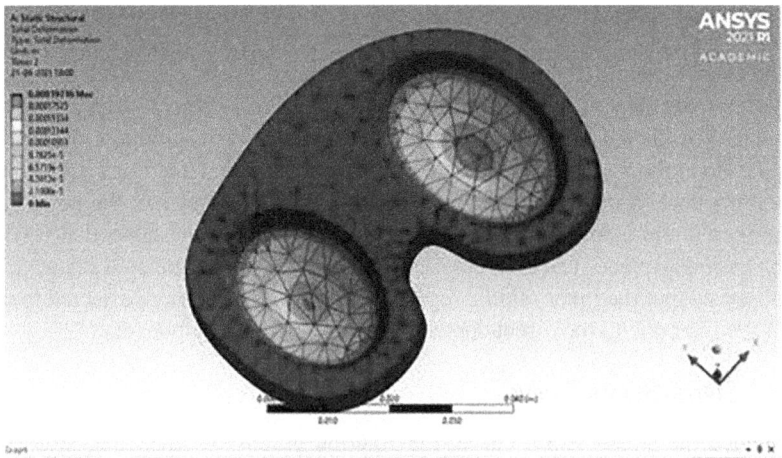

FIGURE 9.12 Solution for total deformation.

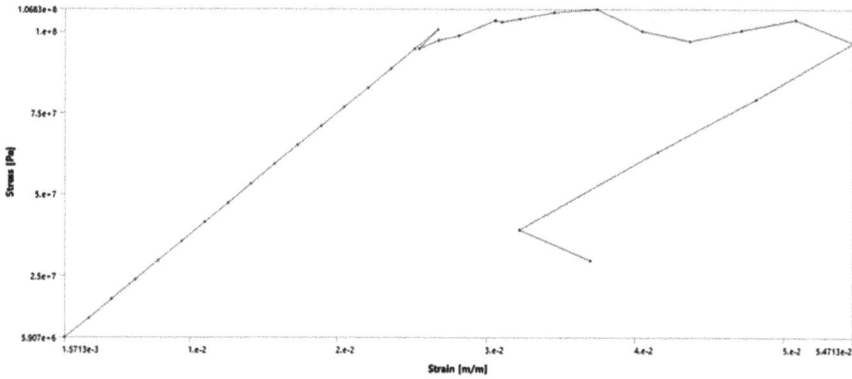

FIGURE 9.13   Stress–strain curve.

Figure 9.13 shows the stress–strain curve, where the system was allowed to increase the stress from zero to 20,000 psi. Here, the stress reaches 16,000 psi or 1.1×10^8 Pa to enter the plastic region and then begins to deform until 0.0054 strain and enters the unloading stage at 14,000 psi. At this stage, the fracture occurs and the liner stops elongation resulting in the spring back of the liner and it attains a final elongation of 3% strain. From the graph, it is noted that ABS has a high tensile strength and can withstand deformation and finally rupture and spring back up to 90 MPa and 5% strain. It is also noted that the liner has a large elastic and plastic region, which is an ideal property of ABS for manufacturing the liner.

9.3.3   COST ESTIMATION OF THE LINER COMPONENT

The different costs required for the manufacture of liner components are classified into four product costs. They are listed as initially the direct cost, where these costs are directly accredited to the manufacturing of the product by the FDM process, for example, cost of the ABS material, final finishing cost, etc. Second, the indirect cost, where these costs are not directly accountable to the cost of the product, for example, labor tax, design cost, etc. Third, the variable cost, where these costs vary depending on the product requirements, for example, support material filament cost, machine-running cost, etc. Finally, the fixed cost, where these costs are independent of the volume produced. Examples are the cost of an FDM printer, software license cost, etc.

Henrique et al. [15] have sub-classified the variable and fixed costs as follows:

Prototype filament material: The usage of a material differs based on the matter and volume of the product to be produced.
Machine work per hour: The time required for the manufacturing is based on finishing and the product's shape configuration requirements.
Energy: The power usage is based on the load needed for the manufacturing of the product and is calculated based on processes such as prototype execution, post-processing of the product, and STL processing.

Labor: The cost of labor is only calculated for the printing of the 3D proto-type and does not change with an increase in the volume and mass of the product.

Maintenance: The maintenance aspect can be linked directly to the entire process by taking certain parameters into account, as the manufacturing of the product is planned based on the calendar. But, it is often applied as execution hours in cost estimation.

Wong et al. [14] propose a particular cost breakdown model for rapid manufacturing processes and the formulated equation [1] is:

1. Processing cost (C_p):

$$C_p = \left(\left(\frac{0.2 \times C_{pc}}{W_{at}} \right) + \omega_d + PC_e \times P_{kh} + \frac{0.2 \times C_{sl}}{W_{at}} \right) \times T_p \qquad (9.2)$$

where

C_{pc} –cost of personal computer −1226 (USD)
C_{sl} – cost of software license −408 (USD).
ω_d – hourly fee of the designer −2 (USD/h).
W_{at} – availability of personal computer per year −2880 (hours).
PC_e – electricity consumption rate of personal computer −0.6 (kWh/h).
P_{kh} – average cost of power −0.026 (USD/kWh).
T_p – time taken by the designer to process the STL model −0.66 (hour).

2. Machine-running cost (r_f):

$$r_f = \left((P_e \times P_{kh}) + \frac{0.2 \times P_{mp}}{W_{at}} + \omega_0 + \left(\frac{M_m}{W_{at}} \right) \times 12 \right) \qquad (9.3)$$

where

ω_0 – hourly fee of the operator −1 (USD/h).
P_e – electricity consumption rate of the machine −0.75 (kWh/h).
P_{kh} – local average energy-specific cost −0.3 (USD/kWh).
M_m – monthly maintenance cost −108 (USD).
P_{mp} – cost of the machine −1361.44 (USD).
W_{at} – availability of machine per year −2880 (hours) – (8 hours a day, 30 days a month, 12 months a year).

3. Execution cost (C_e):

$$C_e = T_e \times r_f \qquad (9.4)$$

where

T_e – time taken to produce the prototype −0.66 (hours).
r_f – cost of running the machine per hour −1.7695 USD.

4. Material cost (C_m):

$$C_m = \frac{(V_m \times P_m)}{V_c} + \frac{(V_s \times P_s)}{V_c} \qquad (9.5)$$

where
V_m – volume of the prototype utilized −151.5 (cm³).
P_m – material cost per cm³ −27.23 (USD).
V_s – volume of the support material utilized −0 (cm³).
V_c – volume of prototype/support material per cartridge −1000 (cm³).
P_s – support material cost per cm³ −0 (USD).

5. Post-processing cost (C_{pp}):

$$C_{pp} = \left(\omega_0 + P_{sm} \times V_{sm} + P_{sp}\right)$$ (9.6)

where
ω_0 – operators fee −2.5 (USD/h).
P_{sm} – cost of solvent −0.014 (USD/mL).
V_{sm} – volume of the solvent material −250 (mL).
P_{sp} – cost of sanding −0.52 (USD).

6. Final cost equation (C_{fp}):

$$C_{fp} = C_p + C_e + C_m + C_{pp}$$ (9.7)

The cost estimation of the liner component is done by taking the sum of various costs involved in the pre and post-processing of the prototype such as processing cost, machine-running cost, execution cost, and post-processing cost. The costs calculated using the formulated equations are given in Table 9.6.

7. Cost Expenditure of prototype from vendor:

Prototype Cost = Weight of Prototype (g) × Cost per gram +

Build time × Cost per hour = 12.5 g × 0.18 + 0.66 × 1.04

= 2.25 + 0.6864
= 2.9364 \$
= 2.9364 + 6.25 (post-processing)
= 9.1864 \$

The error percentage between the theoretical cost and actual cost are listed in Table 9.7. The prototype theoretical cost is the cost calculated by adding the values of processing cost and execution cost. It is compared to the actual cost made by the vendor. The post-processing theoretical cost is calculated using the numerical formula given in equation (9.6) and is compared to the actual cost made by the vendor. The error percentage between the prototype theoretical cost and the actual cost is around 12% and that of post-processing cost is around 4%.

9.3.4 COMPARATIVE STUDY

The total cost of the liner component was estimated as 14.96 \$ using the cost estimation equation. The cost expenditure calculated by the vendor was approximately

TABLE 9.6
Different Types of Costs Required for the Printing of the Prototype

S. No.	Types of Cost	Values ($)
1	Processing cost (C_p)	1.405
2	Machine-running cost (r_f)	1.769
3	Execution cost (C_e)	1.167
4	Material cost (C_m)	4.125
5	Post-processing cost (C_{pp})	6.52
6	Total cost (C_{fp})	14.96

TABLE 9.7
Error Percentage between Theoretical Cost and the Actual Cost

Expenses	Theoretical Cost	Actual Cost (vendor)	Error Percentage
Prototype cost	2.572	2.9364	12.4
Post-processing cost	6.52	6.25	4.3

9 $. The percentage change between the cost calculated by the vendor and the cost determined through the cost estimation equation was 38.63%. When the ABS (acrylonitrile butadiene styrene) liner manufactured by the FDM process was compared with the conventional liner, a huge difference existed between the final cost of the material. The liner made out of conventional methods is time-consuming, which takes around one whole day to finish the prototype, and is more expensive, which costs roughly around 137 $ according to the implant pricing model made by Hiranandhani hospital [16]. The reduction of cost in terms of percentage when the vendor's cost is compared to that of the industrial average cost is around 93.29%.

9.4   CONCLUSION

The stress–strain analysis of the ABS material was performed with the assistance of ANSYS software, where it was observed that the ABS has a high tensile strength to withstand deformation and spring back with a 5% strain and finally rupture. It was also found that the layer thickness plays a major impact compared to other parameters with the build time. The cost estimation indicates that the ABS liner component manufactured by the FDM process is cheaper compared to the conventional method. Currently, the ABS liner is manufactured with a cost of approximately 9 $ compared to the industrial average of 137 $ for the conventional method, which is a cost reduction of 93.29%. Based on the properties, the ABS material is tougher and much lighter than other polymers, especially high-density polyethylene.

REFERENCES

1. Boorla, R., & Prabeena, T. (2019). Fabrication of patient specific knee implant by fused deposition modeling. *Materials Today: Proceedings*, 18, 3638–3642. Doi: 10.1016/j.matpr.2019.07.296.
2. Zammit, R., & Rochman, A. (2017). Development and fabrication of patient-specific knee implant using additive manufacturing techniques. Doi: 10.1063/1.5008037.
3. Williams, D.F. (2008). On the mechanisms of biocompatibility. *Biomaterials*, 29(20), 2941–2953, ISSN 0142–9612, Doi: 10.1016/j.biomaterials.2008.04.023.
4. Markopoulos, A.P., Galanis, N.I., Karkalos, N.E., & Manolakos, D.E. (2018) Precision CNC machining of femoral component of knee implant: A case study. *Machines*, 6, 10. Doi: 10.3390/machines6010010.
5. Guo, N., & Leu, M.C., 2013. Additive manufacturing: Technology, applications and research needs. *Frontiers of Mechanical Engineering*, 8(3), 215–224.
6. Huang, S.H., Liu, P., Mokasdar, A., & Hou, L., 2013. Additive manufacturing and its societal impact: A literature review. *The International Journal of Advanced Manufacturing Technology*, 67(5–8), 1191–1203.
7. Abeykoon, C., Sri-Amphorn, P., & Fernando, A. (2020). Optimization of fused deposition modeling parameters for improved PLA and ABS 3D printed structures. *International Journal of Lightweight Materials and Manufacture*, 3(3), 284–297. Doi: 10.1016/j.ijlmm.2020.03.
8. Chakrabarty, G., Vashishtha, M., & Leeder, D. (2015). Polyethylene in knee arthroplasty: A review. *Journal of Clinical Orthopaedics and Trauma*, 6(2), 108–112. Doi: 10.1016/j.jcot.2015.01.096.
9. Dey, A., & Yodo, N. (2019). A systematic survey of FDM process parameter optimization and their influence on part characteristics. *Journal of Manufacturing and Materials Processing*, 3(3), 64. Doi: 10.3390/jmmp3030064.
10. Wickramasinghe, S., Do, T., & Tran, P. (2020, July 10). FDM-based 3D printing of polymer and associated composite: A review on mechanical properties, defects and treatments. *Polymers*, 12(7), 1529.
11. Mohamed, O. A., Masood, S. H., & Bhowmik, J. L. (2016). Mathematical modeling and FDM process parameters optimization using response surface methodology based on Q-optimal design. *Applied Mathematical Modelling*, 40(23–24), 10052–10073. Doi: 10.1016/j.apm.2016.06.055.
12. Mohamed, O., Masood, S., & Bhowmik, J. (2016). Parametric analysis of the build cost for FDM additive processed parts using response surface methodology. *Reference Module in Materials Science and Materials Engineering*. Published.
13. Nancharaiah, T. (2011). Optimization of process parameters in FDM process using design of experiments. *International Journal on Emerging Technologies*, 2(1), 100–102.
14. Xu, F., Wong, Y.S., & Loh, H.T. (2000). Toward generic models for comparative evaluation and process selection in rapid prototyping and manufacturing. *Journal of Manufacturing Systems*, 19(5), 283–296.
15. Henrique Pereira Mello, C., Calandrin Martins, R., Rosa Parra, B., de Oliveira Pamplona, E., Gomes Salgado, E., & Tavares Seguso, R. (2010). Systematic proposal to calculate price of prototypes manufactured through rapid prototyping an FDM 3D printer in a university lab. *Rapid Prototyping Journal*, 16(6), 411–416.
16. https://www.hiranandanihospital.org/menudetailpage/powai/other-information/total-kneereplacement-implants-pricing/196.

10 Nanostructured Biomaterials for Load-Bearing Applications

Moumita Ghosh and A. Thirugnanam
National Institute of Technology Rourkela Odisha

CONTENTS

DOI: 10.1201/9781003286806-10

10.1 INTRODUCTION

The materials that have been engineered to interact with the biological systems for medical applications are termed biomaterials. Biomaterials have an extensive range of applications in the field of biomedical engineering [1]. They can be defined as a part of any medical alliances used in the medical diagnosis and treatment process. These can be any material either naturally occurring or synthesized artificially. The choice of material or system of materials depends upon the functions. Biomaterials are used in various medical applications such as implants, cardiovascular medical devices, reconstructive surgery, wound healing, drug delivery systems, bioelectrodes and sensors. The most crucial aspect for considering any material as a biomaterial is that it should serve inside the human body without any allergic reactions or adverse effects leading to rejection and implant failure [2]. On the basis of type of body interaction, biomaterials can be classified into bio-tolerant, bioinert and bioactive materials. For orthopedic and dental applications, biomaterials should be bioactive and need to stimulate various biological responses from the body, such as bonding with the adjacent tissues, cartilages or bones [3]. The crucial factors that decide an implant's longevity include the material's resistance to withstand the mechanical forces (predominantly cyclic) to avoid premature failure and a robust interface between the body and the implant for avoiding probable complications including inflammation, implant loosening and allergies [4]. Biocompatibility, high corrosion resistance, better mechanical properties (like hardness, tensile strength, stiffness and shear strength) and high wear resistance are the most important properties, which a biomaterial should possess to achieve the desired lifespan for a load-bearing orthopedic implant [5].

The biomaterials used for medical applications are broadly classified into metals, ceramics, composites and polymers. Metals are used mainly in orthopedics (for load-bearing implants), cardiovascular surgery and dental applications. The most commonly used metals for implants include 316L stainless steel, titanium alloys and Co–Cr alloys [6]. In titanium, beta stabilizers V, Nb, Mo, Zr and Ta are added as alloying elements to reduce Young's modulus. Ceramic biomaterials also exhibit good biocompatibility, low toxicity, high corrosion resistance and better bioactivity. These are mostly used for orthopedic implants, dental applications and other medical applications such as drug delivery. Likewise, polymeric biomaterials are one of the widely preferred materials for medical applications. Synthetic polymeric biomaterials have a wide range of uses as prosthetic materials, clinical disposal materials, implants, drug delivery systems and tissue-engineered products with ceramics and metal substituents. The properties that made biopolymers profoundly used biomaterials are biocompatibility, flexibility, biodegradability, lightweight, and resistance to biochemical attacks. All these properties help them to have unique applications in the biomedical field. Biopolymers also have their applications in clinical inspections, surgical treatments and preventive medicine. Polymer composites have also acquired their place in various medical applications, including tissue engineering, regenerative clinical applications, dental and orthopedic (load-bearing) applications. Due to some favorable properties, metals are preferred over other materials for orthopedic implants. This chapter describes various types of nanostructured materials used for biomedical applications, the methods used to obtain nanostructured features and a comparison study of those methods.

10.2 NANOSTRUCTURED BIOMATERIALS

10.2.1 Metallic Biomaterials

The most widely used biomaterials for load-bearing applications are metallic biomaterials. The load-bearing implant applications include knee implants, hip joint implants and dental applications. The profoundly used metals for medical applications include stainless steel, cobalt–chromium alloys, titanium and its alloys. Metals are preferred as biomaterials for the mentioned load-bearing applications owing to their unique and valuable mechanical properties. The metallic materials should possess apt fatigue strength to withstand the loads and rigors inside the body and avoid implant fracture. The metallic implants used for load-bearing applications suffer from the stress shielding effect, which occurs due to the mismatch in Young's modulus or non-uniform stress distribution between the implant and bone. In the long run, it will lead to bone resorption and eventually will end up in implant loosening. The stress shielding effect can be reduced by choosing a material with a modulus near to that of human bone, which varies in the range of (4–30) GPa. The most famous metallic biomaterials used for medical applications include stainless steel, cobalt–chromium alloys, titanium and its alloys. Stainless steels 316L are used for manufacturing femoral heads and stems as they possess good mechanical properties and high corrosion resistance. Stainless steels are the priority over other metals if compared in terms of cost to outcome ratio. Metal alloys are used because the oxide forms of alloying elements usually form a passive layer on the metal surface, which restricts the corrosion of the implants. Such metal alloys include cobalt and titanium alloys. Cobalt–chromium alloys form the passive layer of Cr_2O_3, which offers good corrosion as well as wear-resistance properties. These alloys are for manufacturing the implants of hip joint replacement applications. Similarly, in titanium alloys, a very robust passive oxide layer of TiO_2 is formed which enhances the corrosion-resistance properties of the implant. Above all, titanium has better biocompatibility properties, low Young's modulus, high strength, better bone adhesion properties, low density and high corrosion resistance as compared to other metallic materials. Due to all these reasons, titanium and its alloys are predominantly used as biomaterials. Few of the load-bearing applications of titanium include hip and knee implants, artificial hip joints, bone screws and plates. In addition to the excellent mechanical properties, metallic biomaterials have some disadvantages as well. They include being highly vulnerable to corrosion and higher chances of toxicity due to the ions released from the alloying elements of the metallic alloys. All these reasons may end up in implant failure. Thereby, the selection of biomaterials should be made accordingly so that the ill effects can be avoided while increasing the longevity and biocompatibility of the implant. To enhance the properties of the implant material, many things can be done such as shaping and surface processing methods. One such method is nanostructuring of materials which is done to get nanostructured materials in the size range of 1–100 nm with a smaller grain size. The smaller grain size ensures the enhancement of mechanical strength as per the Hall–Petch equation. In the case of metallic biomaterials as well as metals like commercially pure titanium, stainless steels are subjected to nanostructuring methods to produce nanostructured materials. The nanostructured metals are then characterized by various characterization techniques like transmission electron microscopy (TEM), scanning electron microscopy (SEM), X-ray diffraction (XRD) and Fourier transform infrared spectroscopy (FTIR) for obtaining the surface morphology, details of crystalline structures and chemical bonding in the metal molecules. They can further be characterized to get the surface wettability property using contact angle, to obtain the microstructures using an optical microscope and to obtain the mechanical properties like tensile strength and hardness. The nanostructured materials are believed to have enhanced mechanical and biocompatibility properties.

10.2.2 Ceramic Biomaterials

Ceramic biomaterials are usually used for dental applications. However, they also have some applications in orthopedic implants. The properties that make ceramic an implant biomaterial include high corrosion resistance, biocompatibility, low toxicity, high rate of bone formation and better bioactivity properties. Some of the bioceramics include hydroxyapatite, tricalcium phosphate and zirconia, which help in better bioactivity and bone regeneration in dental and orthopedic applications. As ceramic materials are bio-degradable, they are also used in drug delivery applications. Ceramic biomaterials such as alumina, zirconia, bioactive glasses, porcelain and carbons have applications in bone replacement, joint replacement, heart valves, dental implants and percutaneous devices. They have been clinically used in load and non-load-bearing implant applications. As conventional bioceramics offer poor mechanical and biodegradability properties, nanostructuring of bioceramics is done to improve the mechanical properties, bioactivity and biodegradability of the material. Nanoceramics are mostly synthesized using the sol–gel methodology due to the feasibility it offers during the synthesis of nanostructures. Nanoceramics can be characterized by TEM, XRD (energy-dispersive X-ray spectroscopy), EDS and FTIR methods. Some of the nanostructured bioceramics include nano-bioglasses, hydroxyapatite and tricalcium phosphate. Ceramics can also be used as a coating material on implants to enhance the bioactivity, corrosion and wear resistance. The profoundly used ceramic coatings include titanium oxide (TiO_2) coating (for example, TiO_2 on stainless steel 316L increases the hemocompatibility and corrosion resistance and exhibits better antibacterial property), alumina (Al_2O_3) coating, which enhances the hardness along with the corrosion and wear resistance of the alloy, silica (SiO_2) coating on alloys that decreases the rate of corrosion, manganese dioxide (MnO_2) which is less costly and at the same time increases the mechanical and chemical stability of the alloys and hydroxyapatite (HA) coating which increases the rate of osseointegration and enhances the bioactivity in implants. The famous technologies used for the ceramic coating process are sol–gel technology, micro-arc oxidation (MAO) technology, chemical vapor deposition (CVD) method, metal–organic chemical vapor deposition (MOCVD) method, laser cladding, dip coating and solution immersion method.

10.2.3 Polymeric Biomaterials

Similar to metals and ceramic biomaterials, polymeric biomaterials have also found their use in biomedical applications. The properties which differentiate them from metals or ceramic biomaterials include ease of manufacturing, low cost and feasible secondary processing steps. They also possess basic properties like biocompatibility, sterilizability, biodegradability and required mechanical properties for body implant applications. Due to ease of manufacturing, they are available in various shapes such as sheets, fibers, films and latex. The most common polymeric biomaterial applications are in dental implants, prosthetic materials, encapsulants, drug delivery, dressings, tissue-engineered products and extracorporeal devices. Primarily used synthetic polymers are polyethylene, polyvinylchloride, polypropylene, polystyrene, polymethylmethacrylate, polyethylene terephthalate and polystyrene [7].

10.2.4 Composite Biomaterials

Materials in which the distinct phases of the material are separated on an atomic scale and some properties like elastic modulus are manipulated as compared to the original homogeneous material are called composite materials. The composite which is used as a biomaterial should have a biocompatible constituent. The interface between the constituents of the composite biomaterial should have resistance to degradation done by the body environment [8]. The most widely used composite applications are dental filling composites, porous orthopedic implants and bone cement (reinforced methyl methacrylate). Flexible composite bone plates have high bone healing properties and are hence highly used in orthopedic load-bearing applications. Mostly, composites are fabricated with natural polymers to achieve a material mimicking the natural bone matrix. The profoundly used combination of such material is the CaP and natural polymer fabrication for orthopedic applications. The addition of coupling agents can further enhance the biocompatibility of composite biomaterials. For possessing properties like `lower density and higher strength, composite materials are considered the apt material for prosthetic limb applications. Likewise, for joint replacement and bone repair applications, carbon-reinforced and carbon–carbon polymer composites are used.

10.3 NANOSTRUCTURING USING SEVERE PLASTIC DEFORMATION (SPD) TECHNIQUES

Metals are extensively used as biomaterials for load-bearing orthopedic implants owing to their excellent mechanical properties and biocompatibility. As the mechanical strength of implants needs to be very high for load-bearing applications, the strength of the material can further be enhanced using methods of grain refinement. As per the Hall–Petch equation, the strength of a material increases with the decrease in the material's grain size [9]. One of the grain refinement techniques is the severe plastic deformation (SPD) technique used for the production of bulk nanostructured materials with enhanced properties in many aspects, including mechanical, corrosion, bioactivity, electrical and texture. These methods are preferred as they keep the other properties of the material unaffected. Severe plastic deformation facilitates the grain refinement of the coarse-grained bulk materials into UFG materials in either the (100 nm–1.0 μm) or the (<100 nm) range. Hence, it is termed as a "top-down" approach [1,10]. Valiev and his co-workers were the first to do research and development in SPD in 1977 in Russia [11]. SPD methods also have their applications for nanostructuring in the field of automobiles and aircraft. The SPD methods must fulfill three following criteria: (i) the UFGs should have high-angle boundaries, (ii) there should be the production of uniform bulk nanostructures and (iii) the materials should avoid mechanical damage when subjected to deformations. The conventional deformation methods do not fulfill these criteria. Various SPD methods like equal channel angular pressing (ECAP), repetitive corrugation and straightening (RCS), accumulative roll bonding (ARB), asymmetric rolling (ASR), ball milling (BM), high-pressure torsion (HPT) and groove pressing (GP) are used to fabricate bulk nanostructured materials.

10.3.1 VARIOUS SEVERE PLASTIC DEFORMATION TECHNIQUES

Nanostructuring of materials has gained importance in biomedical applications over conventional materials as the amount of protein adsorption and rate of cell proliferation and differentiation are much higher on the nanostructured materials. These factors make the biomaterials with nanostructures more favorable for tissue growth than the conventional biomaterials. SPD methods deform the bulk material using mechanical force while avoiding any chemical reactions. These methods involve applying a considerable amount of hydrostatic pressure resulting in the fabrication of UFG metals possessing high-angle grain boundaries [12]. Over the decades, various SPD methods have been evolved for the formation of bulk nanostructured materials. The various SPD techniques vary primarily on the constraints imposed per pass, the deformation pattern of the material and the load applied for processing. SPD techniques are considered an efficient approach for obtaining materials with delicate crystalline structures. The major factors involved in the process of SPD techniques are high strains, huge hydrostatic pressure, nanostructuring of materials with high-angle grain boundaries, homogeneity in the material with uniform properties, material production with almost no pores and reduced mechanical defects or cracks [13].

10.3.1.1 Equal Channel Angular Press Technique

The ECAP method was first introduced in the year 1972. It is one of the SPD techniques, which is used to produce bulk UFG material. It is also known as the pressing technique. In this method, metallic billets are subjected to a higher strain, and they undergo plastic deformation. During the process, there is no alteration in the cross-section of the billet. The methods include the following steps: first, the metallic samples are put into the die through a die channel, and a plunger is placed on the top of the billet. Second, the plunger applies the required load to press the sample through the die channel until the sample gets extruded out of the die. The die channel and billet cross-sectional area can be considered either circular or rectangular based on the application. As mentioned earlier, the extruded samples have whole

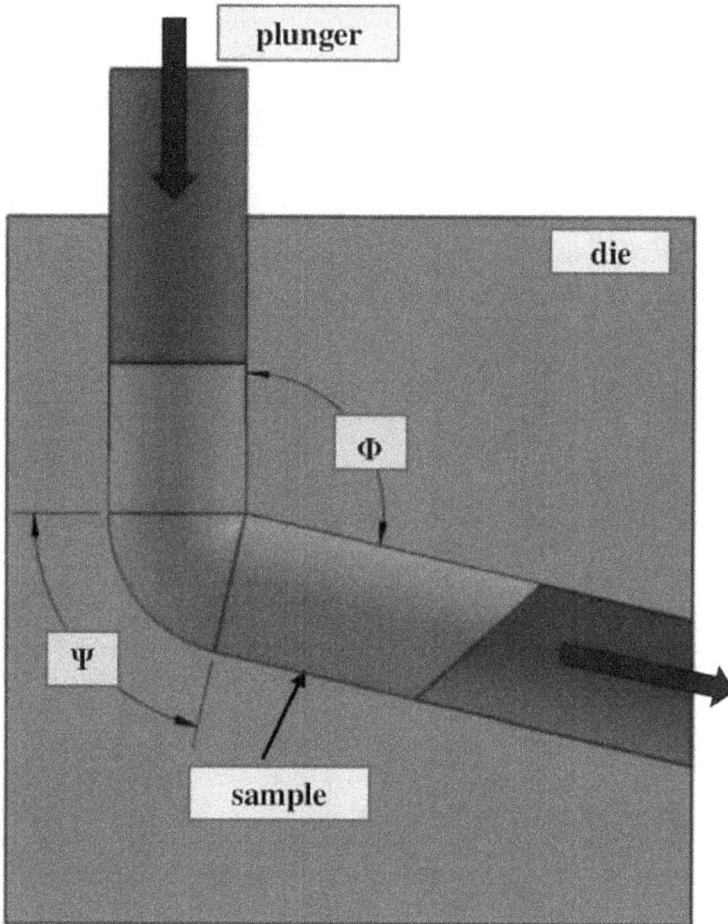

FIGURE 10.1   Schematic diagram representing ECAP die.

dimensions before and after the processing. Figure 10.1 shows the arrangement of the die and plunger for the execution of the ECAP process.

The deformation occurs when the sample passes through the die channel bending part of the die. The level of plastic deformation is dependent on the bend angle of the die. For obtaining a higher plastic strain, the bend angle needs to be low. The ECAP process can be carried out using four passing routes (A, B_a, B_c and C) distinguished based on the rotation angle for achieving desirable strain. The selection of a proper passing route is essential to achieve desirable microstructures of the material. Primarily, route B_c is used to obtain homogeneous microstructures. In route A, there is no alteration in the angle of rotation; in route B_a, for every pressing the angle of rotation is changed by 90° while in route B_c, the sample is rotated by an angle of 90° in the same direction either clockwise or anticlockwise. In route C, the billet is rotated by an angle of 180° for every pressing. Figure 10.2 depicts the processing routes of the ECAP technique.

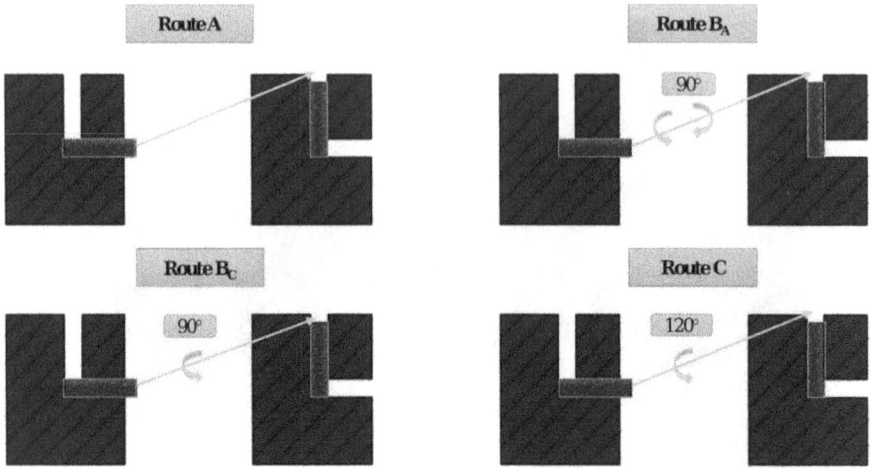

FIGURE 10.2 Schematic showing different processing routes during the ECAP technique.

Since there is no change in the dimension of the sample before and after processing, there can be multiple passes, or the sample can be pushed repeatedly in the die to obtain high strain. Equation 10.1 describes the relationship between the total number of passes and the developed strain in the die [14]:

$$\varepsilon = \left(N/\sqrt{3}\right)\left[2\cot\left\{(\Phi+\Psi)/2\right\} + \Psi\cos ec\left\{(\Phi+\Psi)/2\right\}\right] \qquad (10.1)$$

ECAP has been used widely for industrial applications; however, scale-up production is still not possible. For such purposes, various modifications have been done on the conventional ECAP process to obtain other ECAP methods with advanced outcomes. This is the most preferred SPD technique for obtaining bulk nanostructured materials used in orthopedic implant applications.

10.3.1.2 High-Pressure Torsion (HPT) Technique

The HPT technique was first introduced in the year 1937 by Bridgman. It is also a widely used technique for the nanostructuring of materials for various purposes, including medical applications. Figure 10.3 describes the schematic diagram of the HPT and parts included in it.

In this method, the sample is passed through the two anvils under extremely high pressure. Both the anvils are subjected to counter-rotation throughout the process, such as rotation of one anvil will induce shear stress while the other one will be static. This method is executed at low temperatures for brittle samples. The micro- and nanostructured materials are obtained due to the multiple one-step shears caused by high pressure. The HPT technique is significant for producing nanostructures, while it also has some disadvantages. It has some constraints on the dimensions of the sample like it only allows the processing of small disc-shaped and thin samples. This method is of discontinuous type, which can be overcome by a continuous HPT technique (CHPT) used for either sheets or ring-shaped samples. One more

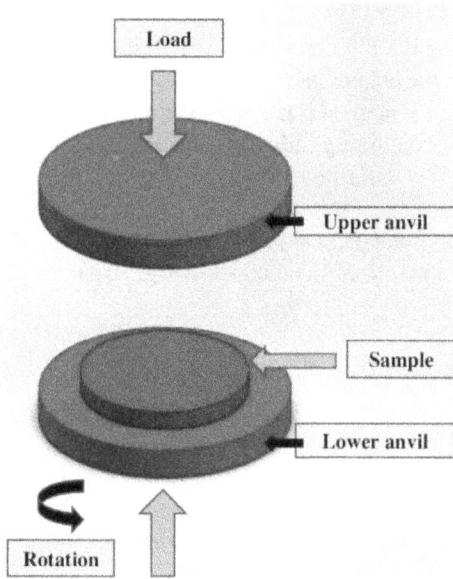

FIGURE 10.3 Schematic diagram for the high-pressure torsion (HPT) technique.

disadvantage of this technique is that it produces a non-uniform microstructure until applying enormous strain to the disc. Moreover, the processing speed of the technique is prolonged and since it involves high pressure, energy and torque, scaling up of the speed becomes very difficult. However, despite all these disadvantages, it has been considered a desirable nanostructuring technique in materials science.

10.3.1.3 Hydrostatic Extrusion (HE)

The hydrostatic extrusion (HE) method was first introduced and patented by James Robertson in 1893 and was first used for experiments in the 1950s by Percy W. Bridgman. This technique is a direct extrusion process performed in a liquid medium and denoted as direct hydraulic extrusion. The billet undergoing the processing is surrounded by a liquid medium (mainly oil), and the extrusion process begins with the piston's movement while the system is sealed by the direct contact between billet and die. The medium is compressed with the movement of the pistons and results in increased hydrostatic pressure inside the chamber. Once the applied stress is more than the yield strength and the friction gets reduced (as the medium restricts the contact between the chamber's wall and piston), plastic deformation of the material begins and eventually, after the processing, the conical-shaped billet is extruded from the die. In comparison with other methods like ECAP and HPT, this method is more suitable for bulk nanostructured production. However, unlike ECAP, it has one disadvantage of reducing the dimensions of the processed sample after processing and hence massive plastic deformation cannot be achieved. Other drawbacks of this method include the trouble of injection and removal of fluid during every extrusion process, loss in the energy during medium compaction and huge requirements for sealed structure and complications while performing extrusion at a high temperature.

10.3.1.4 Twist Extrusion (TE)

Twist extrusion (TE) is the SPD process in which samples are processed under high pressure created with the help of backpressure applied to the specimen while extruding out of the die. The TE method is based on the extrusion of the prism-shaped specimen through the die containing a dual prismatic area separated by the twist part. The specimen is severely deformed without any change in the original cross-section. This technique is beneficial for homogeneous grain refinement in metals like titanium and its alloys for biomedical applications. The grain refinement of the materials at the submicron level increases the metal's strength, making it suitable for orthopedic applications.

10.3.1.5 Friction Stir Processing

The friction stir processing (FSP) was induced from the friction stir welding technology introduced in 1991 by Wayne Thomas. This technique is associated with the surface modifications of the materials. It provides a microstructural modification of the near-surface layers of biomaterials, which quantifies that it offers localized deformation of metals. In this method, a rotating non-consumable cylindrical tool is used that is plunged on the localized area of the sheet or plate. The localized heat application results in softening of sample materials. The processing device also contains a rotating small diameter pin responsible for the heat generation in the area where the pin touches the metal surface. The heat production is basically due to the friction between the sample and the pin. The processed area cools naturally without solidification and leads to the formation of fine-grain microstructures [15]. The promising features of FSP motivated the application of this method for the microstructural modifications in metallic materials like Cu, Fe, Al and Ni alloys with improved modifications.

10.3.1.6 Accumulative Roll Bonding Process

There are a variety of plastic deformation techniques based on the rolling principle introduced for grain refinement up to the UFG level. One such technique is the ARB technique. A conventional rolling device is used in this technique. In this method, after the surface treatment, two metallic strips are placed on top of each other and rolled alike in the conventional rolling method. The rolled strips are then split into two pieces, and again, the obtained strips are surface treated, stacked and roll bonded. Figure 10.4 shows the process of ARB.

The process is usually executed at high temperatures rather than low temperatures. However, the temperature should not exceed the recrystallization temperature to avoid reducing the accumulative strain. Similar to FSP, it is also a solid-state method used to produce a metal-matrix with improved mechanical properties. It is usually processed without any lubricant for achieving better roll bonding. Further, as a comparison to other techniques, it has some limitations. The first limitation is that it is a lengthy process and needs precise technological precision. The second limitation is the direct impact of bonding quality on the mechanical properties of the samples. Still, this method is famous as a nanostructuring SPD technique and produces desirable nanostructures.

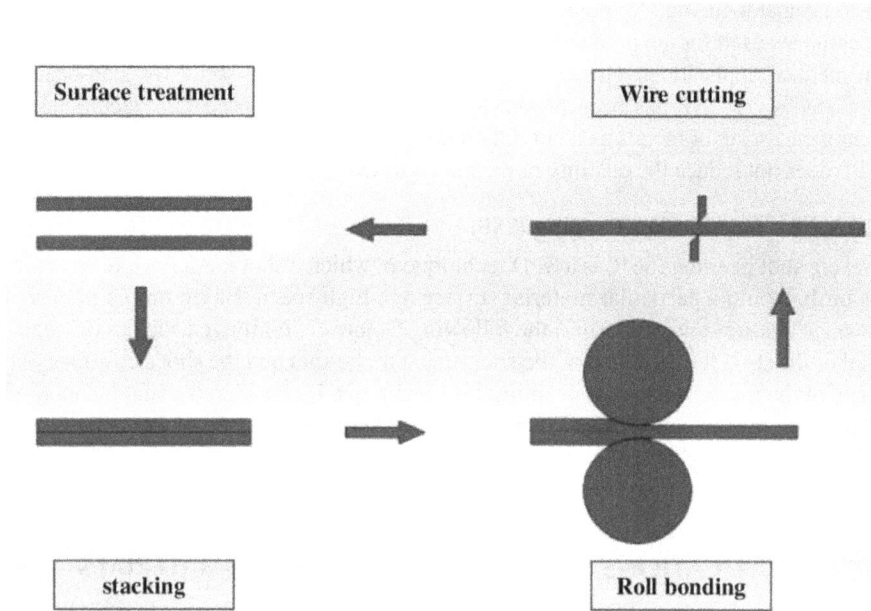

FIGURE 10.4 Schematic diagram of the steps followed in the accumulative roll bonding process.

10.3.1.7 Constrained Groove Pressing

This SPD technique is used to improvise the mechanical properties of UFG metals such as magnesium (Mg), copper (Cu), aluminum (Al), titanium (Ti), and nickel (Ni). without any alterations in the dimensions of the sample. This method involves the use of a groove at either of the three temperatures (room, elevated or cryogenic). It is one of the new forms of SPD techniques in which the specimen is subjected to repetitive deformation of shear-type at different levels of strains with the help of flat dies and a selected groove. In this technique, the sample thickness is similar to the distance between the dies and hence the resulting sample has whole dimensions. This method increases the hardness, strength and fatigue of the metal samples, but unlike ECAP, it decreases the ductility of the metal with the decrease in grain size.

10.3.1.8 Ball Milling (BM)

BM is the SPD method that is used for producing nanostructured materials. This is mostly used for producing metallic and ceramic-based nanomaterials. The system contains a grinding media containing wolfram carbide, or it can also be composed of steel. The balls contained in the container and the material (in the powdered form) are rotated inside the container with very high energy. Eventually, the balls fall on the material with gravity force and crush the material into nanostructured forms. It is used to produce porous materials used for implant applications. This method is used for the production of boron nitride nanotubes and carbon nanotubes. It is also a preferred technique for producing nanocrystals of metal oxides such as zinc oxide (ZnO) and cerium (CEO). Hence, it is a valuable method for porous nanostructured materials. There are many other SPD techniques used for the production of nanostructured materials, which are further used in medical applications. However, considering the most used metal for load-bearing applications, ECAP has been proved to be the most widely used SPD technique for nanostructuring of metals as it not only retains the dimensions of the metal sample but also does not reduce the ductility of the material with the decrease in the grain size.

10.3.1.9 Severe Shot Peening (SSP)

Severe shot peening (SSP) is a SPD technique in which a shot medium-like structure is pushed onto a particular material surface at a high speed. Based on the preferred surface features and properties, the following factors are optimized such as the material of the shot, the direction of the shot, speed of the shot and the shot's coverage and type of the material used for peening. This technique is considered a suitable method that is apt for the complex and intrinsic shapes of materials. The processed material offers special mechanical properties like strain hardening and better hardness compared to the material before processing.

10.4 APPLICATIONS OF NANOSTRUCTURED BIOMATERIALS

Nanostructured biomaterials, including conventional biomaterials and innovatory nanomaterials like nano-hydroxyapatite, protein-based nanostructures and carbon nanotubes (CNTs), play a crucial role in biomedical applications. The different types of applications include tissue engineering, medicine, drug encapsulation or drug delivery, antibacterial applications, dental and orthopedic applications [16].

10.4.1 TISSUE ENGINEERING AND REGENERATIVE MEDICINE

Tissue engineering and regenerative medicine aim to repair tissue and/or regeneration with the help of stem cells, scaffolds, growth and signaling factors. Tissue engineering serves as the alternate way to resolve orthopedic-related problems by reducing the limitations of traditional interventional methods. The effective ways of accomplishing tissue engineering include cell-based therapies, scaffold material implementation, growth factors and bioactive molecules delivery. The notable features of the materials to be used in scaffolds are biocompatibility, bioresorbability, mechanical properties and porosity.

Metal nanomaterials have acquired a higher preference as biomaterials for orthopedic and dental applications. Other than the conventionally used metals and alloys (stainless steel, titanium, TiAlV and Co–Cr alloys), metals like Cu, Mg, Zn, Al and Ag can also be used as biomaterials. However, if used in excess amounts, these materials can lead to cytotoxicity in the human blood. Materials like nHA (nanohydroxyapatite) are widely used for bone regeneration applications due to their morphological and functional similarity with natural bone. It is found to provide improved cellular behavior in terms of better cell adhesion, bone regeneration and cell proliferation compared to micro and macro-sized hydroxyapatite. Biopolymers like chitosan are of great use in preparing artificial bone materials, whereas its composite biomaterials are helpful in orthopedic tissue engineering applications [17]. HA/chitosan is a form of composite biomaterial that is used in orthopedic applications. They mimic the natural structure of the bone, and the addition of HA in chitosan enhances the material's mechanical properties. nHA/ chitosan has also found its use as a scaffold material for being nontoxic and possessing good cytocompatibility properties. Collagen is considered as the main component of bone, and hence a composite of collagen is a preferable material for bone tissue engineering applications. Scaffolds made of the nHA/collagen composite with mechanical properties similar to those of bone are examples of orthopedic applications. Another biopolymer used in bone tissue engineering applications is polylactic acid (PLA) which exhibits outstanding biocompatibility and biodegradability property. Nanohydroxyapatite and polylactic acid (nHA/PLA) composites manifest excellent mechanical, osteoconductive and osteoinductive properties with a good porosity in the scaffolds.

Nanostructured HA has been used so widely compared to its microscale or amorphous forms. It facilitates the bone regeneration process by improving the bone regeneration method's cell attachment, proliferation and differentiation phases. Another nanomaterial that has received quality attention for biomedical applications is protein-based peptide amphiphiles (Pas). PA nanomaterials are self-assembled and very promising nanomaterials for tissue engineering applications. Nanostructured scaffolds formed using PA nanofibers exhibit outstanding cell proliferation, cell adhesion and bone generation properties due to the high surface area-to-volume ratio. The nanostructured scaffolds mimic the architecture of human tissue at the nanoscale level. The high surface area-to-volume ratio of the nanofibers, along with their microporous structure, favors cell adhesion, proliferation, migration and differentiation, all of which are highly desired properties for tissue engineering applications. Due to the high surface energy, cell adhesion and protein adsorption are positively affected in nanostructured biomaterials. Further, this factor helps the nanostructured biomaterials increase wound healing while decreasing the inflammatory response compared to the conventional biomaterials.

10.4.2 DRUG DELIVERY

One of the essential applications of nanostructured materials in biomedical applications is drug delivery. To reduce the chances of bacterial infection, sterilization is usually performed on biomedical instruments. However, forgetting improved results, the drug delivery is associated with the surface modification by introducing coating of nanostructured particles (antibacterial biomaterials) on the drugs or the implants. Metal nanoparticles like titanium (Ti), silver (Ag), zinc (Zn), zinc oxide (ZnO) and zirconia (ZnO_2) are used in implant materials for reducing the bacterial adhesion of the implants. Some metallic, ceramic and polymeric materials are used as drug delivery vehicles or drug carriers in targeted drug delivery systems. The drug delivery system is supposed to enhance the therapeutic efficacy of the drugs along with the safety of therapeutic molecules of drugs.

10.4.3 ANTIBACTERIAL APPLICATIONS

The antibacterial application of nanostructured materials includes preventing bacterial colonization and biofilm formation in the implants or biomedical devices. The methods should solve the purpose of maintaining antibacterial protection for the long term, which is a desirable factor in load-bearing applications such as hip and knee implants. The properties like cytocompatibility and haemocompatibility cannot be compromised to ensure an antimicrobial material as it may end up in implant rejection. Hence, a detailed study regarding the outcomes of the interface between nano-antimicrobial entities and components of the body environment such as cells, tissues and proteins is essential. The metallic nanoparticles, which are based on nano-antimicrobials, are used to include Ag, Au, Cu/CuO, ZnO and chitosan with their nanocomposites. However, every nanomaterial has its own set of advantages and disadvantages, making the development of antimicrobial biomaterials difficult.

10.4.4 LOAD-BEARING APPLICATIONS

The human body consists of some load-bearing sites, such as load-bearing elements, including the skull, spine, joints, neck and pelvis. The implants or devices which are used for these sites come under load-bearing applications. All these sites are exposed to some loads, which are either static or repetitive loads as well; thereby, these elements should be capable of withstanding the load and, at the same time, increase the longevity of the implant. Any ideal load-bearing implants may be either orthopedic or dental, should increase the longevity of the device along with some must-have excellent mechanical properties such as high strength, fatigue and wear resistance, should have high corrosion resistance and should be highly biocompatible with an elastic modulus similar to that of human bone [18]. The mismatch in the elastic modulus of the bone and the implant may give rise to the stress shielding effect and hence need to be avoided as it leads to implant loosening. The need for revision surgery for implants like hip and knee joints is adamant and painful; thereby, selecting the ideal nanostructured biomaterial for such application is required. Considering all these factors, metal nanomaterials are the better option for load-bearing applications, and under that category, pure titanium, titanium alloys and stainless steel are better materials for load-bearing applications [19]. Avoiding alloys is preferable to restrict the adverse effects and allergic reactions caused by the alloying elements. Other materials like calcium phosphate bioceramics and some scaffolds of polymers are also used for these applications.

10.4.5 OTHER APPLICATIONS OF NANOMATERIALS

A wide range of biomedical applications of nanostructured biomaterials includes bioimaging, cancer or virus detection, gene detection and diagnosis [20]. Metallic nanoparticles such as gold nanoparticles are in high demand for bioimaging like MRI and CT scans. Quantum dots are also used for imaging in medical diagnosis. Silicon nanowires can be used to detect specific genes as well as for cancer/virus detection. Other nanomaterials with similar applications, such as disease detection and gene detection, are carbon nanotubes.

10.5 CONCLUSION

Metallic biomaterials are the most widely used biomaterials for biomedical applications due to their mechanical properties and desirable implant applications.

Nanostructuring of materials is crucial to increase the material's strength by grain refinement as per the Hall–Petch equation. Overcoming the drawbacks of many conventional grain-refining techniques, SPD techniques are promising for obtaining nanostructured metals. These methods are an extension of conventional nanostructuring methods to produce bulk nanostructured materials for various medical applications. These techniques are used to synthesize and produce nanostructured biomaterials for implant applications with enhanced mechanical properties. One of the most widely used SPD techniques is the ECAP process, which retains the dimensions of the processing billet and does not reduce the ductility of the material. ECAP is useful for synthesizing and processing biomaterials for load-bearing applications. However, many new SPD techniques have evolved to resolve various problems. Due to the advancement in technology, new biomaterials are also being synthesized for various purposes, and the use of nanomaterials for biomedical applications is the need of the era. As a future scope, the use of these SPD techniques for further enhancing the quality of the biomaterial and increasing the efficiency of the implant material with minimum drawbacks can be a promising area.

REFERENCES

1. Mishnaevsky L. et al., "Nanostructured titanium-based materials for medical implants: Modeling and development," *Mater. Sci. Eng. R Reports*, vol. 81, no. 1, pp. 1–19, (2014).
2. Verma R. P., "Titanium based biomaterial for bone implants: A mini review," *Mater. Today Proc.*, vol. 26, pp. 3148–3151, (2020).
3. Elias C. N., Meyers M. A., Valiev R. Z., and Monteiro S. N., "Ultrafine grained titanium for biomedical applications: An overview of performance," *J. Mater. Res. Technol.*, vol. 2, no. 4, pp. 340–350, (2013).
4. Estrin Y., Lapovok R., Medvedev A. E., Kasper C., Ivanova E., and Lowe T. C., "Mechanical performance and cell response of pure titanium with ultrafine-grained structure produced by severe plastic deformation." In Froes H.F. and Qian M. (Ed.), *Woodhead Publishing Series in Biomaterials, Titanium in Medical and Dental Applications*, Woodhead Publishing., pp. 419–454, (2018).
5. Gang S., Fengzhou F., and Chengwei K., "Tribological performance of bioimplants: A comprehensive review," *Nami Jishu yu Jingmi Gongcheng/Nanotechnology Precis. Eng.*, vol. 1, no. 2, pp. 107–122, (2018).
6. Valiev R. Z., Parfenov E. V., and Parfenova L. V., "Developing nanostructured metals for manufacturing of medical implants with improved design and biofunctionality," *Mater. Trans.*, vol. 60, no. 7, pp. 1356–1366, (2019).
7. Kaur T., Thirugnanam A., and Pramanik K., "Effect of carboxylated graphene nanoplatelets on mechanical and in-vitro biological properties of polyvinyl alcohol nanocomposite scaffolds for bone tissue engineering," *Mater. Today Commun.*, vol. 12, no. June, pp. 34–42, (2017).
8. Saad M., Akhtar S., and Srivastava S., "Composite polymer in orthopedic implants: A review," *Mater. Today Proc.*, vol. 5, no. 9, pp. 20224–20231, (2018).
9. Azushima A. et al., "Severe plastic deformation (SPD) processes for metals," *CIRP Ann. - Manuf. Technol.*, vol. 57, no. 2, pp. 716–735, (2008).
10. Webster T. J. and Ahn E. S., "Nanostructured biomaterials for tissue engineering bone," *Adv. Biochem. Eng. Biotechnol.*, vol. 103, no. June, pp. 275–308, (2006).
11. Valiev R. Z., Islamgaliev R. K., and Alexandrov I. V., "Bulk nanostructured materials from severe plastic deformation", *Progress Mater. Sci.* vol. 45, no. 2. (2000).

12. Kapoor R., "Severe Plastic Deformation of Materials", "Materials under extreme conditions: Recent trends and future prospects", vol. 1, no. February, pp. 717–754, (2017).

13. Kalantari K., Saleh B., and Webster T. J., "Biological applications of severely plastically deformed nano-grained medical devices: A review," *Nanomaterials*, vol. 11, no. 3, pp. 1–24, (2021).

14. Agarwal K. M., Tyagi R. K., Singhal A., and Bhatia D., "Effect of ECAP on the mechanical properties of titanium and its alloys for biomedical applications," *Mater. Sci. Energy Technol.*, vol. 3, pp. 921–927, (2020).

15. Iwaszko J., Kuda K., Fila K., and Strzelecka M., "The effect of friction stir processing (fsp) on the microstructure and properties of am60 magnesium alloy," *Arch. Metall. Mater.*, vol. 61, no. 3, pp. 1209–1214, (2016).

16. Wang M. and Webster T. J., "Nano-Biomaterials and Their Applications," In Narayan R. (Ed.) *Encyclopedia of Biomedical Engineering*, New York, Elsevier, vol. 1–3, pp. 153–161, (2019).

17. Vyas V., Kaur T., and Thirugnanam A., "Chitosan composite three dimensional macrospheric scaffolds for bone tissue engineering," *Int. J. Biol. Macromol.*, vol. 104, pp. 1946–1954, (2017).

18. Thirugnanam A., Sampath Kumar T. S., and Chakkingal U., "Tailoring the bioactivity of commercially pure titanium by grain refinement using groove pressing," *Mater. Sci. Eng. C*, vol. 30, no. 1, pp. 203–208, (2010).

19. Ratna Sunil B., Thirugnanam A., Chakkingal U., and Sampath Kumar T. S., "Nano and ultra fine grained metallic biomaterials by severe plastic deformation techniques," *Mater. Technol.*, vol. 31, no. 13, pp. 743–755, (2016).

20. Siddique S. and Chow J. C. L., "Application of nanomaterials in biomedical imaging and cancer therapy," *Nanomaterials*, vol. 10, no. 9, pp. 1–41, (2020).

11 Improved Biodegradable Implant Materials for Orthopedic Applications

Kundan Kumar, Shashi Bhushan Prasad and Ashish Das
National Institute of Technology Jamshedpur

Mukul Shukla
Motilal Nehru National Institute of Technology Allahabad

CONTENTS

11.1 INTRODUCTION

Bone problems affect millions of people worldwide. Several reasons behind these defects are aging, illness, accidents, and injuries. Orthopedic biomaterials are implanted in the human body to replace or repair defects of different tissues such as bones, ligaments or cartilage, and tendons. In the last 50 years, there has been significant development of biomaterials for orthopedic implant applications. While the first generation of implant materials was of bioinert materials used in physiological environments, the second generation has been the use of bioactive and

DOI: 10.1201/9781003286806-11

biodegradable materials. Two types of implants such as permanent and temporary biomaterials are used to replace or repair these defects. Permanent implants are used as joint and bone replacement as well as in the repair and regeneration of bone. On the other hand, temporary implants are only used to repair and regenerate bone. Permanent implants are nondegradable fixation materials and are very efficient. To prevent any antagonistic effects, the patient's body requires revision surgery to remove these implants after tissue regeneration for orthopedic applications. Temporary implants are biodegradable and require no revision surgery to remove these implants. Therefore, these implants minimize the extra cost of revision surgery, trauma, and complications of a patient. They provide temporary support to the fractured bone and can regenerate new tissue at a rate identical to the degradation rate of implants [1]. The special features of biodegradable implants are their scaffold functions, which are helped in seeded cells and allow new tissue development [2,3]. To design an implant material, the properties needed to keep in mind are mechanical properties, biodegradability, and biocompatibility. One of the foremost requirements of these implants is not to lose their mechanical integrity before complete bone healing. In this chapter, we have studied temporary implants used in orthopedic applications. The biodegradable implant should not lose mechanical integrity before bone healing and allow place for new tissue to form. An initially implanted biomaterial, degraded products, and related products ought not to be toxic, allergenic, and inflammatory [4]. Load is gradually transferred from an implant to newly generated tissue. Three types of biodegradable implant biomaterials are generally used which are metal, polymer, and ceramic.

In the last few decades, a lot of research works have been carried out on the investigation and development of biodegradable implants for orthopedic applications. In this chapter, different types of biodegradable material for orthopedic applications will be discussed and a rigorous insight into the various possible strategies to develop improved biodegradable implant materials for futuristic orthopedic applications is provided.

11.2 BIODEGRADABLE METALLIC IMPLANTS

Titanium and its alloys, cobalt-based alloys, and stainless steels are different metallic biomaterials that have been widely used for orthopedic applications since the mid of the last century. The damages of bone tissues have been continuously repaired or replaced by these implants until now due to the admirable blend of biocompatibility, corrosion resistance, and mechanical properties. However, some drawbacks are there for the development of new biomaterials. The above-mentioned metallic biomaterials have a higher elastic modulus, which causes a stress-shielding effect owing to unmatched elastic modulus that may affect the osseointegration, loosening of the implant, and bone resorption by the body [5–8]. Permanent implants have deprived wear resistance, poor bending ductility, toxicity of their release ions, and allergenicity, which are additional disadvantages [7–12]. Also, nonbiodegradability in the physiological environment is another issue and after bone healing, additional surgery is required to remove these implants from the patient body to avert any antagonistic effects [4,13,14]. Biodegradable metals with matching mechanical properties compared with cortical bone and their better biocompatibility in physiological environments are the best solution for the desired implant. In light of this, biodegradable metals such as iron, zinc, and magnesium are highly desirable. These metals have essential trace elements inside the human body and take part in several biological functions and as implants, they are gradually degraded and completely dissolve in vivo after fulfilling the missions of healing of bone [15–17]. Also, these metals are nontoxic, so their alloys and composites have several biomedical applications.

11.2.1 IRON-BASED IMPLANTS

Compared to Mg, Fe-based materials have a significantly low degradation rate but a higher value of mechanical properties in biological environments. Their elastic modulus is 200 GPa. As biodegradable implants, Fe-based alloys have a strong mechanical strength, which is required for tissue healing [18]. Several in vivo and in vitro studies have shown that Fe-based implants are biocompatible and safe in physiological environments [19–21]; however, excess iron intake causes toxicity [22]. Iron implants have a significantly low degradation rate with an implantation period of 52 weeks and thus their appropriateness as temporary implants become doubtful [23]. The degradation rate of Fe-based biomaterials has been increased by alloying and forming composite. The alloying elements such as manganese, palladium, or silver are added to iron to enhance the degradation rate. Addition of these elements in large amounts hampers the biocompatibility of alloy implants. Recently, to enhance the degradation rate, iron matrix composites have been used as biomaterials for orthopedic implants by incorporating ceramic particles such as hydroxyapatite (HA), β-tricalcium phosphate (TCP), and HA-TCP.

11.2.2 ZINC-BASED IMPLANTS

Zinc shows excellent processability and superior corrosion resistance as compared to magnesium. It does not evolve gases during biodegradation [24,25]. Zinc takes part in several elementary biotic functions. It also interacts with a lot of carbon-based ligands. It plays an important role in the mineralization and growth of bone tissues [26]. It plays an important role in bone mass preservation. Pure zinc has in vivo and in vitro degradation rates of approximately 0.2 mm/year and 0.06–0.08, respectively [5]. Zinc has mechanical integrity of 12–24 weeks in a biological environment that is highly desirable as an implant [27]. However, the low mechanical strength of zinc is a major issue restricting its application as an implant. Alloys and composites of zinc are feasible materials to increase their mechanical strength.

11.2.3 MAGNESIUM-BASED IMPLANTS

Magnesium (Mg) is the lightest structure metal and is the eighth most abundant element found worldwide. It is the fourth most abundant material in the human body. It has a high strength-to-weight ratio and a high damping capacity. It is the easiest structure metal for machines and complex shapes could be easily produced using this. 325 or more enzymatic reactions occur in the human body, which require Mg as a cofactor. Muscles, heart, kidneys, and bones have proper functioning in the presence of an element like Mg [28]. The cortical bone density (1.8–2.1 gm/cm^3) is close to the density of pure Mg (1.74 gm/cm^3) [29]. Young's modulus of cortical bone (10–30 GPa) is close to that of Mg (40–45 GPa), which causes a very little stress-shielding effect. The recommended dosage of Mg for adults is 280–300 mg and that for children is 250 mg daily in the human body. Mg has good mechanical properties, excellent bio-compatibility, as well as biodegradability, which are desirable properties for an ideal orthopedic temporary implant. However, rapid biodegradation is a major issue of Mg as an implant where before bone healing the mechanical integrity is lost. Hydrogen gas evolution takes place as a result of the biodegradation of Mg implants that retard the healing process of tissue. To overcome the issue of high biodegradation rate, engineering approaches such as alloying, surface modification/coating, and compos-ites have been used. Mg-based implants and bone interface are shown in Figure 11.1 [1]. Mg alloys are the most common choice as implants but the main limitations are that not all alloying elements are biocompatible. Surface modifications/coatings are better ways to improve biodegradability but not as desirable as Mg matrix compos-ites. The biodegradation of Mg-based implants and the desired rate of tissue heal-ing are shown in Figure 11.2 [1]. In an Mg matrix composite, the Mg matrix used pure/alloys of Mg, whereas the reinforcements used are hydroxyapatite, graphene nanoplatelets (GNPs), SiO_2, etc. The composite has better properties than any of its constituents. The biocompatibility and applications of reinforcements used in an Mg matrix are listed in Table 11.1 [4,30].

As discussed above, a magnesium matrix composite is the most prominent choice as implants for orthopedic applications. It has two constituents, the matrix and the reinforcement. Matrix is the major constituent (>50%) and reinforcement is the minor constituent (<50%). The composite has better properties than any constitu-ents. Fabrication of a magnesium matrix composite may be classified according to the state of Mg matrices such as liquid state or solid-state or others (including in situ, semi-solid-state, and others). We are discussing some most common methods of fabricating magnesium matrix composites, which are stir casting and powder met-allurgy. Also, we are discussing some typical methods like friction stir processing

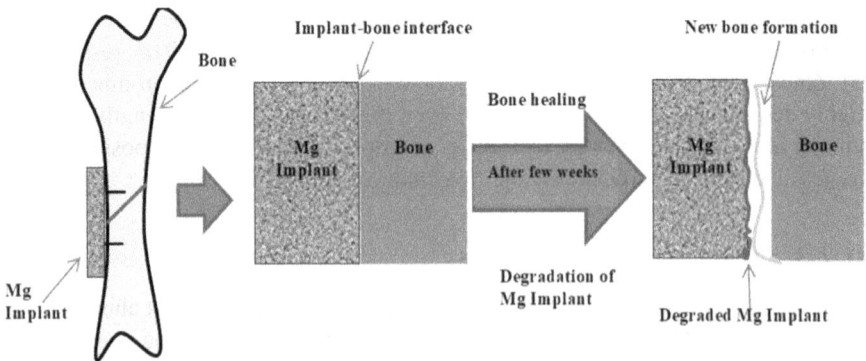

FIGURE 11.1 Mg-based implants biodegradation and tissue healing at the bone–implant interface [1].

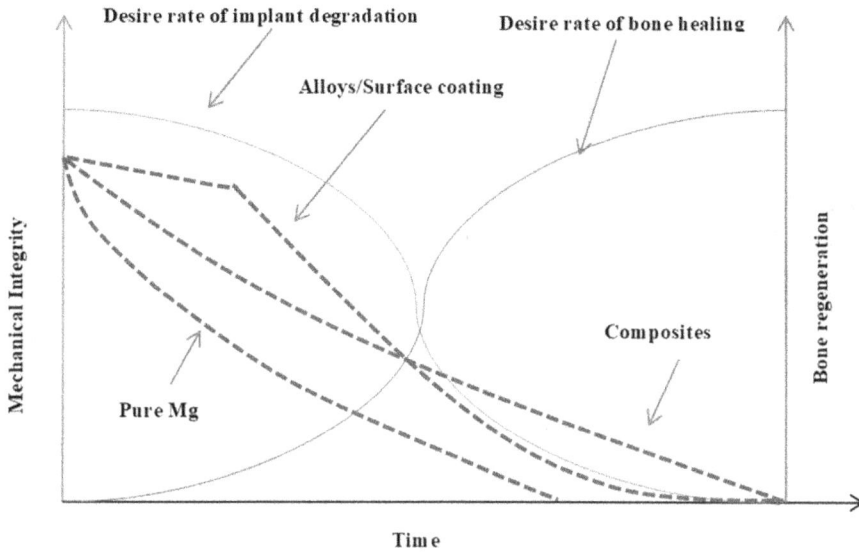

FIGURE 11.2 Biodegradation of Mg-based implants, the desired degradation rate of an ideal implant, and the desired rate of healing of fractured bone [1].

TABLE 11.1
Some Common Reinforcements Used in the Mg Matrix [4]

Reinforcement	Biocompatibility	Applications
ZnO_2	Improves cell viability, greater bone stability, bioinert to blood, and nontoxic	Artificial knee, femoral head, bone screw
Al_2O_3	Cell adhesion, proliferation, and protein adsorption improvement	Knee prosthesis, bone plate, bone screws
GNPs	Biocompatible even in blood contact, no tissue reaction, and nontoxic to cells	Bone screws, bone plates, endovascular materials
Y_2O_3	Cell viability improvement	Dental implant
HA	Nontoxic and bioactive, reduction in the release of the Mg ion, excellent cell proliferation, and osteoblastic differentiation	Bone joint, bone pins, and screw
FA	Enhance cell viability and osteoconductivity	Bone screw, bone pins, bone plate
Si_3N_4	Promotes bone fusion in spinal surgery and bone–cell adhesion	Knee joints, prosthetic hip, spinal fusion devices
CPC	Do not cause inflammation. Bioinert, higher protein adsorption and nontoxic to tissues, excellent proliferation, and osteoblastic differentiation induction	Bone tissue, joint replacements, and dental implant
SiC	Slightly toxic, durable coating for bone prosthetics	Hip replacement, bone plate, bone screw

(FSP) to fabricate surface or bulk composites. Stir casting is a liquid state method whereas powder metallurgy and FSP are solid-state methods. Other fabrication methods are semi-solid casting [31], sol–gel method [32], disintegrated melt deposition [31], ultrasound-assisted particle dispersion method [33], FSP [31], accumulative roll bonding [31], and vacuum cold spraying [34].

11.2.3.1 Fabrication of Magnesium Matrix Composite by Stir Casting

In stir casting, Mg matrix is heated first and reinforcement is mixed uniformly in the molten matrix using a stirrer driven by a motor as shown in Figure 11.3. Then the mixture of molten Mg matrix and reinforcement is poured into the mold. After solidification, the specimen is removed from the mold and that specimen is Mg matrix composite.

11.2.3.2 Fabrication of Magnesium Matrix Composite by Powder Metallurgy

Powder metallurgy is a solid-state method of fabrication of Mg matrix composites where steps of manufacturing are the production of powders, blending, compaction, sintering, and secondary finishing operations as shown in Figure 11.4. There are several methods of production of powder such as milling, atomization, chemical reduction, and electrolytic deposition. Blending is used for the uniform mixing of Mg matrix and reinforcement particles. Desired shapes and sizes are obtained using the die and punch to produce a green compact in the comparison process.

The green compact is heated in a controlled environment in the furnace to tie the particles in the sintering process. The sintering temperature is below the melting

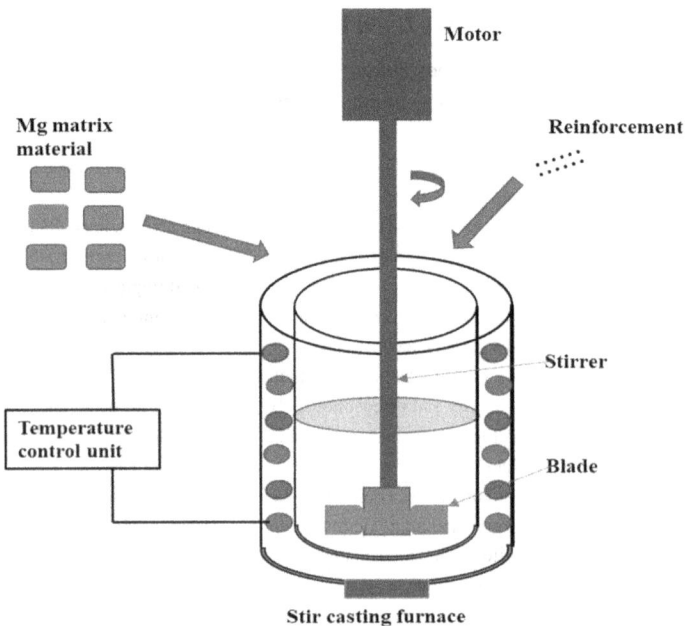

FIGURE 11.3 Furnace of stir casting for the fabrication of composites.

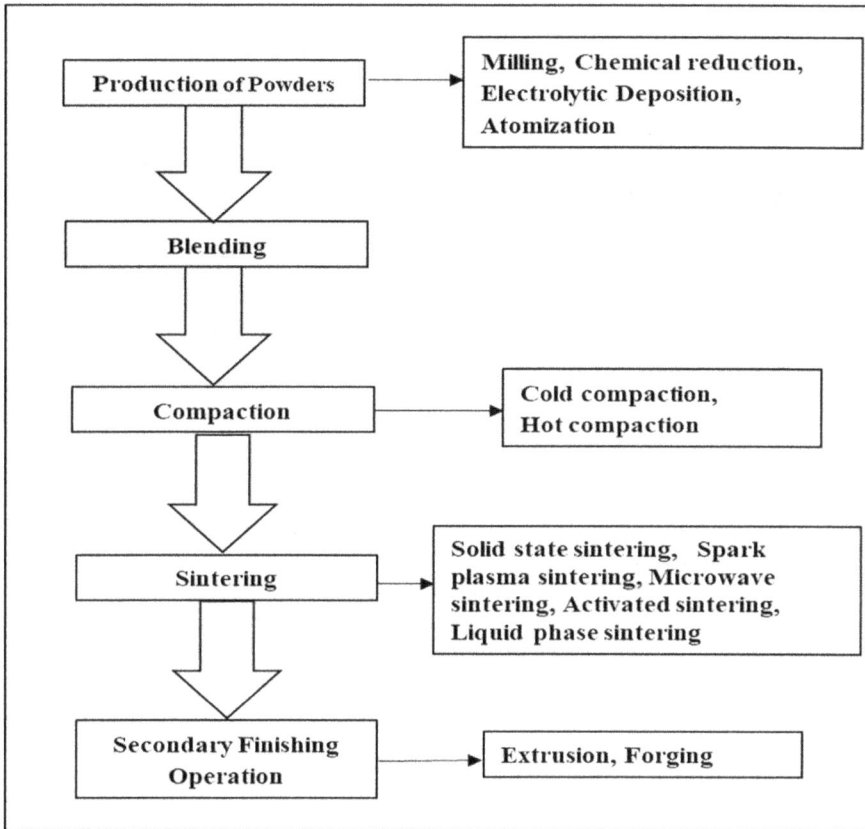

FIGURE 11.4 Fabrication of composites by powder metallurgy.

temperature of powder particles. Finally, secondary operations are used for finishing if required.

11.2.3.3 Friction Stir Processing (FSP)

FSP is the solid-state process of fabrication of surface composites or bulk composites. Generally, a milling machine with special attachments is used for these purposes. In this process, a groove is made in workpieces as shown in Figure 11.5, and the groove is filled with reinforcement particles. The workpiece is clapped by a fixture in a vertical milling machine. The FSP tool without pin is used to seal the grooves to prevent scattering of the reinforcement particles. Then, the FSP tool with pin is used to incorporate and disperse reinforcement particles into the Mg plate to make surface or bulk composites.

11.3 POLYMER-BASED IMPLANTS

Biodegradable polymers are broadly classified into natural- and synthetic-based polymers. Some natural-based polymers are starch, chitosan, collagen, and hyaluronic

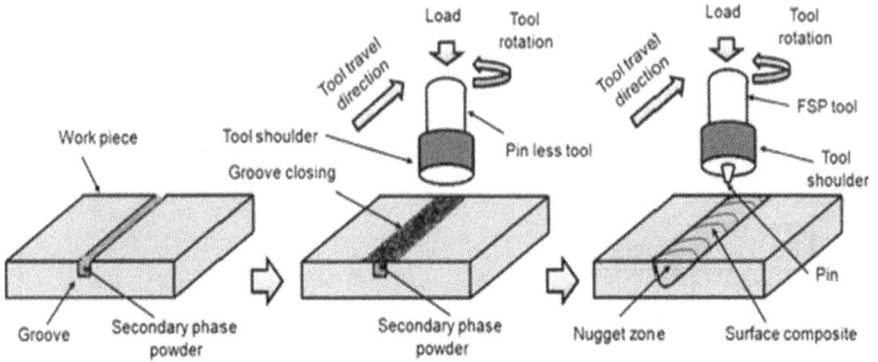

FIGURE 11.5   Fabrication of composites by friction stir processing [35,36].

acid derivatives. Owing to high biological activity, low mechanical strength, repellence, and unidentified rate of degradation, natural-based polymers have limited use of a temporary implant. In light of this, synthetic polymers have been shown to have a lot of potentials to overcome these challenges. Synthetic biodegradable polymers have been the subject of the most widely researched. In this row, poly (α-hydroxy acids) also known as polyesters are used as biodegradable implants. The most commonly used polyesters are poly(glycolic acid) (PGA), poly(lactic acid) (PLA), and poly(lactic-co-glycolide) as a copolymer of two [37,38]. These polymers are used as candidate biomaterial implants for the repair and rebirth of bone tissue because of their biodegradability and biocompatibility in a biological environment [39].

11.4   CERAMIC-BASED IMPLANTS

As a substitute for metallic biomaterials, ceramic-based biomaterials were initially examined and used for orthopedic implant applications owing to their biocompatibility, bioactivity, and biodegradability. Zirconia (ZrO_2) [40] and alumina (Al_2O_3) [41] were, initially, developed as bioinert bioceramics to fabricate femoral heads. Ceramic biomaterials are presently used for the repair of bone fracture and bone defect filling as well as the replacement and stabilization of defected bone tissues [42,43]. Periodontal, dental, maxillofacial, cochlear, otolaryngology, and spinal discs are the area where presently bioceramics are used. The risk of disease immunogenicity and transmission is avoided by the use of bioceramic implants. The physical and chemical composition of bioceramics is used to determine their biological response. The drawbacks of bioceramics are brittleness, poor fracture toughness, and very high stiffness [44] that limit their orthopedic implant applications.

11.5   CONCLUSION

The field of biomaterial developments has a series of journey to come to the present state and has enormous chances to further develop for orthopedic implant applications. The first generation of development of biomaterials is bioinert. The second generation of their development is biodegradable, bioactive, and biocompatible materials. The molecular level is designed to stimulate specific responses in the development of their third generation. Still now, the second and third generation are under development stages. In light of this, biodegradable implants are temporary fixations and require no revision surgery to remove from the patient body. Biodegradable biomaterials are biometals, biopolymers, and bioceramics. Biopolymers are biocompatible and biodegradable but have low mechanical strength that impedes their application. Bioceramics are brittle that limits their applications. Biodegradable metals are conventional choices where magnesium-based materials are most widely accepted owing to admirable mechanical and biocompatibility properties.

REFERENCES

1. K. Kumar, A. Das, and S. B. Prasad, "Recent developments in biodegradable magnesium matrix composites for orthopaedic applications: A review based on biodegradability, mechanical and biocompatibility perspective," *Mater. Today Proc.*, vol. 44, pp. 2038–2042, 2021, doi: 10.1016/j.matpr.2020.12.133.
2. C. A. Heath, "Cells for tissue engineering," *Trends Biotechnol.*, vol. 18, no. 1, pp. 17–19, Jan. 2000, doi: 10.1016/S0167-7799(99)01396-7.
3. J. J. Marler, J. Upton, R. Langer, and J. P. Vacanti, "Transplantation of cells in matrices for tissue regeneration," *Adv. Drug Deliv. Rev.*, vol. 33, no. 1–2, pp. 165–182, Aug. 1998, doi: 10.1016/S0169-409X(98)00025-8.
4. M. Shahin, K. Munir, C. Wen, and Y. Li, "Magnesium matrix nanocomposites for orthopedic applications: A review from mechanical, corrosion, and biological perspectives," *Acta Biomater.*, vol. 96, pp. 1–19, 2019, doi: 10.1016/j.actbio.2019.06.007.
5. D. Vojtěch, J. Kubásek, J. Šerák, and P. Novák, "Mechanical and corrosion properties of newly developed biodegradable Zn-based alloys for bone fixation," *Acta Biomater.*, vol. 7, no. 9, pp. 3515–3522, Sep. 2011, doi: 10.1016/j.actbio.2011.05.008.
6. F. Witte et al., "Degradable biomaterials based on magnesium corrosion," *Curr. Opin. Solid State Mater. Sci.*, vol. 12, no. 5–6, pp. 63–72, Oct. 2008, doi: 10.1016/j.cossms.2009.04.001.
7. A. Biesiekierski, J. Wang, M. Abdel-Hady Gepreel, and C. Wen, "A new look at biomedical Ti-based shape memory alloys," *Acta Biomater.*, vol. 8, no. 5, pp. 1661–1669, May 2012, doi: 10.1016/j.actbio.2012.01.018.
8. K. Yang, L. Tan, P. Wan, X. Yu, and Z. Ma, "Biodegradable metals for orthopedic applications," in *Orthopedic Biomaterials*, Cham: Springer International Publishing, 2017, pp. 275–309.
9. A. M. Ribeiro, T. H. S. Flores-Sahagun, and R. C. Paredes, "A perspective on molybdenum biocompatibility and antimicrobial activity for applications in implants," *J. Mater. Sci.*, vol. 51, no. 6, pp. 2806–2816, Mar. 2016, doi: 10.1007/s10853-015-9664-y.
10. M. Cramers and U. Lucht, "Metal sensitivity in patients treated for tibial fractures with plates of stainless steel," *Acta Orthop. Scand.*, vol. 48, no. 3, pp. 245–249, Jan. 1977, doi: 10.3109/17453677708988763.
11. R. Radha and D. Sreekanth, "Insight of magnesium alloys and composites for orthopedic implant applications – a review," *J. Magnes. Alloy.*, vol. 5, no. 3, pp. 286–312, Sep. 2017, doi: 10.1016/j.jma.2017.08.003.
12. L. C. Lucas, R. A. Buchanan, J. E. Lemons, and C. D. Griffin, "Susceptibility of surgical cobalt-base alloy to pitting corrosion," *J. Biomed. Mater. Res.*, vol. 16, no. 6, pp. 799–810, Nov. 1982, doi: 10.1002/jbm.820160606.

13. H. Windhagen et al., "Biodegradable magnesium-based screw clinically equivalent to titanium screw in hallux valgus surgery: Short term results of the first prospective, randomized, controlled clinical pilot study," *Biomed. Eng. Online*, vol. 12, no. 1, p. 62, 2013, doi: 10.1186/1475-925X-12-62.

14. C. Castellani et al., "Bone–implant interface strength and osseointegration: Biodegradable magnesium alloy versus standard titanium control," *Acta Biomater.*, vol. 7, no. 1, pp. 432–440, Jan. 2011, doi: 10.1016/j.actbio.2010.08.020.

15. M. Saini, "Implant biomaterials: A comprehensive review," *World J. Clin. Cases*, vol. 3, no. 1, p. 52, 2015, doi: 10.12998/wjcc.v3.i1.52.

16. X. Tong et al., "Microstructure, mechanical properties, biocompatibility, and in vitro corrosion and degradation behavior of a new Zn–5Ge alloy for biodegradable implant materials," *Acta Biomater.*, vol. 82, pp. 197–204, Dec. 2018, doi: 10.1016/j.actbio.2018.10.015.

17. M. S. Dargusch et al., "Exploring the role of manganese on the microstructure, mechanical properties, biodegradability, and biocompatibility of porous iron-based scaffolds," *ACS Biomater. Sci. Eng.*, vol. 5, no. 4, pp. 1686–1702, Apr. 2019, doi: 10.1021/acsbiomaterials.8b01497.

18. C. G. Finkemeier, "Bone-grafting and bone-graft substitutes," *J. Bone Jt. Surgery-American Vol.*, vol. 84, no. 3, pp. 454–464, Mar. 2002, doi: 10.2106/00004623-200203000-00020.

19. B. Liu and Y. F. Zheng, "Effects of alloying elements (Mn, Co, Al, W, Sn, B, C and S) on biodegradability and in vitro biocompatibility of pure iron," *Acta Biomater.*, vol. 7, no. 3, pp. 1407–1420, Mar. 2011, doi: 10.1016/j.actbio.2010.11.001.

20. H. Hermawan, A. Purnama, D. Dube, J. Couet, and D. Mantovani, "Fe–Mn alloys for metallic biodegradable stents: Degradation and cell viability studies☆," *Acta Biomater.*, vol. 6, no. 5, pp. 1852–1860, May 2010, doi: 10.1016/j.actbio.2009.11.025.

21. M. Peuster et al., "Degradation of tungsten coils implanted into the subclavian artery of New Zealand white rabbits is not associated with local or systemic toxicity," *Biomaterials*, vol. 24, no. 3, pp. 393–399, Feb. 2003, doi: 10.1016/S0142-9612(02)00352-6.

22. G. Papanikolaou and K. Pantopoulos, "Iron metabolism and toxicity," *Toxicol. Appl. Pharmacol.*, vol. 202, no. 2, pp. 199–211, Jan. 2005, doi: 10.1016/j.taap.2004.06.021.

23. T. Kraus et al., "Biodegradable Fe-based alloys for use in osteosynthesis: Outcome of an in vivo study after 52weeks," *Acta Biomater.*, vol. 10, no. 7, pp. 3346–3353, Jul. 2014, doi: 10.1016/j.actbio.2014.04.007.

24. T. Kraus, S. F. Fischerauer, A. C. Hänzi, P. J. Uggowitzer, J. F. Löffler, and A. M. Weinberg, "Magnesium alloys for temporary implants in osteosynthesis: In vivo studies of their degradation and interaction with bone," *Acta Biomater.*, vol. 8, no. 3, pp. 1230–1238, Mar. 2012, doi: 10.1016/j.actbio.2011.11.008.

25. P. K. Bowen, J. Drelich, and J. Goldman, "Zinc exhibits ideal physiological corrosion behavior for bioabsorbable stents," *Adv. Mater.*, vol. 25, no. 18, pp. 2577–2582, May 2013, doi: 10.1002/adma.201300226.

26. C. J. Frederickson, J.-Y. Koh, and A. I. Bush, "The neurobiology of zinc in health and disease," *Nat. Rev. Neurosci.*, vol. 6, no. 6, pp. 449–462, Jun. 2005, doi: 10.1038/nrn1671.

27. Y. F. Zheng, X. N. Gu, and F. Witte, "Biodegradable metals," *Mater. Sci. Eng. R Reports*, vol. 77, pp. 1–34, Mar. 2014, doi: 10.1016/j.mser.2014.01.001.

28. V. V. R, P. R, and G. M, "Synthesis and characterization of magnesium alloy surface composite (AZ91D - SiO_2) by friction stir processing for bioimplants," *Silicon*, vol. 12, no. 5, pp. 1085–1102, 2020, doi: 10.1007/s12633-019-00194-6.

29. W. Ding, "Opportunities and challenges for the biodegradable magnesium alloys as next-generation biomaterials," pp. 79–86, 2016, doi: 10.1093/rb/rbw003.

30. K. Kumar, A. Das, and S. B. Prasad, "Biodegradable metal matrix composites for orthopedic implant applications: A review," 2021, pp. 557–565.

31. M. Malaki et al., *Advanced Metal Matrix Nanocomposites*, vol. 9, no. 3. 2019.

32. M. Ashuri, F. Moztarzadeh, N. Nezafati, A. Ansari Hamedani, and M. Tahriri, "Development of a composite based on hydroxyapatite and magnesium and zinc-containing sol-gel-derived bioactive glass for bone substitute applications," *Mater. Sci. Eng. C*, vol. 32, no. 8, pp. 2330–2339, 2012, doi: 10.1016/j.msec.2012.07.004.

33. H. Dieringa, "Processing of magnesium-based metal matrix nanocomposites by ultrasound-assisted particle dispersion: A review," *Metals (Basel).*, vol. 8, no. 6, 2018, doi: 10.3390/met8060431.

34. Y. Liu, Z. Dang, Y. Wang, J. Huang, and H. Li, "Hydroxyapatite/graphene-nanosheet composite coatings deposited by vacuum cold spraying for biomedical applications: Inherited nanostructures and enhanced properties," *Carbon N. Y.*, vol. 67, pp. 250–259, 2014, doi: 10.1016/j.carbon.2013.09.088.

35. P. K. Nakka et al., "Developing composites of ZE41 Mg alloy - naturally derived hydroxyapatite by friction stir processing: Investigating in vitro degradation behavior," *Mater. Technol.*, vol. 33, no. 9, pp. 603–611, 2018, doi: 10.1080/10667857.2018.1483470.

36. B. Ratna Sunil, T. S. Sampath Kumar, U. Chakkingal, V. Nandakumar, and M. Doble, "Friction stir processing of magnesium-nanohydroxyapatite composites with controlled in vitro degradation behavior," *Mater. Sci. Eng. C*, vol. 39, no. 1, pp. 315–324, 2014, doi: 10.1016/j.msec.2014.03.004.

37. B. Seal, "Polymeric biomaterials for tissue and organ regeneration," *Mater. Sci. Eng. R Reports*, vol. 34, no. 4–5, pp. 147–230, Oct. 2001, doi: 10.1016/S0927-796X(01)00035-3.

38. J. F. Mano, R. A. Sousa, L. F. Boesel, N. M. Neves, and R. L. Reis, "Bioinert, biodegradable and injectable polymeric matrix composites for hard tissue replacement: State of the art and recent developments," *Compos. Sci. Technol.*, vol. 64, no. 6, pp. 789–817, May 2004, doi: 10.1016/j.compscitech.2003.09.001.

39. L. S. Nair and C. T. Laurencin, "Biodegradable polymers as biomaterials," *Prog. Polym. Sci.*, vol. 32, no. 8–9, pp. 762–798, Aug. 2007, doi: 10.1016/j.progpolymsci.2007.05.017.

40. U. Lohbauer, M. Zipperle, K. Rischka, A. Petschelt, and F. A. Müller, *J. Biomed. Mater. Res. Part B Appl. Biomater.*, vol. 87B, no. 2, pp. 461–467, Nov. 2008, doi: 10.1002/jbm.b.31126.

41. I. Wittenbrink et al., "Low-aspect ratio nanopatterns on bioinert alumina influence the response and morphology of osteoblast-like cells," *Biomaterials*, vol. 62, pp. 58–65, Sep. 2015, doi: 10.1016/j.biomaterials.2015.05.026.

42. L. L. Hench, "The story of Bioglass®," *J. Mater. Sci. Mater. Med.*, vol. 17, no. 11, pp. 967–978, Nov. 2006, doi: 10.1007/s10856-006-0432-z.

43. Z. Sheikh, M. Geffers, T. Christel, J. E. Barralet, and U. Gbureck, "Chelate setting of alkali ion substituted calcium phosphates," *Ceram. Int.*, vol. 41, no. 8, pp. 10010–10017, Sep. 2015, doi: 10.1016/j.ceramint.2015.04.083.

44. M. S. Hasan, I. Ahmed, A. J. Parsons, C. D. Rudd, G. S. Walker, and C. A. Scotchford, "Investigating the use of coupling agents to improve the interfacial properties between a resorbable phosphate glass and polylactic acid matrix," *J. Biomater. Appl.*, vol. 28, no. 3, pp. 354–366, Sep. 2013, doi: 10.1177/0885328212453634.

12 Fracture Performance Evaluation of Additively Manufactured Titanium Alloy

Manvendra Tiwari and Pankaj Kumar
National Institute of Technology Goa

CONTENTS

12.1 INTRODUCTION

This work received impetus from the growing demand for orthopedic implants and degenerative diseases. Dependency on these implants has been forecasted to have the highest compound annual growth rate of 7.2% until 2020 [1]. It has been reported that up to 80% of implants belong to the metallic biomaterials domain. Earlier, metals and their alloys were considered promising bio-implants to repair/replace human bone fracture owing to their good mechanical properties. In recent years, the development of biomedical titanium alloys has emerged as one of the frontiers in research for contemporary materials scientists and engineers, as these materials can enhance fineness and longevity and ameliorate patient health care. Moreover, these health care products are indispensable because of high health hazards namely degenerative diseases, musculoskeletal system pathological conditions, trauma caused by accidents (traffic, sports, and domestic), and risk-taking practices. It is well known that orthopedic biomaterials have gained valuable attention in both clinical applications and the biomedical industry especially metallic implants [2]. Humans have been looking for metallic materials to replace fractured body parts and to treat fractures for over a century. Stainless steel and alloys of magnesium, titanium, and cobalt are preferred materials for human bone implants. The persistent demand for

DOI: 10.1201/9781003286806-12

engineering materials has been observed, requiring the combination of excellent strength-to-density ratio, elevated temperature strength, and corrosion resistance for modern aerospace, automobile, marine, and medical applications. Such requirements are well effectuated by Ti alloys for several decades now. Titanium is the fourth most abundant metal in the universe after Al, Fe, and Mg whereas, 9th on earth's crust and lithosphere in the form of various minerals such as ilmenite ($FeTiO_3$), rutile (TiO_2), titanite ($CaTiSiO_5$), perovskite ($CaTiO_3$), and arizonite ($Fe_2Ti_3O_9$). Recently, several Ti alloys have been studied concerning additive manufacturing such as Ti–5Al–5Mo–5V–1Cr–1Fe, Ti–3Al–8V–6Cr–4Mo–4Zr, Ti–6.5Al–1Mo–1V–2Zr (TA15), Ti–6.5Al–3.5Mo–1.5Zr–0.3Si (TC11), Ti–5Al–4Mo–2Zr–2Sn–4Cr (TC17), and Ti–3Al–10V–2Fe (TB6) for product development in various applications. These alloys are boon for fabricating biomedical implants, man-made extra-terrestrial, and aerospace structural components with a proper surface treatment to provide core strength. This is because of its lightweight and multifunctional properties like high fatigue strength, high fracture toughness, low thermal expansion, high melting point, high thermal stability, and excellent cryogenic properties, while being recyclable, machinable, nonmagnetic, high shock resistant, high ballistic resistant, non-toxic, and non-allergic, with good biocompatibility and a low radioactive half-life. In modern days, the industry 4.0 revolution supports Ti alloys well and pushed them miles ahead for premium and critical applications.

Among these, Ti–Nb–Ta–Zr titanium alloy (TNTZ) is considered a promising candidate because it exhibits good mechanical and fatigue strengths besides high corrosion resistance and excellent biocompatibility [3]. Several authors [2,4] reported that Ti alloys have been satisfactorily used for orthopedic fixation devices as well as knee and shoulder replacements. The major challenge encountered by the researchers in using metallic implants was to match the elastic properties (elastic modulus) to avoid premature failure of the implant during its service. This phenomenon is named as the "stress shielding effect". Further, a large difference in elastic modulus can lead to an unstable interface between human bone and implant due to bone resorption during the bone remodeling process. Hence, to nail down these issues, lattice-structured materials are proposed as one of the possible structures because they bear elastic properties close to those of human bone. Further, lattice structures are a kind of cellular material consisting of an interconnected network of struts/plates by virtue of which they are capable of absorbing high energy during dynamic loading. Therefore, potentially it can be beneficial to operate bone defects; however, its mechanical stability and biomechanics repair process understanding are still in the infant stage. The fabrication of these lattice-structured materials involves creating porosities in bulk materials considering repetitive building blocks, often called unit cells. These innovative mechanical designs of lattice structures could potentially enhance implant–bone contact and durability of the femoral component by exhibiting the extraordinary property of auxetic behavior or negative Poisson's ratio effect (expand laterally in response to uniaxial extension). These auxetic materials facilitate improved mechanical properties such as more energy absorption, bending stiffness, toughness, and enhanced fatigue resistance. Besides this, they have greater flexibility in the adjustment of mechanical properties, increased surface area that could be used for bio-functionalization and infection prevention, and controlled pore space that facilitates bone ingrowth and drug delivery from within the implants.

Fabrication of lattice-structured metallic materials is possibly accomplished by a variety of means, including investment casting methodology, a combination of extrusion and electro-discharge machining, or various composite fabrication methods including textile weaving, interlacing, interlocking, hot-press, or filament winding. However, since the proliferation of AM in the early 2000s, much research attention has been paid to the AM fabrication of lattice structures. Therefore, to print an ordered layer of lattice-structured materials, the selective laser melting (SLM) process is preferred, which enables the fabrication of complex 3D auxetic structures directly from CAD. The flexibility in design through the SLM process is associated with various process parameter complexities. Henceforth, to ensure the quality of printed lattice structures and dimensional accuracy, the process parameter must be optimized. In this proposed work, process parameter optimization of SLM processing and subsequently design optimization of the lattice-structured titanium alloy are performed with the expectation to improve the mechanical stability and biocompatibility with bone.

The novelty of the work lies in the fact that in the prevailing situation, the usage of a metallic implant is leading to premature failure of the repaired/replaced bones on account of different elastic properties of human bone and the implant material. This premature failure has increased the resurgical procedure exponentially. The proposed work focuses on reducing this resurgery frequency by adopting the SLM process for developing a new lattice structure design that will be potentially more biocompatible and will be able to withstand a higher dynamic load. In the present scenario, the SLM powder-based additive manufacturing technology is preferred to produce lattice-structured materials. The latest investigation, focusing on the SLM process, revealed that due to its flexibility in feedstock and shapes, it is a preferred methodology to print cellular lattice structures with extraordinary features directly from metal powder. To the best of the author(s) knowledge, topology optimization and its performance characteristics of SLM-processed lattice-structured material against orthopedic fixations are still in the developing stage and the research is going on. In this work, the printing of triply periodic minimal surface (TPMS) lattice-structured metallic materials is executed by the SLM technique for orthopedic applications. SLM offers processing of a lattice-structured material with high resolution by selecting suitable processing parameters easily. Therefore, SLM processing will be utilized to fabricate the TPMS lattice structures.

SLM processing is convenient in producing the varying inclination angle of cell walls in a TPMS lattice structure, which provides strong interconnection with the subsequent layers to improve the processing technique. It is also suggested that varying the inclination angle leads to the surface curvature of cell walls and, therefore, helps in stimulating bone ingrowth easily. Additionally, the pores present in the printed material promote uniform stress distribution during stimulating the bone healing process. Some typical TPMS-based structures are shown in Figure 12.1. The selected 3D haptic physical lattice-structured material is primarily applicable for orthopedic fixation; therefore, resistance against bending and compressive loading dominated structures should be preferred. Hence, topology optimization inevitably generates concepts

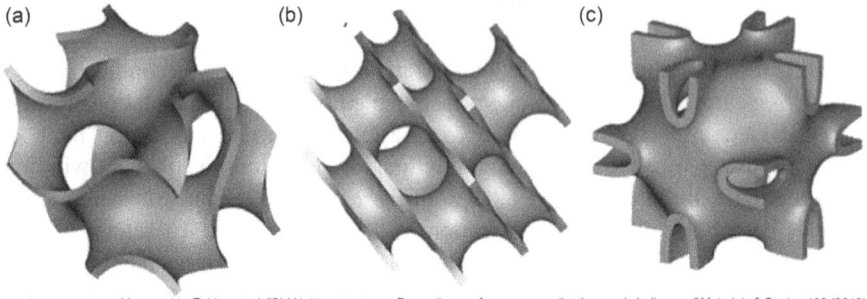

Image courtesy: Maconachie, Tobias, et al. "SLM lattice structures: Properties, performance, applications and challenges." Materials & Design 183 (2019)

FIGURE 12.1 Typical TPMS-based unit cells: (a) Schoen gyroid, (b) Schwarz diamond, and (c) Neovius.

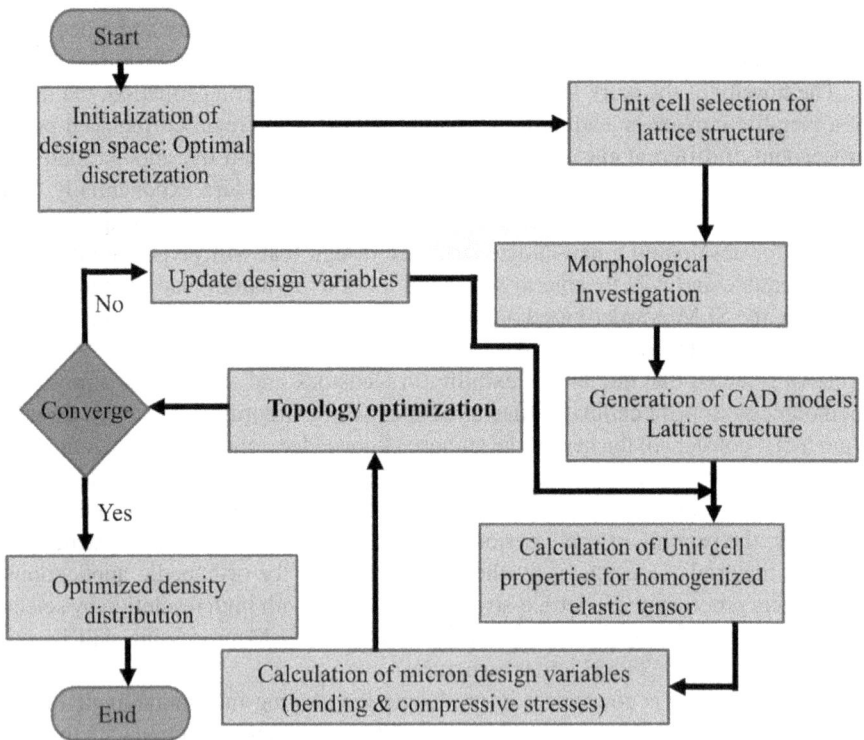

FIGURE 12.2 Flowchart for topology optimization of the lattice structure.

in designing the optimized lattice-structured material, which can offer optimal osseo-integration, stiffness close to bone (negligible stress shielding effect) and enhanced mechanical properties. A topologically optimized structure would exhibit optimal material distribution within unit cells, which can be effectively applied for orthopedic surgery. A detailed flow chart for topology optimization is described in Figure 12.2.

The human bone encounters fatigue load during its daily activities, and this situation/condition recommends carrying out analysis of the implants under cyclic loading. Since post bone transplant, these materials suffer direct cyclic loads, which may affect the fatigue durability and consequently, second surgery becomes essential due to loosening of the implant by repeated cyclic loads, leading to early fracture of implants, which comprises risk-associated surgery along with longer hospitalization time and higher health care costs. Therefore, high fatigue strength along with long fatigue life is desirable to avoid catastrophic failure. There are no detailed numerical studies reported in the literature for mechanical characterization and crack growth analysis of SLM-processed lattice-structured orthopedic implants.

12.2 EXTENDED FINITE ELEMENT METHOD FORMULATION

Extended finite element method (XFEM) is an advanced form of FEM having distinct advantages because of ease in the modeling of any crack or discontinuous domain [5]. In XFEM, the approximation of FEM is enriched with additional functions to capture the discontinuities present in the displacement field. These enrichment functions in the FE solution are added by a partition of unity (PU) property [6,7]. In XFEM, modeling of cracks is independent of mesh as shown in Figure 12.3. In the provided figure, the crack tip and crack surface have been taken care by enriched nodes through Heaviside and asymptotic crack tip enrichment functions. The mathematical derivations are also explained in detail.

The enriched displacement approximation at any point can be written as [8]:

$$u^h(x) = \sum_{k=1}^{n} N_k(x) \left[u_k + \left(H(x) - H(x_k)\right)a_k + \sum_{\alpha=1}^{4} \left(\phi_\alpha(x) - \phi_\alpha(x_k)\right)b_k^\alpha \right] \quad (12.1)$$

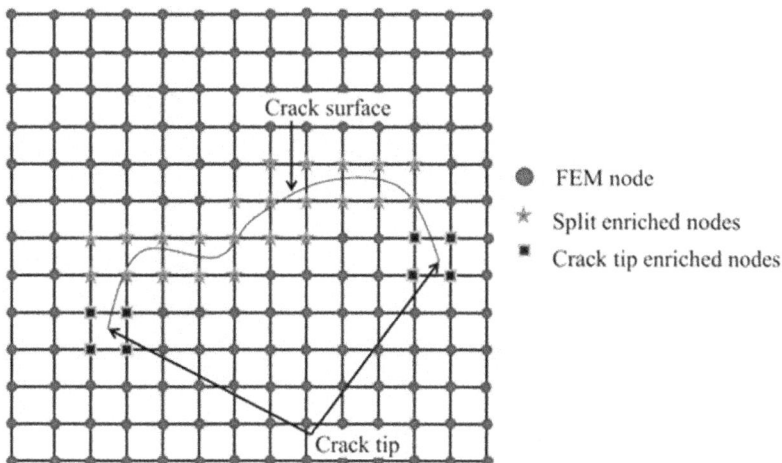

● FEM node

* Split enriched nodes

■ Crack tip enriched nodes

Crack surface

Crack tip

FIGURE 12.3 Extended finite element approximation with discontinuity.

where $N_k(x)$ is the Lagrange interpolation function and $u^h(x)$ is the nodal displacement vector associated with a continuous part of the domain. $H(x)$ is the Heaviside function across the crack surface; a_k is the additional degree of freedom associated with the Heaviside function; $\varphi_a(x)$ is the asymptotic enrichment function taken from the Westergaard–William solution for displacement field at the crack tip and b_k^α is the enriched nodal degree of freedom associated with the crack tip enrichment function:

$$H(\mathbf{x}) = \begin{cases} 1 \text{ if } (x - x^*)\, n \geq 0 \\ -1 \text{ otherwise}, \end{cases} \tag{12.2}$$

where x is the sample Gauss point; x^* is the point on the crack closest to x and n is the unit outward normal to the crack at x^*.

In the above relation, $\varphi_a(\mathbf{x})$ functions are used to model the radial as well as the angular characteristics of asymptotic stress fields near the crack front [6]:

$$\phi_\alpha(\mathbf{x}) = \left[\ \sqrt{r}\cos\frac{\theta}{2}, \quad \sqrt{r}\sin\frac{\theta}{2}, \quad \sqrt{r}\cos\frac{\theta}{2}\sin\theta, \quad \sqrt{r}\sin\frac{\theta}{2}\sin\theta \ \right] \tag{12.3}$$

where (r, θ) represents the polar coordinate system where the origin is considered at the crack tip.

During simulation, the displacement fields λ (trial function) proposed by Belytscko and Black [5] is given as:

$$\lambda = (\mathbf{v} \in \delta \,|\, \mathbf{v} = \bar{\mathbf{u}} \quad \text{on} \quad \Gamma_u) \tag{12.4}$$

In the above relation, $\mathbf{v}$ is discontinuous on Γ_u, whereas space δ is related to the uniformity of the solution.

The weak formulation for the equilibrium equation is as follows:

$$\int_\Omega \sigma(\mathbf{u}):\varepsilon(\mathbf{v})\, d\Omega = \int_\Omega \mathbf{b}.\mathbf{v}\, d\Omega + \int_{\Gamma_t} \bar{\mathbf{t}}.\mathbf{v}\, d\Gamma \tag{12.5}$$

The constitutive relation $\sigma = \mathbf{C}:\varepsilon$ is substituted in equation (12.5). We get:

$$\int_\Omega \varepsilon:\mathbf{C}:\varepsilon\, d\Omega = \int_\Omega \mathbf{b}.\mathbf{v}\, d\Omega + \int_{\Gamma_t} \bar{\mathbf{t}}.\mathbf{v}\, d\Gamma \tag{12.6}$$

The trial and test functions are substituted in equation (12.6) and using the randomness of the nodal variations, a discrete equation is obtained as:

$$[\mathbf{K}]\{\mathbf{d}\} = \{\mathbf{f}\} \tag{12.7}$$

where $\mathbf{d}$ is the unknown nodal vector, $\mathbf{K}$ and $\mathbf{f}$ are the global stiffness matrix and external force vector, respectively.

In the post-processing phase, stress intensity factors (SIFs) have been extracted using a domain-based interaction integral approach. By using SIFs, fatigue crack growth simulation has been performed under quasi-static crack growth conditions. The fatigue crack growth simulations assume an incremental crack increment process in which a sequence of linear elastic fracture mechanics steps are repeated to describe the evolution of the crack tip/front. After evaluating the SIFs using the domain-based interaction integral approach, the range of SIFs for constant amplitude cyclic loading is defined as:

$$\Delta K = K_{\max} - K_{\min} \tag{12.8}$$

where $K_{\max}$ and $K_{\min}$ are the values of SIFs corresponding to the defined stress ratio range.

To get the direction of crack growth, the maximum principal stress criterion is implemented. Thus, at each crack increment step, the direction of crack growth θ_c is obtained by equating the local shear stress to zero [7]:

$$K_{\mathrm{I}} \sin\theta_c + K_{\mathrm{II}}(3\cos\theta_c - 1) = 0 \tag{12.9}$$

The solution of the above equation gives

$$\theta_c = 2\tan^{-1}\left(\frac{K_{\mathrm{I}} - \sqrt{K_{\mathrm{I}}^2 + K_{\mathrm{II}}^2}}{4K_{\mathrm{II}}}\right) \tag{12.10}$$

where angle θ_c is calculated in the orthogonal plane.

12.2.1 IMPACT TOUGHNESS AS A CRACK GROWTH CRITERION

Impact toughness plays a major role while simulating crack growth properties. Here, impact energy evaluated from experiments preferably by the Charpy test is considered as the crack progression criterion during simulating the crack advancement via XFEM. Previously, authors [9] have already described how to predict the crack progression problems for various materials employing the below provided mathematical relation:

$$I_T = I_i + I_p \tag{12.11}$$

Here, I_T = total energy; I_i = energy needed for crack initiation; and I_p = energy required for stable growth

The above-provided relation (8) is equivalent to Griffith's fracture criterion [10] and can be expressed as:

$$T_r = \frac{\partial}{\partial S}\left(W_F - E_e - E_p - U_S\right)$$

$$\begin{bmatrix} T_r > I_T \text{ Crack propagation} \\ T_r = I_T \text{ Critical condition} \\ T_r < I_T \text{ Crack does not propagate} \end{bmatrix} \tag{12.12}$$

In the provided relation, T_r = final strain energy; E_e = elastic strain energy; and E_p = inelastic strain energy. On the other hand, W_F = work performed by external load; U_s = surface energy; and S = total crack surface area. As suggested by the Griffith criterion, the energy release rate (G) is estimated from ($W_F - E_e$), whereas the last two terminologies, i.e. ($E_p - U_s$) of relation (9) denotes the inelastic dissipation and surface dissipation energy rates of newly formed crack tips.

Using the above XFEM, a step-by-step crack propagation and ductile rupture simulations are performed. This method has provided ease in modeling any discontinuity or crack present in the domain along with its crack growth. The purpose of the simulation is to get better insight into the existing problem; it helps in visualizing critical areas of stress distribution in the selected alloy. Fracture mechanics experiments (like in the present case, FCG) are always resource intensive. They need costly machines and time-consuming procedures for each set of parameters. Therefore, in the present work, crack growth behavior under two various crack lengths is predicted for a lattice-structured Ti-alloy.

12.3   RESULTS AND DISCUSSION

12.3.1 Tension Test Simulation

The extended finite element method is used to simulate the ductile fracture and the corresponding stress–strain response of the SLM-processed TNTZ alloy. In this simulation work, a full-scale model of the test specimen is developed in an ABAQUS environment and the model is discretized using eight-noded quadrilateral elements. This approach of discretization resulted in the usage of 447 elements and 1140 nodes, respectively. The boundary conditions are kept similar to actual experimental conditions. During XFEM simulation, all the degrees of freedom of one end of the computational model (test specimen) are completely arrested while the other end is displaced by the same magnitude as crossheads were displaced during the real-time experiment. Now, a combined XFEM and experimental tensile plastic data points are selected (source, [4]) for smoothening of the experimental stress–strain curves to simulate the entire stress–strain curve till ductile separation of the material.

In the XFEM framework, the plastic straining along with classical nucleation and coalescence of cavities for the crack initiation and its subsequent development has been traced. This approach helps in modeling the crack initiation once the ultimate tensile stress (UTS) is reached, using the maximum principal stress criterion.

Figure 12.4a represents the simulated tensile test results in which zoomed view represents the crack initiation, propagation, and ductile fracture near gauge length. It is a well-established fact that at the onset of necking, clusters of micro-voids and interfacial non-connected cracks get accumulated near secondary phase particles or inclusions, which results in small sized crack formation [11]. Furthermore, with an increase in plastic straining, cracks propagate and are essentially responsible for weakening the specimen and result in necking formation centrally. This phenomenon is nicely captured in the current XFEM simulation work as shown in Figure 12.4a. Various stages of crack propagation and ductile rupture phenomenon has been

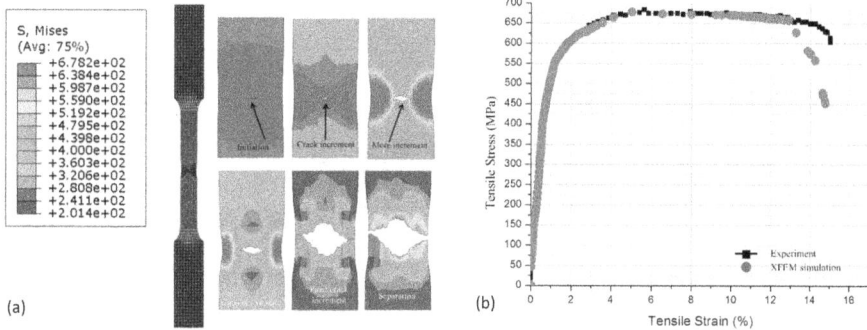

FIGURE 12.4 XFEM simulated (a) von-Mises stress contour plot and (b) comparative stress–strain curve.

described in the zoomed view of an SLM-processed TNTZ alloy, by arrow indications in the 2D model (Figure 12.4a). From these observations, it is clear that in the tensile curve, plasticity is accompanied with plastic straining and this phenomenon of ductile tearing is also confirmed in the zoomed view of the fractured specimen. In addition to this, comparison is carried out between the simulated and experimentally recorded stress–strain curves for TNTZ alloys (Figure 12.4b). It is observed that the simulated curve is almost coinciding with the experimental curve up to the UTS value (678 MPa). However, there is a deviation between the curves post UTS value. The probable reason may be the unseen factors, which are induced during the real-time experiment. But this study gives perfect information related to the onset of crack initiation, which is paramount.

12.3.2 Crack Growth Simulation

XFEM is adopted for simulating the crack advancement during the brittle fracture toughness test. Experimental fracture toughness value and its corresponding force versus crack opening displacement (COD) travel curve are taken from the available literature (source [12]) for simulating the fracture toughness and crack growth curves. The computational domain is replicated using ABAQUS software, the same as that of test specimen used in real-time experiments. The discretization is performed with optimized 14,016 elements and 32,476 nodes by eight-noded brick elements to perform crack growth simulation as shown in Figure 12.5a.

The upper section of the circular hole of a computational compact tension (CT) specimen is displaced vertically with the same magnitude as that given during the experiment while arresting the axial motion of the lower end of the specimen. For modeling the crack path, impact energy crack growth principle has been used. In the fracture toughness simulation, brittle fracture toughness value, K_{Ic}, is calculated numerically using the ASTM E399 standard and governing equations as discussed in the below equations from 13 to 16.

A schematic of a CT specimen is used for evaluation of plane strain fracture toughness (K_{Ic}) of the material, as shown in the computational domain of Figure 12.5a. The

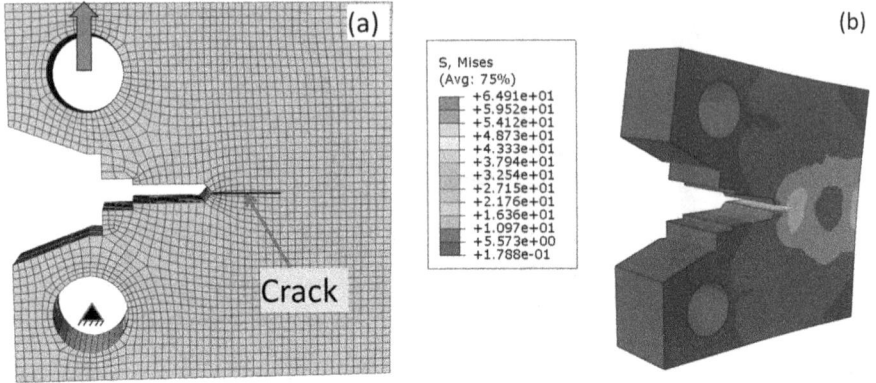

FIGURE 12.5 Computational compact tension specimen with (a) discretized and boundary conditions and (b) von-Mises stress contour plot.

following relations are used to estimate the apparent fracture toughness, K_Q, which after satisfying some validity criteria becomes K_{Ic} of the specimen [9]:

$$K_Q = \frac{P_Q}{B\sqrt{W} f\left(\frac{a}{W}\right)} \tag{12.13}$$

$$f\left(\frac{a}{W}\right) = \frac{\left(2 + \frac{a}{W}\right)}{\left(1 - \frac{a}{W}\right)^{3/2}} \left[0.866 + 4.64\left(\frac{a}{W}\right) - 13.32\left(\frac{a}{W}\right)^2 \right. $$
$$\left. + 14.72\left(\frac{a}{W}\right)^3 - 5.60\left(\frac{a}{W}\right)^4\right] \tag{12.14}$$

where 'B' and 'a' symbolize the specimen thickness and crack size, respectively.

The below-mentioned criteria substantiate the apparent fracture toughness K_Q into brittle fracture toughness (K_{Ic}) of the specimen.

$$B, a \geq 2.5 \left(\frac{K_Q}{\sigma_Y}\right)^2 \tag{12.15}$$

$$P_{\max} \leq 1.1 P_Q \tag{12.16}$$

Here, σ_Y represents the yield stress of the specimen, and $P_{\max}$ is the highest load attained during post-quasi-static loading.

The simulation study includes tracing of the crack path, which is represented in the form of force versus COD travel curve and the comparison of simulated and experimental work is depicted in Figure 12.6a. Both experimental and simulated curves demonstrate close agreement with each other. In the plot (Figure 12.6a), the

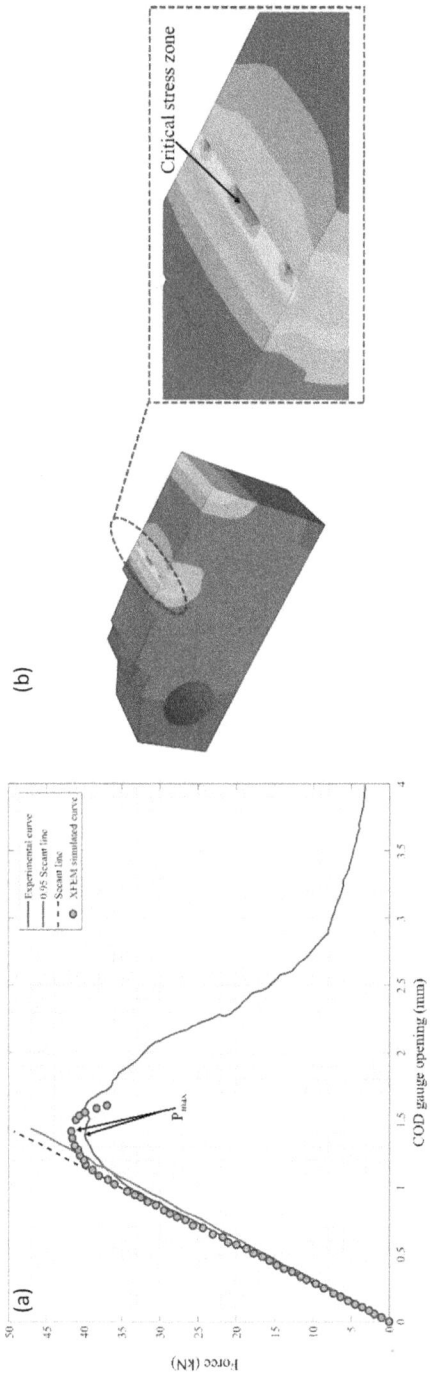

FIGURE 12.6 Experimental and simulated (a) force versus COD travel curve and (b) critical stress contour plot and its location in a sectional compact tension specimen.

values of maximum load (39.7 and 41.8 kN) from the experiment and simulation, respectively, are indicated with the help of arrow heads, which is achieved during application of load with respect to COD opening. The difference between the simulated and experimental maximum load is due to non-consideration of change in stiffness while performing simulation over the range of plastic deformation. Apart from this, the von-Mises stress contour plot is also presented (Figure 12.6a), and for better visualization, a sectional view is also presented to observe critical stress variation near crack tip along the thickness. As seen from the force versus COD travel curve (refer Figure 12.6a), there is sudden drop or kink in the magnitude of load with COD increment at the highest loading point. This sudden drop phenomenon is well captured by simulation, which is shown in Figure 12.6a. The critical stress zone (refer zoomed view of Figure 12.6b) at the mid-section of the CT specimen is visible at the crack vicinity, which signifies that the crack is likely to grow from the crack tip and becomes unstable if it crosses its fracture toughness value.

12.4   CONCLUSION

In this work, a novel numerical technique, XFEM is utilized to simulate the ductile rupture and crack growth behavior of orthopedic TNTZ alloys. The following inferences have been drawn from the present work:

a. Lattice-structured TNTZ alloys are recommended for orthopedic surgery to minimize the stress shielding effect, thereby reducing the resurgery procedure owing to the premature failure of the implants.
b. The validated in-house developed XFEM simulations performed on finite element software are found to be quite conducive for simulating the step-by-step ductile rupture from crack nucleation till fracture during uniaxial tensile loading.
c. XFEM simulation accurately predicted the uniform elasto-plastic deformation during tensile loading.
d. XFEM simulations captured critical stress in the CT specimen at the crack vicinity, which mimic the experimental observations.
e. The differences in the value of maximum load, i.e. 39.7 kN from experiment and 41.8 kN from simulation, are very small and within the acceptable regime.
f. The numerically predicted K_{Ic} value is in close agreement with the experimentally evaluated results.
g. The XFEM simulated results are found to be in good agreement with the experimentally recorded observations and fracture characteristics of the lattice-structured TNTZ alloy.

REFERENCES

1. Niinomi M. Recent metallic materials for biomedical applications. *Metall Mater Trans A*, vol. 55, pp. 477–486, (2002).
2. Liu H, Niinomi M, Nakai M, Obara S, Fujii H. Improved fatigue properties with maintaining low Young's modulus achieved in biomedical beta-type titanium alloy by oxygen addition. *Mater Sci Eng A*, vol. 704, pp. 100–107, (2017).

3. Banerjee R, Nag S, Fraser HL. A novel combinatorial approach to the development of beta titanium alloys for orthopaedic implants. *Mater Sci Eng C*, vol. 25, pp. 282–289, (2005).

4. Luo JP, Sun JF, Huang YJ, Zhang JH, Zhao DP, Yan M, et al. Low-modulus biomedical Ti–30Nb–5Ta–3Zr additively manufactured by selective laser melting and its biocompatibility. *Mater Sci Eng C*, vol. 97, pp. 275–84, (2019).

5. Belytschko T, Black T. Elastic crack growth in finite elements with minimal remeshing. *Int J Numer Methods Eng*, vol. 45, pp. 601–620, (1999).

6. Kumar P, Pathak H, Singh A, Singh IV. Failure analysis of orthotropic composite material under thermo-elastic loading by XFEA. *Mater Today Proc*, vol. 26, pp. 2163–2167, (2019).

7. Kumar P, Pathak H, Singh A. Fatigue crack growth behavior of thermo-mechanically processed AA 5754: Experiment and extended finite element method simulation. *Mech Adv Mater Struct*, vol. 28, pp. 88–101, (2018).

8. Gajjar M, Pathak H, Kumar S. Elasto-plastic fracture modeling for crack interaction with XFEM. *Trans Indian Inst Met*, vol. 73, pp. 1679–87, (2020).

9. Kumar P, Singh A. Investigation of fatigue and fracture behaviour of sensitized marine grade aluminium alloy AA 5754. *Fatigue Fract Eng Mater Struct*, vol. 42, pp. 2625–43, (2019).

10. Das P, Jayaganthan R, Singh I V. Experimental finding of initiation fracture toughness and fem simulation of fracture behaviour of UFG 7075 al alloy. *Adv Mater Lett*, vol. 4, pp. 668–81, (2013).

11. Kumar P. Experimental and extended finite element simulations for tensile fracture phenomenon of cryorolled aluminium alloy 5754. *Proc Inst Mech Eng Part C J Mech Eng Sci*, (2021). DOI:10.1177/09544062211028270

12. Zhang X, Martina F, Ding J, Wang X, Williams SW. Fracture toughness and fatigue crack growth rate properties in wire plus arc additive manufactured Ti-6Al-4V. *Fatigue Fract Eng Mater Struct*, Vol. 40, pp.790–803, (2017).

13 Design of a Low-Cost Prosthetic Leg Using Magnetorheological Fluid

Ganapati Shastry, T. Jagadeesha and Ashish Toby
National Institute of Technology Calicut

Seung-Bok Choi
The State University of New York Korea

Vikram G. Kamble
Technical University Dresden Germany

CONTENTS

13.1 INTRODUCTION

In today's world where the pace of life has significantly accelerated, amputations are no exceptions. Be it an urban region or a rural region, people get to hear cases of amputations everywhere. According to a consensus of 2017, there are over 1 million annual limb amputations globally, around one every 30 seconds. The causes of

DOI: 10.1201/9781003286806-13

amputations are many, including accidents, diseases, snake bites, surgery to remove tumors, etc. Transfemoral or above-knee (AK) amputees account for 27% of the total lower limb amputees. This is a huge number [1,2]. India is a country with a high count of around 23,500 amputees each year, with 29% being post-femoral amputees. Approximately 70% of the amputees in our country hail from rural areas with low incomes [3]. Active prosthesis, generally being expensive, cannot be afforded by a considerable section of society. Although less expensive, a passive prosthesis cannot outperform or provide enough aid for regular human activities or work [4–6]. Therefore, it is essential to develop a prosthetic leg that is not as expensive as an active leg but can provide adequate torque for walking.

It is essential, especially for the lower limb amputees, to use artificial devices to be able to perform daily activities with as much ease as possible. Therefore, the demand for prosthetic devices is quite high. This has also led to a surge in the prices of these prosthetic devices, curtailing the poor section of humanity from the benefit of those. However, there are passive devices available for a much cheaper rate, but seldom do they satisfy the requirements of amputees. This has led to increased research in the area of prosthetic devices, with the intent of making the product more and more affordable for everyone.

The main objective of designing any prosthetic device is to make it mimic the natural human limb as closely as possible so that the amputee feels comfortable. This can be easily achieved by electronic systems (known as active controllers), but as mentioned above, these are very expensive. Therefore, one has to make sure the manufacturing cost of the material involved has to be minimum and simultaneously, the device should perform like a natural limb. Use of smart materials like MR fluid is one such way.

MR fluid or magnetorheological fluid is a smart material that changes its viscosity and shear stress according to its magnetic field [7]. A piston-cylinder mechanism can provide adequate damping force and the torque at the knee necessary for walking properly when used inside a damper. Apart from this, the MR damper serves another purpose. Fluid is present inside the knee in a natural human leg that provides damping or shocking absorption while walking. An amputated leg would not have this. Therefore, with the help of an MR damper, this can also be achieved [4–6,8–11]. The semi-active prostheses are more flexible than the passive ones and are also not as expensive as the active ones. Such prostheses can be made using semi-active controllers like MR dampers.

An MR damper can be easily controlled with the help of a **PID: Proportional Integral Derivative** controller. A relationship between current and required torque must be found, stabilized by tuning suitable control gains [12–21].

13.1.1 MAGNETORHEOLOGICAL FLUIDS

MR fluids are smart materials that vary in their viscosity and shear stress depending on the magnetic field acting on them [22]. MR materials include MR fluids, MR foam and MR elastomers [23]. They usually consist of a carrier fluid with ferromagnetic particles. The fluid quality depends on various factors, the cost, the density, the sensitivity to the magnetic field, the sedimentation rate, etc. MR fluids are a suspension of ferromagnetic particles in a carrier fluid. Under the action of a magnetic field, they aggregate and align themselves with the magnetic field, leading to a change of state from a Newtonian fluid to a non-Newtonian fluid, like toothpaste. Under normal conditions, it acts as a carrier fluid with suspended particles in it. The magnetic field changes the viscosity and yield stress of the fluid, depending on the direction and magnitude of the field applied. A vast number of models have been defined to explain the working of the MR fluid. From Buoc-Wen and Bingham models to Dahl and visco-elastic-plastic models, many models theorized to numerically quantify the variations of properties of MR fluids [24].

Compared to their counterpart electrorheological fluids, MR fluids have shorter response times, a broader working temperature range, a higher maximum yield stress and a higher maximum field and have tolerance to impurities and changes after the application of magnetic fields are visible almost instantly [25,26]. Due to their control over mechanical properties, they quickly became a part of many devices, mainly as dampers, in brakes, clutches, and now in prosthesis [27,22]. Modern medicine is currently researching the use of MR materials for multiple ways of treatment [28]. Due to its property variation, the damping coefficients and the damping forces can be easily controlled by changing the magnetic field.

13.1.2 WORKING OF AN MR DAMPER

An MR damper is essentially a piston-cylinder mechanism that performs reciprocating motion. However, unlike other hydraulic dampers, the piston is provided with an electrical circuit in it so that current could be passed through it, thereby inducing a magnetic field and changing the properties of the fluid instantaneously [9,12,29,30]. There are various designs of MR dampers available, most of which have holes or orifices in the piston to let the fluid flow through them. As the name suggests, the primary purpose of the MR damper is to provide adequate damping force for the intended purpose. It does so by exploiting the property of the MR fluid that its yield stress increases significantly when under a magnetic field. As mentioned earlier, MR fluid, under the influence of a magnetic field, behaves like a Bingham plastic or a non-Newtonian liquid. The equation governing its behavior is:

$$\tau_s = \pm\tau_y + \eta\gamma \tag{13.1a}$$

where τ_s represents the shear stress, τ_y represents the yield stress, η represents the coefficient of dynamic viscosity and γ represents the shear rate.

Figure 13.1 clearly shows that only after the shear stress increases to a particular value under magnetic field, the fluid shear increases. The damping force produced can be divided into two components: (i) force due to viscosity and (ii) force due to the yield stress [23,26–28,31,32]. The yield stress of the MR fluid is a property of the magnetic field strength, which in turn depends upon the current flowing through the coil in the piston. Therefore, by controlling the current flowing through the coil, one can easily get the required damping force.

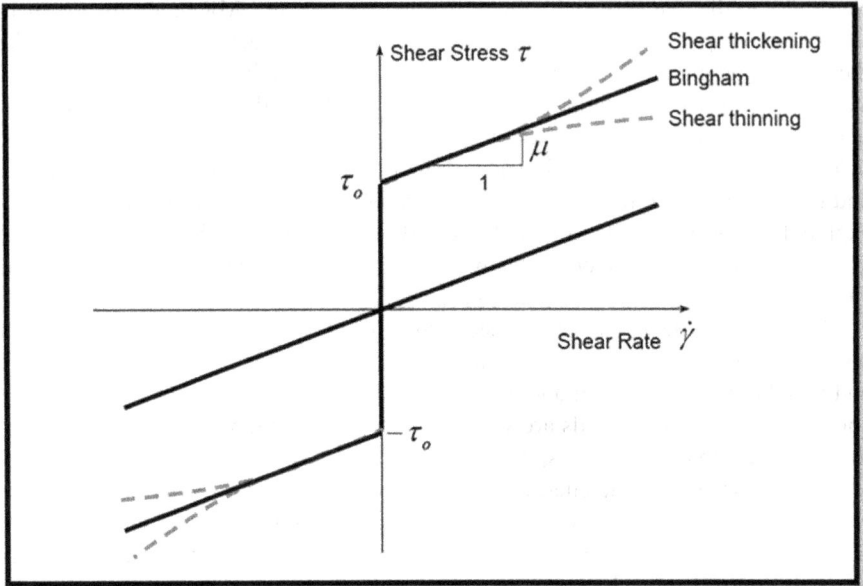

FIGURE 13.1 Behavior of MR fluid under magnetic field.

13.1.3 TWIN-TUBE MR DAMPER

One major problem that most of the damper's face is that their magnetic core is fixed at a particular location in the cylinder (usually centralized). This problem can be overcome by designing a piston so that the armature core and the coil can be fitted in it so that they move along with the piston as one unit. The final assembly of the MR damper in a sectioned view is shown in Figure 13.2. The various parts of the twin-tube MR damper are discussed below:

  i. **Inner shock tube**: The inner shock tube is a hollow cylinder that houses the MR fluid and the assemble of piston and armature core. The design of the inner shock tube is shown in the figure below.
 ii. **Outer shock tube**: The outer shock tube is the damper's outermost part o, which houses all the parts inside it. Toward the end of the piston's forward stroke, the MR fluid is contained in the outer shock tube.
iii. **Piston**: The piston is one of the most critical parts of the MR damper. It reciprocates and makes the fluid flow inside the damper. The damper force is experienced by the piston, which is translated to the knee via the piston rod. The piston contains the armature. Three holes are provided in the piston so that fluid can flow through the piston as well.
 iv. **Piston rod**: The piston rod is attached to the piston. It is made hollow to reduce its weight.
  v. **Piston cap**: This is a plate that is attached at the top end of the piston. This also serves the purpose of preventing any magnetic flux leakages from the piston's outer surface.

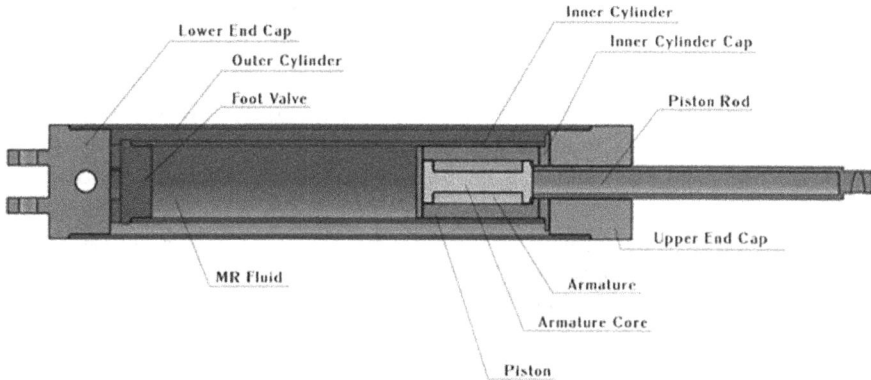

FIGURE 13.2   Assembled sectioned view of the twin-tube MR damper.

vi. **Armature core**: The armature core is inside the piston. It contains the coil windings through which the current flows and induces the magnetic field.

vii. **Inner cylinder cap**: This is like a seal provided at the rear end of the inner shock tube. This is necessary to prevent any leakage of MR fluid to the outside of the damper.

viii. **Foot valve**: This part is like a connection between the inner and outer shock tubes. The fluid flows through the inner shock tube to the foot valve and then to the outer shock tube during the piston's forward stroke. It follows the exact path in the reverse direction during the backward stroke.

ix. **Lower end cap**: This is the lower-most part of the MR damper. It closes the outer shock tube. It has an appendage that attaches to the shank of the prosthetic leg.

x. **Upper-end cap**: This is the uppermost part of the MR damper. It also closes the outer shock tube but on the upper end.

13.1.4   APPLICATION OF MR DAMPER IN THE BIOMEDICAL FIELD

The MR damper finds its application in the field of biomedicals, specifically in the field of prosthetics. One such application is the use of an MR damper in the prosthetic leg for AK amputees. Passive prosthetic legs available can provide the adequate torque at the knee required for walking. Therefore, amputees using passive prosthetic legs walk awkwardly. Although it can provide the required torque at the knee, the active legs are way too expensive for everyone to afford [5]. Therefore, a semi-active control of the knee joint, which is readily achieved by the MR damper, will serve the purpose of providing the right amount of torque as well as being less expensive. It is a semi-active control because it controls the knee joint only during the stance phase (60%) of the gait cycle [4,33].

To model the prosthetic leg with an MR damper, we first need to understand the basics of human walking dynamics. The hip angle and the knee angle vary in relation to each other. This relation can be experimentally found out by noting down many values of the hip and the knee angle at various points of time in the gait cycle, then plotting them to get a relation. This relation will be different in the swing and the stance phase. The relation of stance phase is shown below:

$$\theta = 29.25 + 4.16\varnothing + 0.057\varnothing^2 - 0.022\varnothing^3 - (5.0e - 5)\varnothing^4 + (4e - 5)\varnothing^5 \quad (13.1b)$$

where θ is the knee angle and $\varnothing$ is the hip angle. Now, the next step is to find out the torque acting at the knee of the natural human leg as a function of hip angle. This torque can be taken as the torque that the MR damper is supposed to apply (by producing a suitable damping force) on the prosthetic knee. This is a highly complex task and has to be performed in steps.

   i. **Step 1**: Make a model of the prosthetic leg (entire assembly including the MR damper) and give inputs to its various joints as taken from the natural gait cycle to make the prosthetic leg move like a natural one. Note down the velocities and accelerations of various parts.
   ii. **Step 2**: Make a free-body diagram (FBD) of a natural human leg and analytically calculate the torque at the knee. This will require the velocities and accelerations obtained in step 1.
   iii. **Step 3:** Using the obtained torque, find out the required damping force.
   iv. **Step 4**: Perform magnetic and CFD analysis on the damper to obtain the yield stress v/s current graph.
   v. **Step 5**: Combine the results of steps 3 and 4 to get the damping force v/s current graph.

13.2   DESIGN AND ANALYSIS

13.2.1   Designing the Prosthetic Leg

Prosthesis legs are usually simple passive attachments. Prosthetic knees are of various types, usually controlled through a lot of mechanisms [34]. The two most used important mechanisms are a four-bar mechanism and a single joint mechanism. Many actuator options are available, with the most widely used one being the servo motor. Servo motors are expensive options but are simple to implement with high accuracy. A cheaper option is the use of an MR damper with a four-bar mechanism. In a design by Xie et al., the knee joint is four-bar mechanisms with the MR damper attached between the superior and inferior links. It works very effectively with very little error at low walking speeds, but the error increases with the walking speed [8]. A design by Kim et al. showed that a rotary MR damper controlling knee joint be used for post-femoral amputees. The error seen on the first few cycles is high, which reduces later to match the actual gait cycle [11]. Borijan used myoelectric sensors with servo motors as actuators and a fuzzy PID controller as the control mechanism. Using all these, the achieved result is exceptionally compliant with the actual gait cycle [34]. Another design using electric–hydraulic actuators to control the knee with the help of motors is made by Sup et al., showing outstanding performance during the stance phase at all speeds and moderate performance in swing phase at higher walking speeds [35].

There are many prosthetic ankle designs, primarily passive [36,37]. Prosthetic ankles are usually 1 DOF part, with a compliant mechanism like flexible struts to store and release energy [38]. But with the help of 2 DOF prosthetic ankle, it is more flexible in adhering to the actual gait cycle torques and ankle angles. With a 2 DOF, the non-linearity in the torque variation can be controlled, making it a more complex system to design [39,40]. Many active ankle designs use electric actuators directly via DC motors or servo motors, allowing for a faster response time and a higher power consumption [35,41–43]. Modern developments in intelligent materials and prosthetic technology have enabled more complex and robust designs that will enable more flexible changes for different users and closely resemble an actual ankle in terms of the torque produced. Through MR fluids, it is possible to design active ankle prosthesis and exoskeletons with less power consumption [44–48]. Although more complex and expensive, MR fluid-controlled ankles via dampers, brakes and actuators are relatively cheaper than motor-controlled ankles while providing similar performance and reliability. An element called the "robotic tendon" allows for changes in the lever arm length, which aids in reducing the power consumption for the overall ankle design [49]. One way to control an ankle shown by Yu et al. is using an electro hydrostatic actuator. This actuator can be turned off and on, allowing for both passive and active mode of control [50]. A complex design controlled by a four-bar mechanism, actuated by an electric motor, shows a polycentric prosthetic ankle that can allow changes in moments produced without changing the dimensional properties of the overall prosthesis [51]. Another great way to control the ankle is using a cam controlled by motors. It is very complex in design but offers a higher degree of accuracy [52]. A great way to reduce energy consumption is to use regenerative systems to reuse the spent energy [42].

A model of the prosthetic leg can be efficiently designed using the available commercial software. In this example, the model shown is designed using SOLIDWORKS. This prosthetic leg has a four-bar mechanism as its knee joint, to which the twin-tube MR damper (shown in Figure 13.3) is attached. The objective of performing motion analysis is to determine whether the designed leg can move like a natural human leg when given inputs from the gait cycle. A duplicate of this leg can also be connected using a rod, the length of which is the average length of the human waist. This configuration is shown in Figure 13.3a and b.

The gait cycle duration for a normal human being is anywhere between 1.2 and 1.5 seconds. However, since the amputee would not walk as swiftly, the gait cycle is stretched to about 3 seconds, making a stance phase of about 1.7 seconds.

13.2.1.1   Inputs for Simulation

To simulate the leg like a natural human leg, we need to give inputs following the natural human gait cycle. In the configuration shown above, the legs are fixed at the extreme position of their respective phases (swing phase-left and stance phase-right) so that when the simulation begins, the left leg starts its stance phase. Angles from the gait cycle of each joint should be taken. The angle at which various joints are fixed in the above configuration should be noted down and should be subtracted from the gait angles so that the present configuration becomes 0°. These data points should be given as inputs to the six joints. Apart from this, a force should be given at the

(a)   (b)

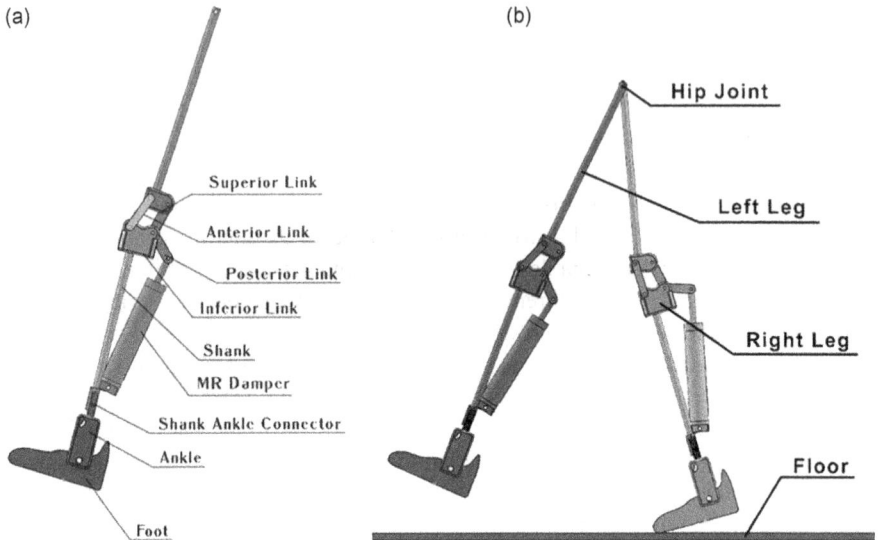

FIGURE 13.3   (a) and (b) Configurations for simulating the entire gait cycle.

top of the rod joining the two legs, equal to 490.5 N (equivalent to upper body mass, 50 kg). Gravity should also be switched on in the simulation, and contact should be established between the two legs and the floor so that the reaction force while walking also comes into the picture. The curves of inputs are shown in Figures 13.4–13.9.

13.2.1.2   Outputs of the Simulation

As mentioned in the earlier sections, the angular displacements, velocities and accelerations of various parts required should be noted to move to step 2. Here, the required outputs are velocity and acceleration of hip and knee joints, the linear velocity of a piston, the angular velocity of the posterior part of the knee joint (to which the MR damper is attached) and the angular displacement between the posterior part and the piston. The obtained outputs are shown in Figures 13.10–13.16.

This completes step 1 of our process. Using these results, we now head to step 2 of our process.

13.3   ANALYTICAL MODEL OF THE HUMAN LEG

The next step is to make an analytical model of the human leg to obtain the torque acting at the knee joint. The FBD of the human leg is shown in Figure 13.17.

The torque acting at the human leg can be divided into three components: the inertial torque, the Coriolis torque and the gravitational torque. Since the amputee for whom the prosthetic leg is being designed is an AK amputee, it is assumed that he/she will control the hip joint, and therefore the computations of torque at the hip joint can be ignored. From the FBD, the following equations can be obtained:

$$\tau_k = I_\theta \cdot \ddot{\theta} + I_\varnothing \, \ddot{\varnothing} + V + G \tag{13.2}$$

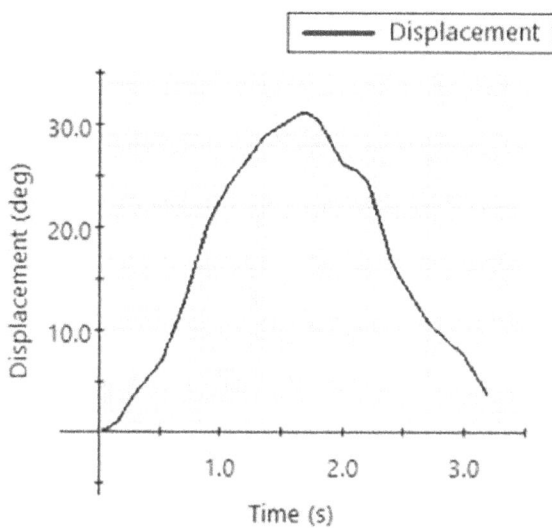

FIGURE 13.4 Input for left hip joint.

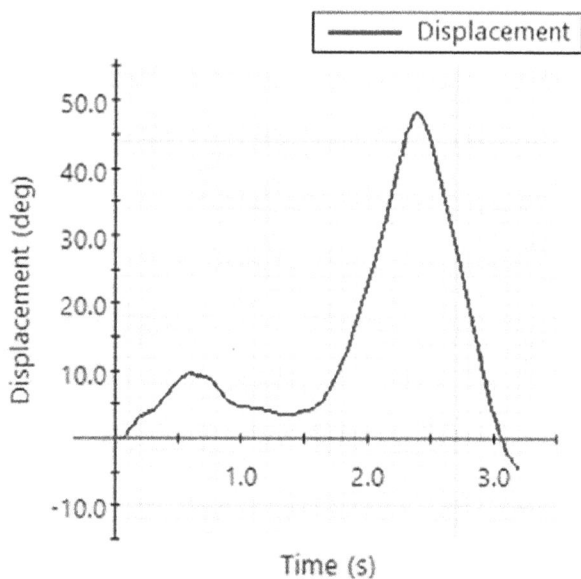

FIGURE 13.5 Input for left knee joint.

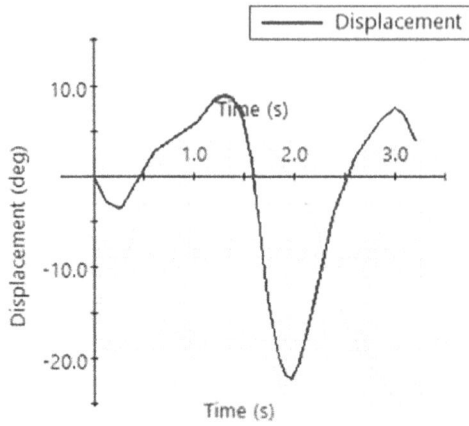

FIGURE 13.6   Input for left ankle joint.

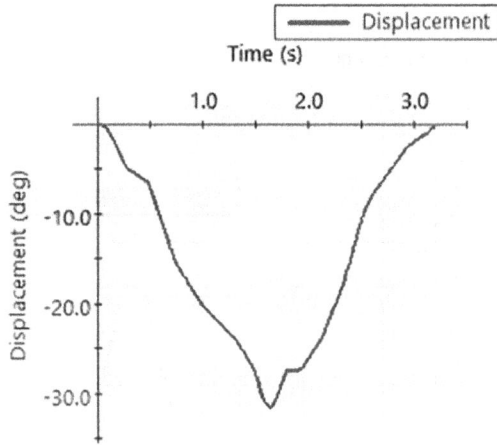

FIGURE 13.7   Input for right hip joint.

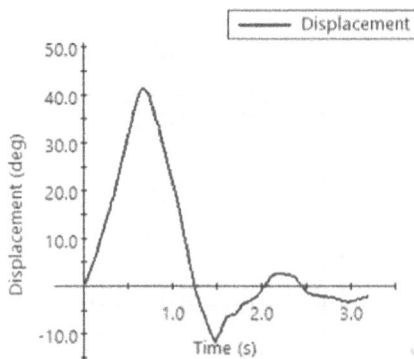

FIGURE 13.8   Input for right knee joint.

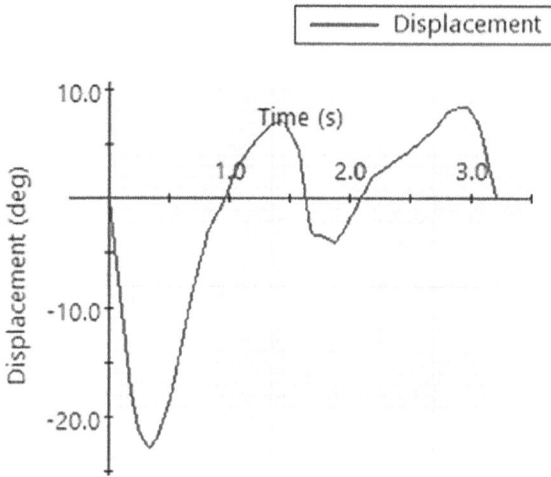

FIGURE 13.9 Input for right ankle joint.

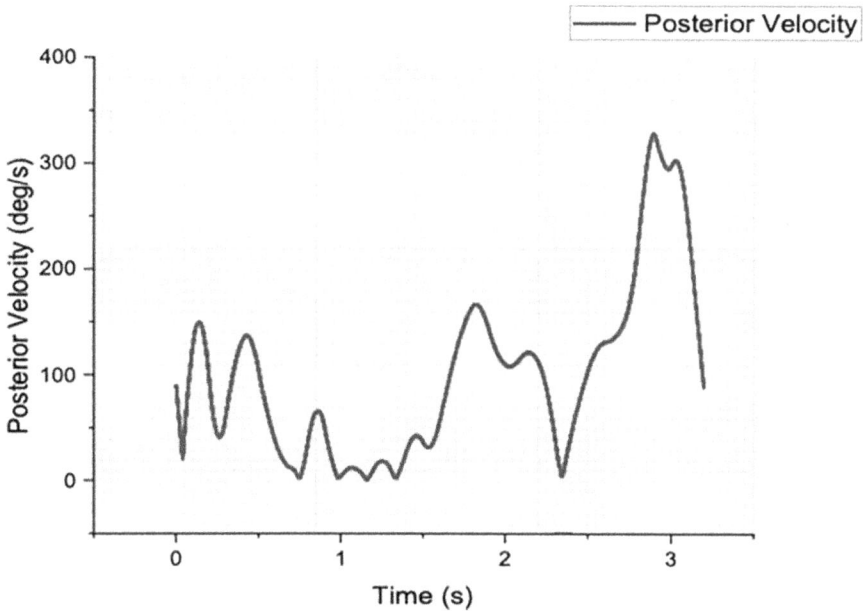

FIGURE 13.10 Angular velocity of posterior part.

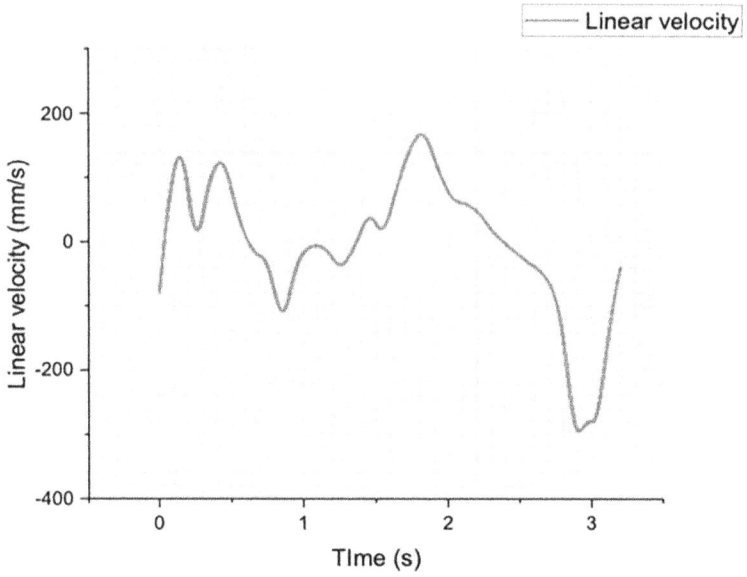

FIGURE 13.11   Linear velocity of piston with respect to cylinder.

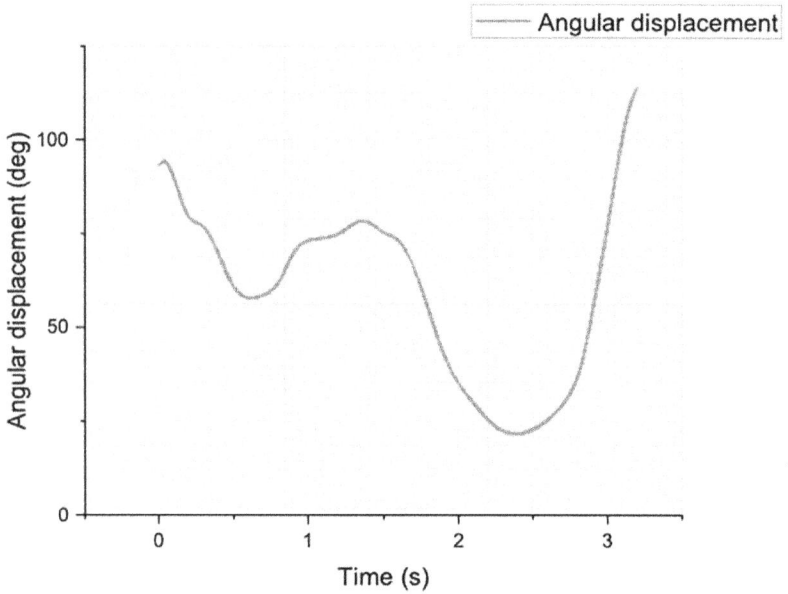

FIGURE 13.12   Angular displacement of piston with respect to posterior.

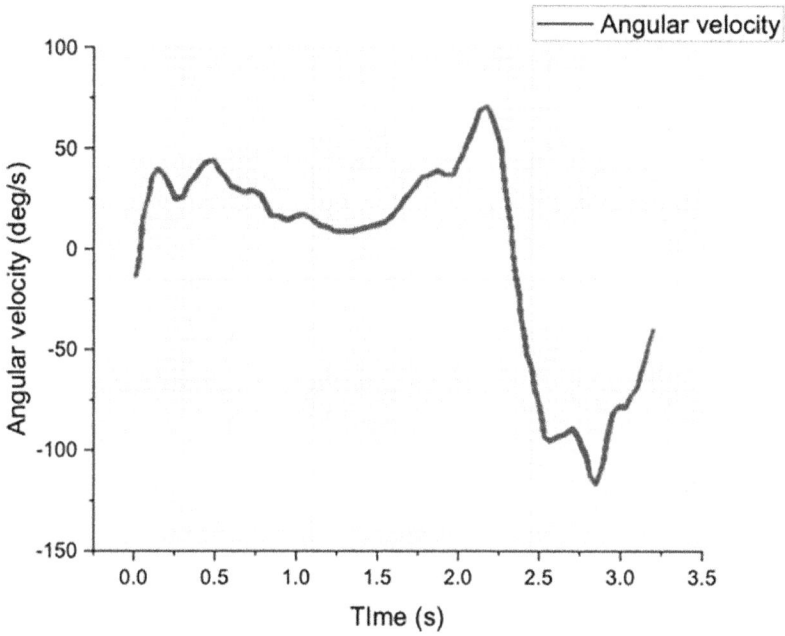

FIGURE 13.13 Angular velocity of inferior part of knee.

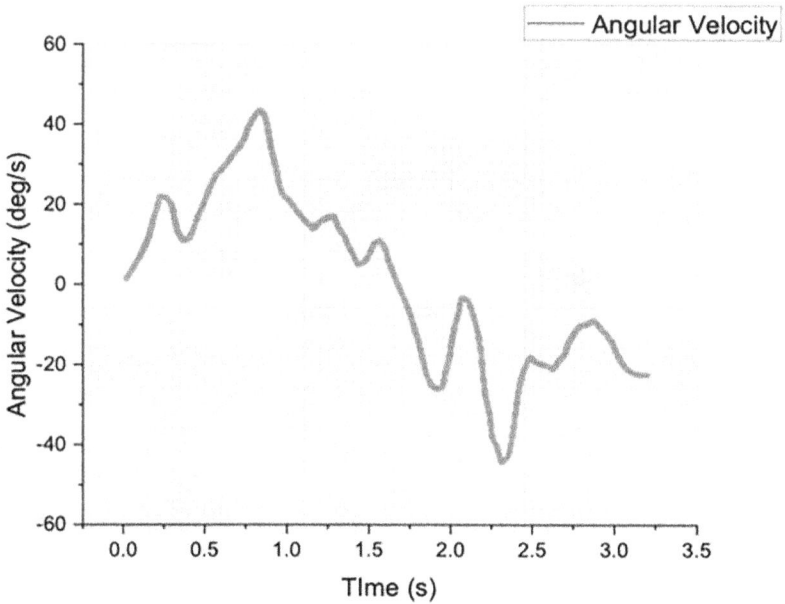

FIGURE 13.14 Angular velocity of hip joint.

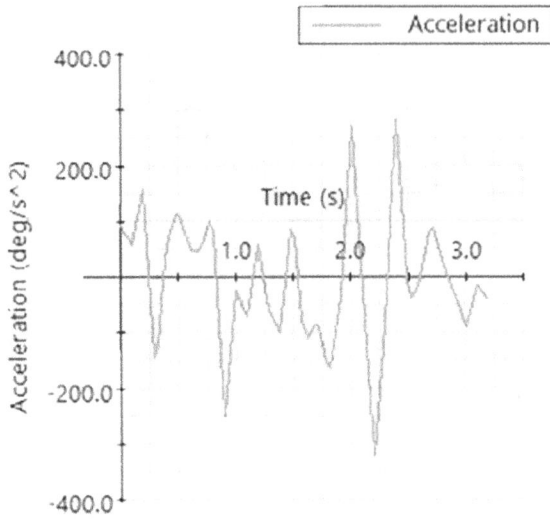

FIGURE 13.15   Angular acceleration of hip joint.

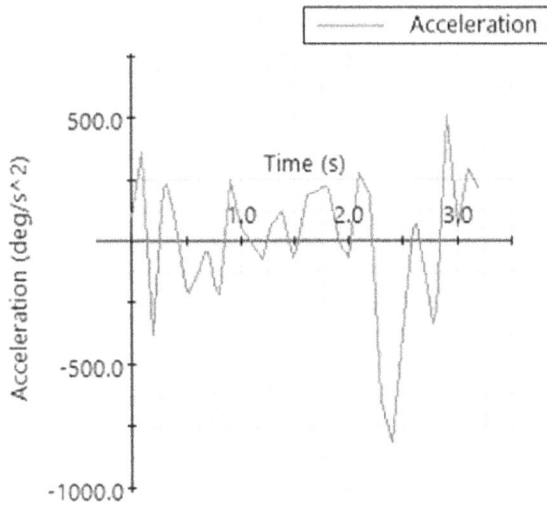

FIGURE 13.16   Angular acceleration of knee joint.

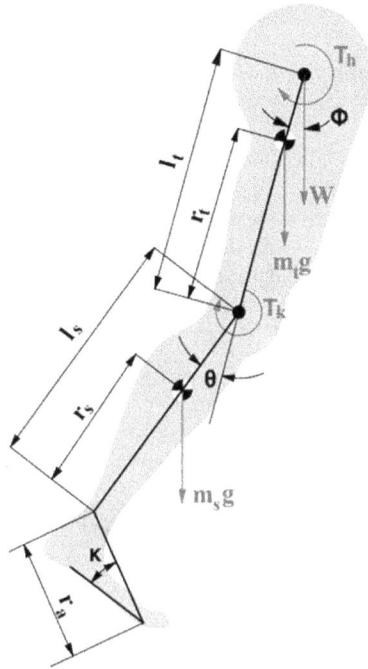

FIGURE 13.17 Free-body diagram of the human leg.

The various terms in the above equation, again obtained from FBD, can be written as follows:

$$I_\theta = I_s + m_t l_s^2 + m_s r_a^2 + m_t r_a^2 + m_s r_s^2 + 2(m_s l_s + m_t r_s) r_a \sin(k) \quad (13.3)$$

$$I_\emptyset = I_s + m_t l_s^2 + m_s r_a^2 + m_t r_a^2 + m_s r_s^2 + m_t l_s r_i \cos(\theta)$$
$$+ 2(m_t l_s + m_s r_s) r_a \sin(k) + m_t r_i r_a \sin(k+\theta) \quad (13.4)$$

$$V = -m_t r_i (r_a \cos(k+\theta) - l_s \sin(\theta)) \emptyset^2 \quad (13.5)$$

$$G = g((m_s r_a + m_t r_a)\cos(k+\theta+\emptyset) - (m_t l_s + m_s r_s)\sin(\theta+\emptyset))$$
$$-Wg(r_a \cos(k+\theta+\emptyset) - l_s \sin(\theta+\emptyset)) \quad (13.6)$$

The various parameters that can be taken for the calculations are listed in Table 13.1.
'k' is the angle that the sole makes with the ankle joint, assumed to be constant at 15°. Using equations (13.2–13.6), the torque at the knee joint was obtained. As mentioned earlier, the knee joint is a four-bar mechanism; hence the torque obtained using equations 13.2–13.6 is the torque at the inferior part of the knee joint. However, the MR damper is attached to the posterior part of the knee joint;

TABLE 13.1

Various Parameters for Calculations

Parameters	Unit	Values
Length of thigh (l_t)	m	0.43
Length of shank (l_s)	m	0.41
Distance of center of mass of the thigh (r_t)	m	0.19
Distance of center of mass of the shank (r_s)	m	0.18
Distance of point of contact of the ankle and joint (r_a)	m	0.275
Mass of thigh (m_t)	kg	5.7
Mass of shank (m_s)	kg	5
Moment of inertia of the thigh (I_t)	kg/m²	0.0982
Moment of inertia of the shank (I_s)	kg/m²	0.0402
Upper body weight of person (W)	kg	50

therefore, we need the torque acting at the posterior part. For this, we use the following equation:

$$T_1\omega_1 = T_2\omega_2 \tag{13.7}$$

The subscript '1' refers to inferior, and the subscript '2' refers to posterior. Using equation (13.7), the curve of torque at the posterior v/s hip angle is obtained, as shown in Figure 13.18.

13.4 CALCULATION OF DAMPING FORCE

Now that we have obtained the torque acting at the posterior part of the knee, we are in a position to calculate the damping force acting on the posterior link. We use the basic torque equation:

$$\vec{T}_p = \vec{r_d} X \vec{F_d} = r_d.F_d.\sin(\alpha)\hat{k} \tag{13.8}$$

where r_d is the length of the appendage of posterior to which the MR damper is attached (75 mm), F_d is the damping force and α is the angle between the piston and posterior, which has already been obtained in Section 13.2.1.2. The curve of damping force v/s hip angle is shown in Figure 13.19.

13.5 DAMPING FORCE ANALYSIS OF MR DAMPER

13.5.1 CFD ON TWIN-TUBE MR DAMPER

Now the next step is to perform CFD and magnetic analysis on the MR damper to understand MR fluid's behavior (MRF 140 CG by Lord corp. in this case). Many commercial software is available to perform CFD. However, ANSYS Fluent is

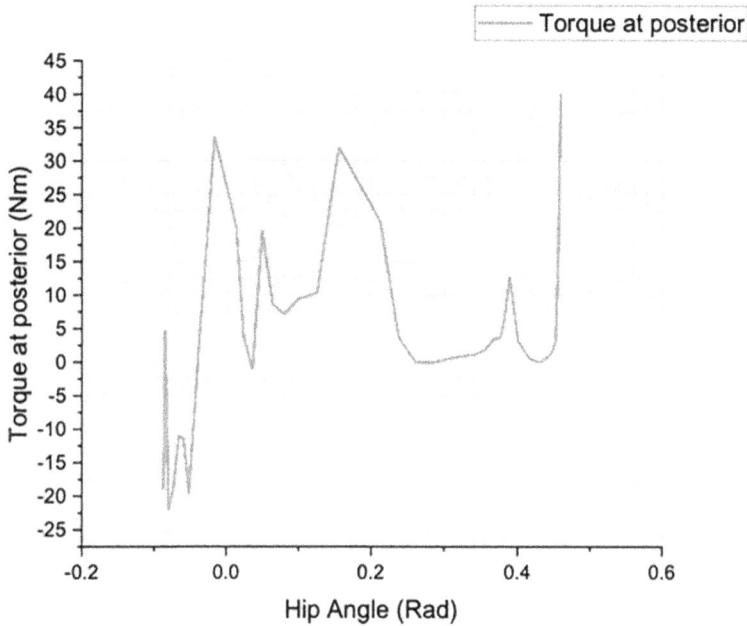

FIGURE 13.18   Variation of torque at the knee (posterior) with hip angle.

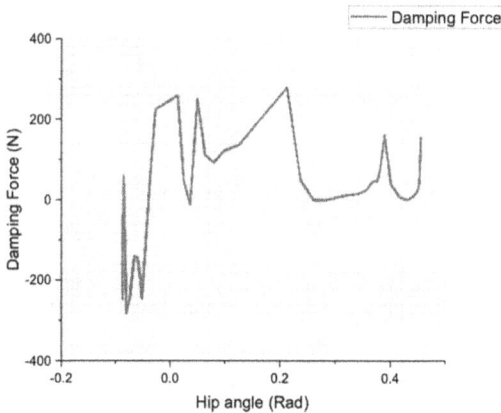

FIGURE 13.19   Variation of damping force with hip angle.

one of the most commonly used. The main aim of CFD is to understand the flow of MR fluid inside the damper and to find out the variation of pressure and velocity of the fluid. This is a transient analysis, and the result shown is valid only for that particular instant. The flow pattern can also be seen; the fluid moves from the inner shock tube to the outer via the foot valve. The obtained results are shown in Figure 13.20.

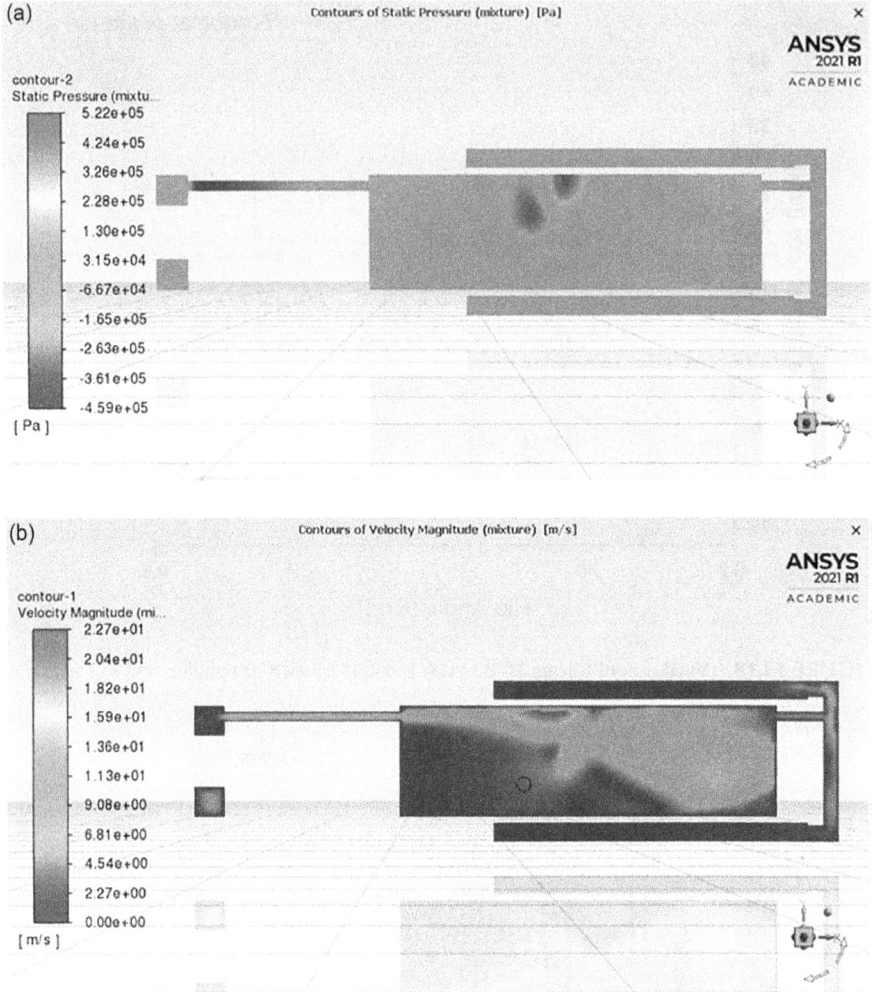

FIGURE 13.20   Variation of pressure (a) and velocity (b) of the MR fluid in the damper.

13.5.2   MAGNETIC ANALYSIS OF MR DAMPER

To understand the behavior of the MR fluid under the influence of a magnetic field, we need to perform magnetic simulation on it. The main aim of magnetic simulation is to obtain the curve of yield stress v/s current. We first need to find out the relationship among magnetic field induced in the MR fluid, current and the coil wire area. The governing equations of the magnetic analysis are:

$$\nabla X H = J \tag{13.9}$$

$$B = \nabla X A \tag{13.10}$$

$$J = \sigma E + \sigma B \ X \ V + J_e \tag{13.11}$$

TABLE 13.2

List of Materials in Piston and Armature

Part	Material
Iron core	Iron
MR fluid	MRF 140CG
Armature coil windings	Copper
Outer piston body	Stainless steel

H is the magnetic field intensity, J is the current density, B is the magnetic field strength and σ is the conductivity. The materials used for simulation are listed in Table 13.2.

The results obtained from the magnetic analysis are shown in Figure 13.21:

The curves obtained from the magnetic analysis showing the variable magnetic flux density with current and coil wire diameter are shown in Figures 13.22 and 13.23.

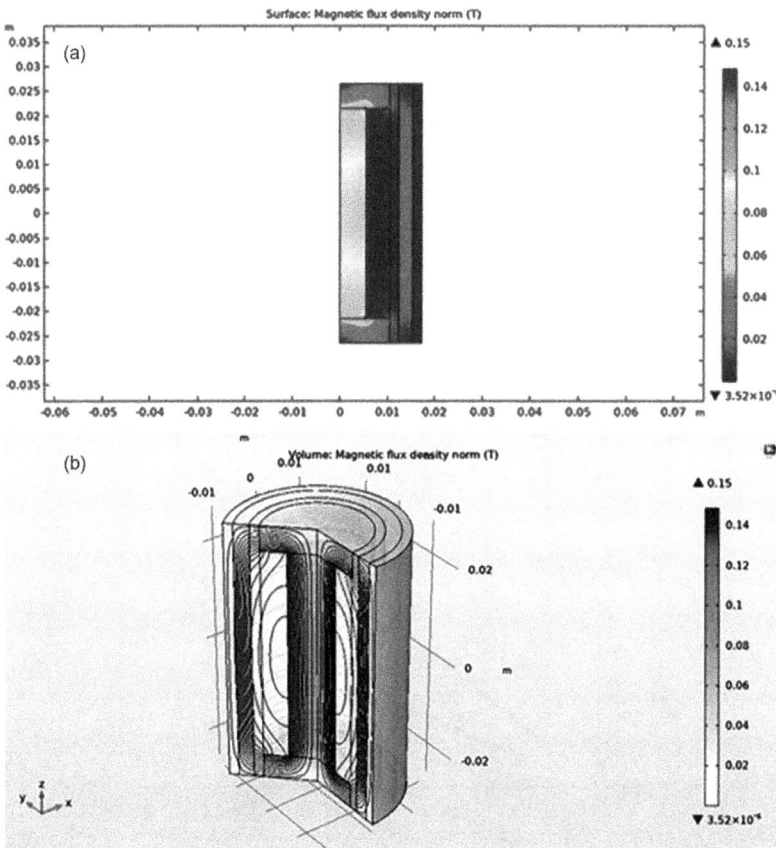

FIGURE 13.21 Variation of magnetic flux density: (a) 2D and (b) 3D (A = 1 mm²).

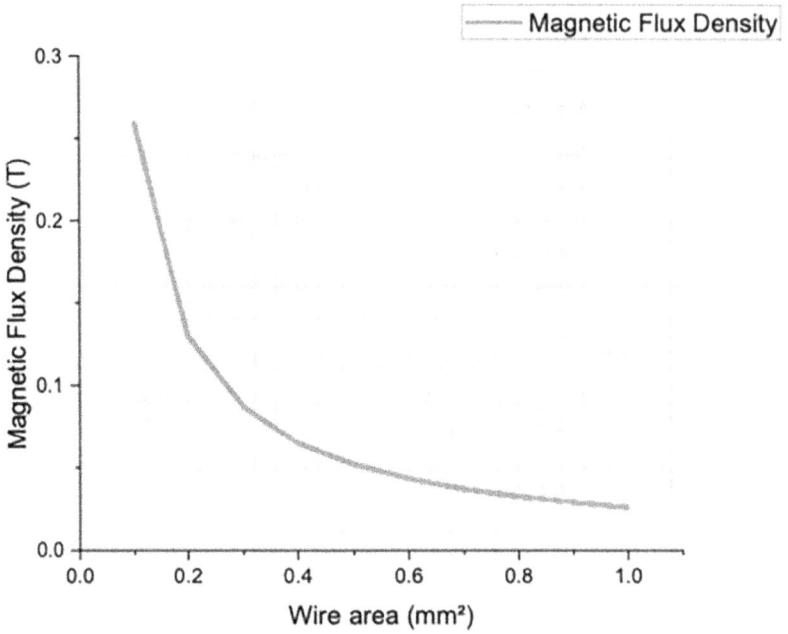

FIGURE 13.22   Variation of magnetic flux density with wire area (Current = 1A).

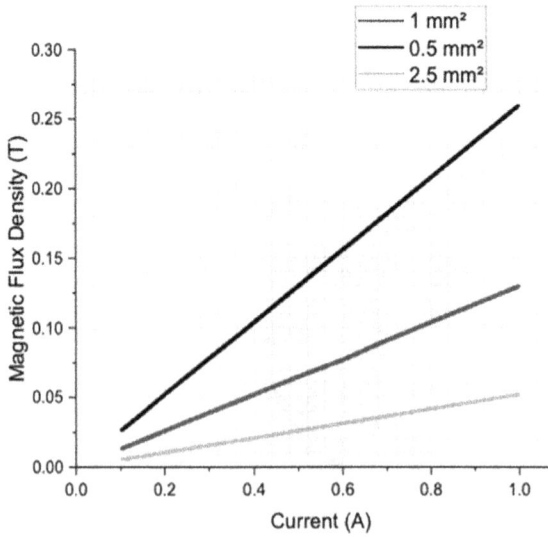

FIGURE 13.23   Variation of magnetic flux density with the current for various wire areas.

These results obtained from the magnetic analysis can be used to find the relationship between the yield stress of MRF 140CG and the current. The hysteresis curve and the yield stress v/s magnetic field strength curves, being standard for the chosen MR fluid, can be taken from the Lord corporation website. Combining these two curves with the obtained curve of magnetic flux density v/s current, yield stress v/s current has been obtained as shown in Figures 13.24 and 13.25:

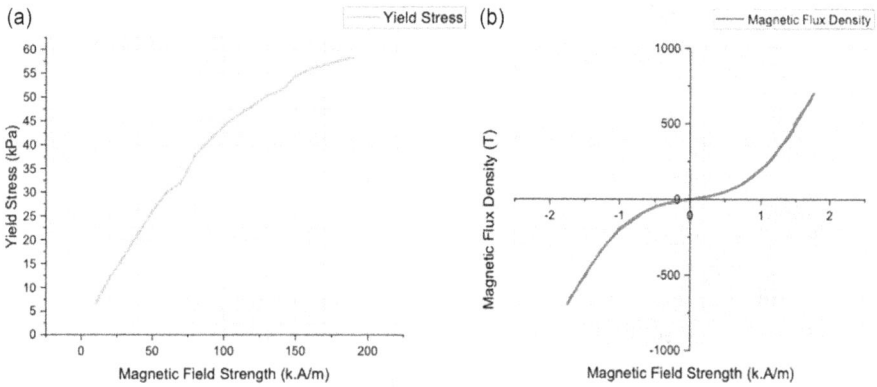

FIGURE 13.24   Shear stress v/s magnetic field (a) and hysteresis curve (b) of MRF 140CG.

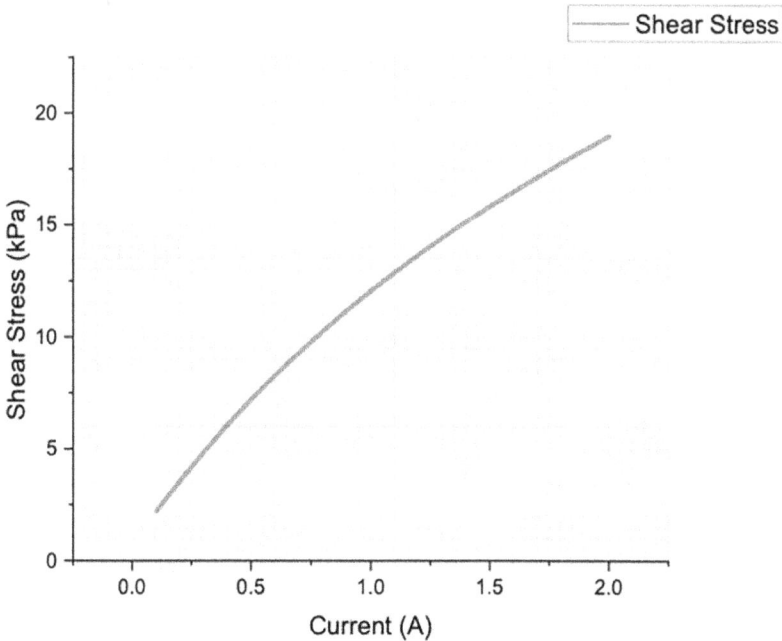

FIGURE 13.25   Variation of yield stress v/s current.

13.6   SUMMARY

1. More and more research on prosthetic devices has led to the use of smart materials like MR fluid. MR fluid is a smart material whose properties vary with change in the magnetic field. It changes its yield stress and viscosity in the direction of the magnetic field, allowing it to be used in various designs. It is used in brakes, dampers, fluid valves, prosthesis, medical industries, etc.
2. An MR damper is a simple yet effective device that provides damping force under its working fluid's rheological properties. It is used in prosthetic devices to a) absorb shocks and b) provide necessary damping force and torque at the specific joint.
3. A simple design of a prosthetic leg for AK amputees was shown in this chapter. Kinematic and dynamic analysis was shown to understand the various velocities, accelerations, forces, and torques on the human leg during the gait cycle. CFD and magnetic analysis were performed to understand the flow patterns and rheological properties of the MR fluid. A damping force v/s current curve was established, and it was seen that the MR damper could be easily controlled to provide the necessary damping force.
4. Prosthetic knees and ankles have various kinds of mechanisms and actuators. MR damper is a cheap actuator that can also act as a vibration control. A practical design for the knee joint is a four-bar mechanism that perfectly serves the purpose due to its wide range of motion.
5. There are many control strategies for the MR damper and many MR damper models defining the working principle of MR fluids. One of the most common controllers is the PID controller, which is very easy to design and simple to implement and improves the device's performance. A PID controller stabilizes the entire system by minimizing the error between the desired and the actual knee angle and hence the torque too.

REFERENCES

1. "15 limb loss statistics that may surprise you - access prosthetics." https://accessprosthetics.com/15-limb-loss-statistics-may-surprise/ (accessed Jun. 10, 2021).
2. "Physical therapy guide to above-knee amputation (transfemoral amputation) - ChoosePT.com."https://www.choosept.com/symptomsconditionsdetail/physical-therapy-guide-to-aboveknee-amputation (accessed Jun. 10, 2021).
3. D. Mohan, "A report on amputees in India," *Orthot. Prosthetics*, vol. 40, no. 1, pp. 16–32, 1986, [Online]. Available: http://www.oandp.org/jpo/.
4. B. Daniele, *Evolution of Prosthetic Feet and Design Based on Gait Analysis Data*, 2nd Ed. Elsevier Inc., (2019).
5. P. K. Kumar, M. Charan, and S. Kanagaraj, "Trends and challenges in lower limb prosthesis," *IEEE Potent.*, vol. 36, no. 1, pp. 19–23, (2017).
6. A. F. Azocar, L. M. Mooney, J. F. Duval, A. M. Simon, L. J. Hargrove, and E. J. Rouse, "Design and clinical implementation of an open-source bionic leg," *Nat. Biomed. Eng.*, vol. 4, no. 10, pp. 941–953, (2020).
7. G. Shastry, A. Toby, M. B. Kumbhar, V. G. Salunkhe, and T. Jagadeesha, "Simulation and optimization of materials used for prosthetic leg for above-knee amputees using MR fluid," *Mater. Today Proc.*, vol. 45, no. 6, pp. 5292–5298, (2021).

8. H. L. Xie, Z. Z. Liang, F. Li, and L. X. Guo, "The knee joint design and control of above-knee intelligent bionic leg based on magneto-rheological damper," *Int. J. Autom. Comput.*, vol. 7, no. 3, pp. 277–282, (2010).

9. J. Park, G.-H. Yoon, J.-W. Kang, and S.-B. Choi, "Design and control of a prosthetic leg for above-knee amputees operated in semi-active and active modes," *Smart Mater. Struct.*, vol. 25, no. 8, p. 085009, Aug. (2016).

10. O. Baser, H. Kizilhan, and E. Kilic, "Employing variable impedance (stiffness/damping) hybrid actuators on lower limb exoskeleton robots for stable and safe walking trajectory tracking," *J. Mech. Sci. Technol.*, vol. 34, no. 6, pp. 2597–2607, (2020).

11. J. H. Kim and J. H. Oh, "Development of an above knee prosthesis using MR damper and leg simulator," *Proc. - IEEE Int. Conf. Robot. Autom.*, vol. 4, pp. 3686–3691, (2001).

12. H. Metered, A. Elsawaf, T. Vampola, and Z. Sika, "Vibration control of MR-damped vehicle suspension system using PID controller tuned by particle swarm optimization," *SAE Int. J. Passeng. Cars - Mech. Syst.*, vol. 8, no. 2, pp. 426–435, (2015).

13. M. R. Mataušek and T. B. Šekara, "PID controller frequency-domain tuning for stable, integrating and unstable processes, including dead-time," *J. Process Control*, vol. 21, no. 1, pp. 17–27, (2011).

14. M. H. A. Talib and I. Z. M. Darus, "Self-tuning PID controller with MR damper and hydraulic actuator for suspension system," *Proceedings - International Conference on Intelligent Systems, Modelling and Simulation*, pp. 119–124, (2013).

15. M. H. Ab Talib et al., "Vibration control of semi-active suspension system using PID controller with advanced firefly algorithm and particle swarm optimization," *J. Ambient Intell. Humaniz. Comput.*, vol. 12, pp. 1119–1137, (2020).

16. G. Q. Zeng, X. Q. Xie, M. R. Chen, and J. Weng, "Adaptive population extremal optimization-based PID neural network for multivariable nonlinear control systems," *Swarm Evol. Comput.*, vol. 44, pp. 320–334, (2019).

17. W. W. Choe, "Intelligent PID controller and its application to structural vibration mitigation with MR Damper," *Trans. Korean Inst. Electr. Eng.*, vol. 64, no. 8, pp. 1224–1230, (2015).

18. B. Kasemi, A. G. A. Muthalif, M. M. Rashid, and S. Fathima, "Fuzzy-PID controller for semi-active vibration control using magnetorheological fluid damper," *Procedia Eng.*, vol. 41, no. Iris, pp. 1221–1227, (2012).

19. M. H. A. Talib and I. Z. M. Darus, "Self-tuning PID controller with MR damper and hydraulic actuator for suspension system," in *2013 Fifth International Conference on Computational Intelligence, Modelling and Simulation*, Sep. 2013, pp. 119–124, (2013).

20. G.-Q. Zeng, X.-Q. Xie, M.-R. Chen, and J. Weng, "Adaptive population extremal optimization-based PID neural network for multivariable nonlinear control systems," *Swarm Evol. Comput.*, vol. 44, pp. 320–334, Feb. (2019).

21. H. L. Li, C. Yong, H. Qi, and L. I. Jian, "Fuzzy PID control for landing gear based on magneto-rheological (MR) Damper," *2009 International Conference on Apperceiving Computing and Intelligence Analysis ICACIA 2009*, pp. 22–25, (2009).

22. J. D. Carlson, D. M. Catanzarite, and K. A. St. Clair, "Commercial magneto-rheological fluid devices," *Int. J. Mod. Phys. B*, vol. 10, no. 23n24, pp. 2857–2865, Oct. (1996).

23. J. D. Carlson and M. R. Jolly, "MR fluid, foam and elastomer devices," *Mechatronics*, vol. 10, no. 4–5, pp. 555–569, Jun. (2000).

24. M. Braz Cesar and R. de Barros, "Properties and numerical modeling of Mr Dampers," *15th International Conference on Experimental Mechanics*, pp. 1–17, (2012).

25. B. K. Kumbhar and S. R. Patil, "A study on properties and selection criteria for magneto-rheological (MR) fluid components," *Int. J. ChemTech Res.*, vol. 6, no. 6 SPEC. ISS., pp. 3303–3306, (2014).

26. T. Data, "MRF-140CG magneto-rheological fluid," *Lord Prod. Sel. Guid. lord Magnetorheol. fluids*, vol. 74, pp. 5–6, 2008, [Online]. Available: www.lord.com (2008).

27. J. S. Kumar, P. S. Paul, G. Raghunathan, and D. G. Alex, "A review of challenges and solutions in the preparation and use of magnetorheological fluids," *Int. J. Mech. Mater. Eng.*, vol. 14, no. 1, (2019).

28. C. Guerrero-Sanchez, T. Lara-Ceniceros, E. Jimenez-Regalado, M. Raşa, and U. S. Schubert, "Magnetorheological fluids based on ionic liquids," *Adv. Mater.*, vol. 19, no. 13, pp. 1740–1747, (2007).

29. S. Jain et al., "Performance investigation of integrated model of quarter car semi-active seat suspension with human model." *Appl. Sci.* Vol.10 no. 9, p. 3185, (2020).

30. Z. Q. Gu and S. O. Oyadiji, "Application of MR damper in structural control using ANFIS method," *Comput. Struct.*, vol. 86, no. 3–5, pp. 427–436, (2008).

31. J. D. Carlson, "What makes a good MR fluid?" *J. Intell. Mater. Syst. Struct.*, vol. 13, no. 7–8, pp. 431–435, (2002).

32. P. Kulkarni, C. Ciocanel, S. L. Vieira, and N. Naganathan, "Study of the behavior of MR fluids in squeeze, torsional and valve modes," *J. Intell. Mater. Syst. Struct.*, vol. 14, no. 2, pp. 99–104, (2003).

33. V. M. Akhil, M. Ashmi, P. K. Rajendrakumar, and K. S. Sivanandan, "Human gait recognition using hip, knee and ankle joint ratios," *IRBM*, vol. 41, no. 3, pp. 133–140, Jun. (2020).

34. R. Borjian, *Design, Modeling, and Control of an Active Prosthetic Knee*. University of Waterloo, (2008).

35. F. Sup, H. A. Varol, J. Mitchell, T. Withrow, and M. Goldfarb, "Design and control of an active electrical knee and ankle prosthesis," in *2008 2nd IEEE RAS & EMBS International Conference on Biomedical Robotics and Biomechatronics*, pp. 523–528, (2008).

36. A. K. Lapre, *Semi-Active Damping for an Intelligent Adaptive Ankle Prosthesis*. University of Massachusetts Amherst, (2012).

37. S. G. Bhat, *Design and Development of a Passive Prosthetic Ankle*. Arizona State University, (2017).

38. W. Li, *Development and Evaluation of a Quick Release Posterior Strut Ankle Foot Orthosis*. Univeristy of Ottawa, Ottawa, (2020).

39. S. Huang and J. M. Schimmels, "Design of a 2 DOF prosthetic ankle using coupled compliance to increase ankle torque," *Volume 4: 36th Mechanisms and Robotics Conference, Parts A and B*, pp. 27–34, (2012).

40. E. M. Ficanha, M. Rastgaar, and K. R. Kaufman, "Control of a 2-DOF powered ankle-foot mechanism," *2015 IEEE International Conference on Robotics and Automation*, pp. 6439–6444, (2015).

41. S. K. Au and H. M. Herr, "Powered ankle-foot prosthesis," *IEEE Robot. Autom. Mag.*, vol. 15, no. 3, pp. 52–59, (2008).

42. J. K. Hitt, T. G. Sugar, M. Holgate, and R. Bellman, "An active foot-ankle prosthesis with biomechanical energy regeneration," *J. Med. Devices, Trans. ASME*, vol. 4, no. 1, pp. 1–9, (2010).

43. J. Geeroms, L. Flynn, R. Jimenez-Fabian, B. Vanderborght, and D. Lefeber, "Energetic analysis and optimization of a MACCEPA actuator in an ankle prosthesis: Energetic evaluation of the CYBERLEGs alpha-prosthesis variable stiffness actuator during a realistic load cycle," *Auton. Robots*, vol. 42, no. 1, pp. 147–158, (2018).

44. D. Adiputra, Ubaidillah, S. A. M. H. Zamzuri, and M. A. A. Rahman, "Jurnal Teknologi fuzzy logic control for ankle foot equipped with," *J. Teknol.*, vol. 11, pp. 25–32, (2016).

45. C. Khazoom, C. Veronneau, J. P. L. Bigue, J. Grenier, A. Girard, and J. S. Plante, "Design and control of a multifunctional ankle exoskeleton powered by magnetorheological actuators to assist walking, jumping, and landing," *IEEE Robot. Autom. Lett.*, vol. 4, no. 3, pp. 3083–3090, (2019).
46. T. Kikuchi, S. Tanida, K. Otsuki, T. Yasuda, and J. Furusho, "Development of third-generation intelligently controllable ankle-foot orthosis with compact MR fluid brake," *Proc. - IEEE Int. Conf. Robot. Autom.*, pp. 2209–2214, (2010).
47. C. Li et al., "Research and development of the intelligently-controlled prosthetic ankle joint," *2006 IEEE Int. Conf. Mechatronics Autom. ICMA 2006*, vol. 2006, pp. 1114–1119, (2006).
48. H. Naito, Y. Akazawa, K. Tagaya, T. Matsumoto, and M. Tanaka, "An ankle-foot orthosis with a variable-resistance ankle joint using a magnetorheological-fluid rotary damper," *J. Biomech. Sci. Eng.*, vol. 4, no. 2, pp. 182–191, (2009).
49. M. A. Holgate, J. K. Hitt, R. D. Bellman, T. G. Sugar, and K. W. Hollander, "The SPARKy (spring ankle with regenerative kinetics) project: Choosing a DC motor based actuation method," *Proceedings of the 2nd Biennial IEEE/RAS-EMBS International Conference on Biomedical Robotics and Biomechatronics, BioRob 2008*, pp. 163–168, (2008).
50. T. Yu, A. R. Plummer, P. Iravani, J. Bhatti, S. Zahedi, and D. Moser, "The design, control, and testing of an integrated electrohydrostatic powered ankle prosthesis," *IEEE/ASME Trans. Mechatronics*, vol. 24, no. 3, pp. 1011–1022, (2019).
51. M. Cempini, L. J. Hargrove, and T. Lenzi, "Design, development, and bench-top testing of a powered polycentric ankle prosthesis," *IEEE Int. Conf. Intell. Robot. Syst.*, vol. 2017-Sept, pp. 1064–1069, (2017).
52. T. Lenzi, M. Cempini, L. J. Hargrove, and T. A. Kuiken, "Design, development, and validation of a lightweight nonbackdrivable robotic ankle prosthesis," *IEEE/ASME Trans. Mechatronics*, vol. 24, no. 2, pp. 471–482, (2019).

14 FEA of Humerus Bone Fracture and Healing

Ashwani Kumar
Technical Education Department Uttar Pradesh

Yatika Gori and Brijesh Yadav
Graphic Era University Dehradun

Sachin Rana
ABES Institute of Technology Ghaziabad

Neelesh Kumar Sharma
Indian Institute of Technology Patna

CONTENTS

14.1 INTRODUCTION

Many research works have been carried out over the past 20 years in the field of whole-body vibration (WBV) and hand vibration. Femur bone and humerus bone were studied by various researchers. Finite element analysis (FEA) [1] method was also used earlier for bone analysis [2,3]. Pedestrian and seat-induced vibration was studied for proper investigation of WBV [4,5]. They have analyzed transmission of vibrations from the seat to the human head and procured its mechanical and psychological aspects on the whole body. WBV causes lower back pain. From the study, it was established that there exists a direct relation

DOI: 10.1201/9781003286806-14

between WBV and back pain. Methods that could be used to reduce the back pain caused by external vibrations were also discussed in the review. In earlier studies, authors have done a limited study of WBV or hand vibration to find natural frequencies [6]. Tiemessen et al. [7] have studied different strategies for reducing WBV in drivers. They have conducted a study to reduce hazards caused by WBV. Vibrational characteristics of the femur and human tibia were studied by a researcher to find natural frequencies [8,9]. Khalil et al. [9] carried out an experiment based on Fourier analysis to deduce the resonance frequency and mode shape results of the femur bone. An analytical approach was also used for the same purpose. The mathematical model generated used 59 elements for performing the analysis. The frequency used in the experiments was within the range of 250–7300 Hz. Oliver et al. [10] have performed case studies for improving WBV attenuation in the lab and field.

Pelker et al. [11] have investigated the femur bone dynamic conditions. Holmlund et al. [12] performed an experiment to deduce the effect of vibrations on the human body in sitting posture. The results show that the impedance increases with the frequency up to 5 Hz and then starts to decrease in a complex manner. Valentini et al. [13] have studied the human spine and vibration impact on the human spine using the dynamic spline approach. Huiskes et al. [14] have studied the biomechanics of the hand-arm system. Dong et al. [15,16] have introduced a method to determine the vibration energy absorbed in the palm and fingers of the hand-arm vibration (HAV) system. The experiment was performed for frequencies ranging from 16 to 1000 Hz. They have performed various tests to find the resonance frequency of a hand-arm system. It was found that resonance frequency for the human hand-arm system varies from 20 to 50 Hz. They have used the finite element method to study the HAV system and accomplished that most of the vibrations are confined at the fingers and the palm. Kumar et al. [17] have studied HAV and identified the first ten natural frequencies using modal analysis for different boundary conditions. Kumar et al. [18–20] have studied cortical, femur bone and identified different modes of vibration using FEA. From the literature survey, it was concluded that fracture in humerus bone can occur under two conditions, first across the shaft and second across the elbow and shoulder joints. Fracture across the shaft occurs under high pressure and loading conditions or under continuous vibrations for example as in a road accident. The 3D analysis of humerus bone is difficult to perform due to its intricate alignment. Therefore, for this research work, we consider a simple profile of the humerus bone using solid works [21]. A. Kumar et al. have studied the grid independency test for better meshing results and biomechanical aspects of femur bone was studied using finite element analysis [22]. In continuation Gangwar et. al. [23] has performed the FEA design and analysis of Femur bone. They have performed the structural and modal analysis for finding the crack location. After identifying the crack, they have suggested suitable healing method.

14.2   RESEARCH METHODOLOGY

Figure 14.1 shows a step-by-step research methodology that has been adopted for the design and analysis of humerus bone and its fracture healing.

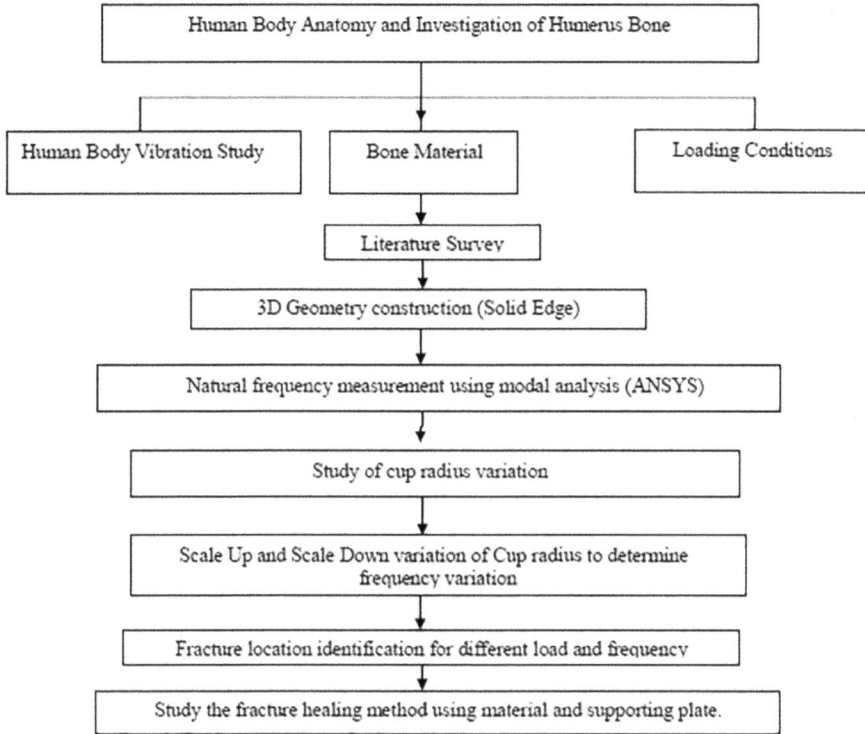

```
┌─────────────────────────────────────────────────────────────────────┐
│         Human Body Anatomy and Investigation of Humerus Bone          │
└─────────────────────────────────────────────────────────────────────┘

┌──────────────────────────┐  ┌──────────────────┐  ┌──────────────────┐
│ Human Body Vibration Study│  │  Bone Material   │  │ Loading Conditions│
└──────────────────────────┘  └──────────────────┘  └──────────────────┘

                      ┌──────────────────────┐
                      │   Literature Survey   │
                      └──────────────────────┘

              ┌────────────────────────────────────────┐
              │ 3D Geometry construction (Solid Edge)   │
              └────────────────────────────────────────┘

        ┌──────────────────────────────────────────────────────┐
        │ Natural frequency measurement using modal analysis (ANSYS)│
        └──────────────────────────────────────────────────────┘

           ┌────────────────────────────────────────────┐
           │       Study of cup radius variation          │
           └────────────────────────────────────────────┘

        ┌──────────────────────────────────────────────────┐
        │ Scale Up and Scale Down variation of Cup radius to determine│
        │                  frequency variation              │
        └──────────────────────────────────────────────────┘

        ┌──────────────────────────────────────────────────┐
        │ Fracture location identification for different load and frequency│
        └──────────────────────────────────────────────────┘

     ┌──────────────────────────────────────────────────────────┐
     │ Study the fracture healing method using material and supporting plate.│
     └──────────────────────────────────────────────────────────┘
```

FIGURE 14.1   Systematic representation of the research methodology adopted.

14.3   MODELING AND BOUNDARY CONDITIONS

CT scan data collected from the hospital were analyzed and used to construct the CAD model of the humerus bone (Figure 14.2). The modeling of the bone is done using the software Solid Works [21]. To perform the vibrational analysis of the bone, the humerus bone shaft is considered to be cylindrical and the shoulder and elbow joints are modeled as hemispherical cups, keeping the elbow cup smaller than the shoulder cup. This is done to simplify the design as well as the analysis procedure as the actual geometry of the bone is complex. However, the properties of the bone are kept the same to predict the actual bone results. The dimensions of the humerus bone are as follows: length (L) of bone shaft = 250 mm and cylindrical shaft radius (r) = 8.33 mm. Shoulder cup radius ($R1$) = 33.32 mm, elbow cup radius ($R2$) = 24.99 mm, L/r = 30, $R1/r$ = 4, and $R2/r$ = 3 [2].

The software used for modeling the humerus bone is Solid Works and the analysis is performed using Ansys 16.2. The .*IGES file of the model designed in Solid Works is imported into Ansys. To carry out the FEA simulation, the model is divided into smaller parts called elements and these elements are connected at nodes. Figure 14.3 shows the meshed model of the humerus bone. The number of elements in the meshed model of the bone is 24,644 and the number of nodes is 8647. Meshing is done by using linear tetrahedral elements. Humerus bone analysis

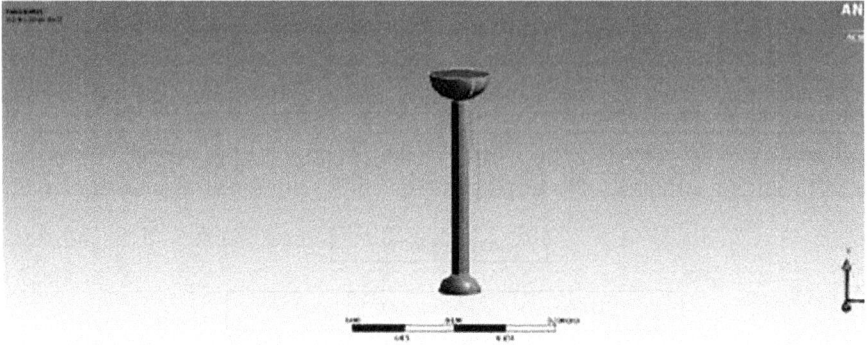

FIGURE 14.2 Humerus bone shown as CAD model.

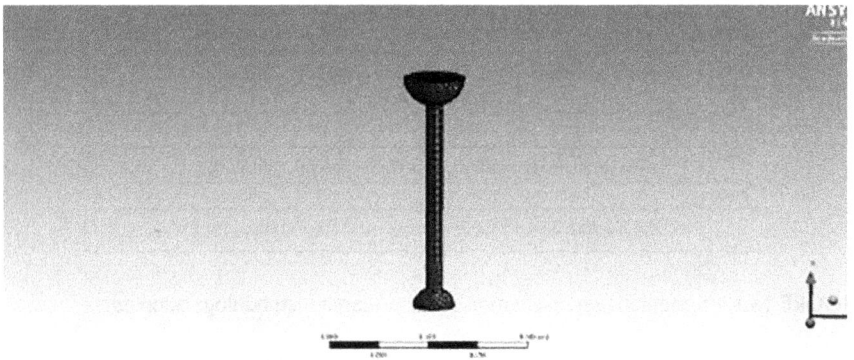

FIGURE 14.3 Meshed model of the humerus bone.

was performed for three boundary conditions. The first condition of analysis is the free-free boundary condition. The second boundary condition is fixed-fixed. The last boundary condition used for analysis is one side fixed and one side free. For the free-free condition, the degree of freedom (DOF) is allowed variations, i.e., both the shoulder and elbow cups are free at the joints. For fixed-fixed boundary conditions, the cups at the shoulder and elbow are constrained. Under the third boundary condition of one side fixed and one side free, the shoulder cup is kept fixed and the elbow cup is free for variations. The results of all three boundary conditions are analyzed and compared. It is found that the second boundary condition (fixed-fixed) gives the more accurate outcomes and also explains the human hand-arm biodynamics precisely. Vibration mode shapes for the first ten modes are considered in our analysis. The two boundary conditions applied are free-free and fixed-fixed. The DOF under free-free conditions is exposed to variations and in the case of fixed-fixed ones, all DOF are obliged in boundaries. The mechanical properties of the humerus bone are shown in Table 14.1 [2].

TABLE 14.1
Mechanical Properties of the
Humerus Bone Material [2]

Mechanical Properties	Mathematical Value
Young's modulus	17.2 GPa
Poisson's ratio	0.30
Density	1900 kg/m³

TABLE 14.2
Mode and Natural Frequency Variation

Mode	Both Sides Fixed (N.F) (Hz)	Both Sides Free (N.F) (Hz)	One Side Fixed-One Side Free (N.F) (Hz)
1	565.47	0	53.133
2	573.49	0	53.454
3	1573.2	7.8953e-004	423.61
4	1587.1	1.4904e-003	425.79
5	3063.9	15.468	527.72
6	3081.2	15.832	1200.5
7	3452.2	276.87	1209.2
8	4971.8	277.24	1855.7
9	4988.1	600.43	2194.2
10	5321.2	805.9	2229.5

14.4 FEA RESULTS

Table 14.2 shows the resonance frequencies for all three boundary conditions. The simulated results when compared with the experimental results show that the fixed-fixed (Figure 14.4) condition gives more precise results for humerus bone analysis. Therefore for further analysis, we choose this condition. The natural frequency for this condition for mode one is 565.67 Hz. Of the many reasons for a fracture in the humerus bone, we consider external excitation as the main reason for fracture. A fracture may occur in the bone when the natural frequency is paired with the external excitation frequency. The resonance frequency of the humerus bone lies between 565.67 and 5321.2 Hz (Table 14.2). The analysis results are compared with the experimental results deduced by Khalil et al. [9] and validated. The experimental value for the frequency is given between 250 and 7239 Hz. The natural frequency deduced from the modal simulation is in the range of 0–805.9 Hz for free-free conditions (Figure 14.5). Under both side fixed conditions, the range of frequency is 565.47–5321.2 Hz. For the one side fixed and one side free condition, the frequency is between 53.133 and 2229.5 Hz (Figure 14.6). The results match with those of Khalil et al. [9].

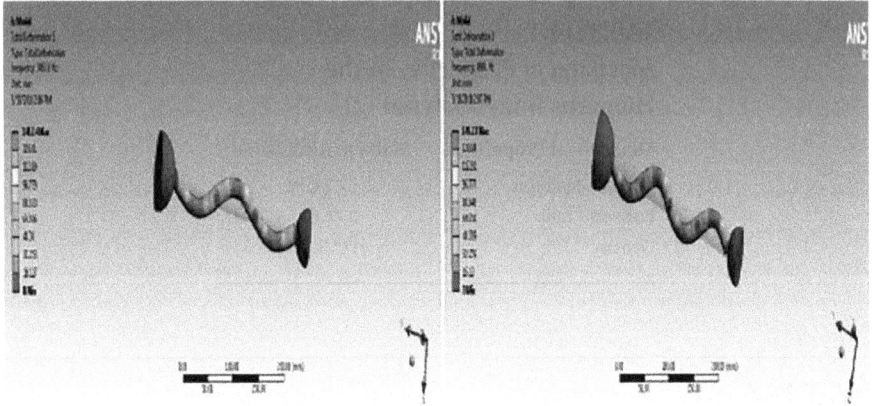

FIGURE 14.4   Different modes of the humerus bone model (both sides fixed boundary condition).

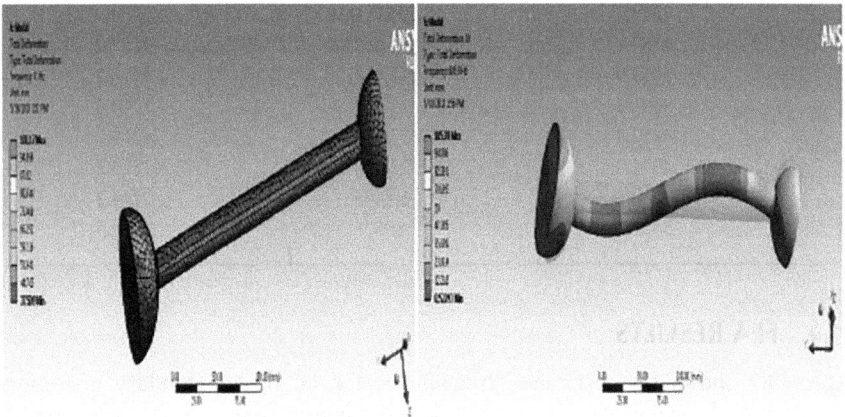

FIGURE 14.5   Different mode shapes of the humerus bone model (both sides free boundary condition).

Figure 14.7 shows that boundary conditions fixed-fixed have better results in comparison to other conditions. For this condition, deformation requires more natural frequency compared to other boundary conditions. For further analysis, only fixed-fixed conditions will be considered.

14.5   CUP RADIUS VARIATION

The simulation is carried out for different size humerus bones. First, the geometry parameters (length of shaft and cup radius) are scaled down by 0.85. For the second

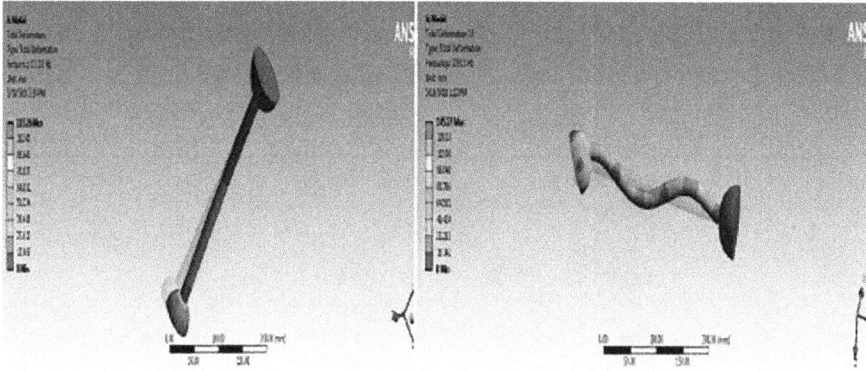

FIGURE 14.6 Different mode shapes (one side fixed and one side free boundary condition).

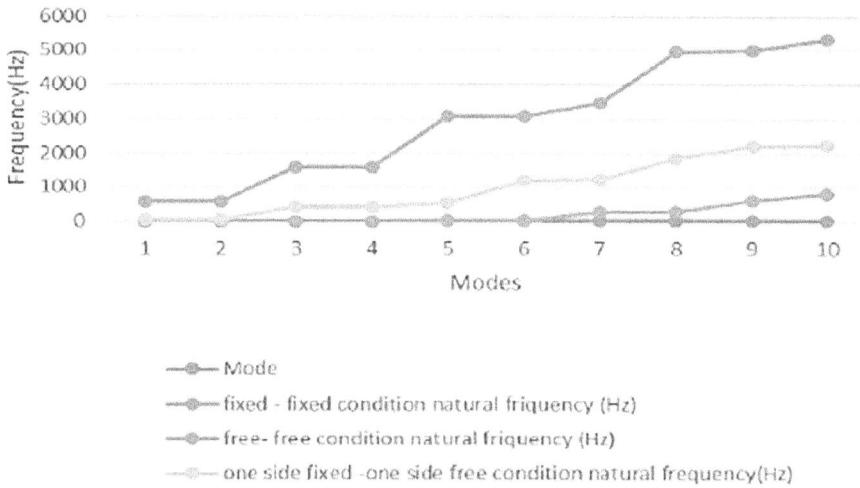

FIGURE 14.7 Frequency variation plot for different boundary conditions.

analysis, the geometry parameters (length of shaft and cup radius) are scaled up by 1.5. The scaling of the geometry is done because the bone size varies from person to person. By scaling down 0.85, the geometry size is reduced and the size of geometry increases by scaling up 1.5. Body height, age, nutrition, etc. affect the bone size. The modal analysis for these two geometries is performed. All three boundary conditions are studied. The dimensions of the two profiles used for analysis are: for scaling down, the shaft length and radius are 0.2125 and 0.00708 m, respectively, the shoulder cup radius is 0.02832 m, and the elbow cup radius is 0.02124 m. For scaling up, the shaft length and radius are 0.3750 and 0.01249 m and shoulder and elbow cup radius are 0.0498 and 0.03748 m, respectively.

TABLE 14.3

For Scaling 0.85 Natural Frequency Variation and Mode No.

Mode	Both Sides Fixed Condition (Natural Frequency, Hz)	Both Sides Free Condition (Natural Frequency, Hz)	Fixed-Free Condition (Natural Frequency, Hz)
1	757.08	0	71.189
2	771.17	0	72.097
3	2041	1.091e-003	538.26
4	2072.7	7.5442e-003	539.62
5	3884.7	31.176	639.15
6	3933.4	32.695	1523.9
7	4272.3	339.84	1528.7
8	6194.4	341.23	2229.6
9	6254.6	720.44	2884.2
10	6563.3	989.07	2917.3

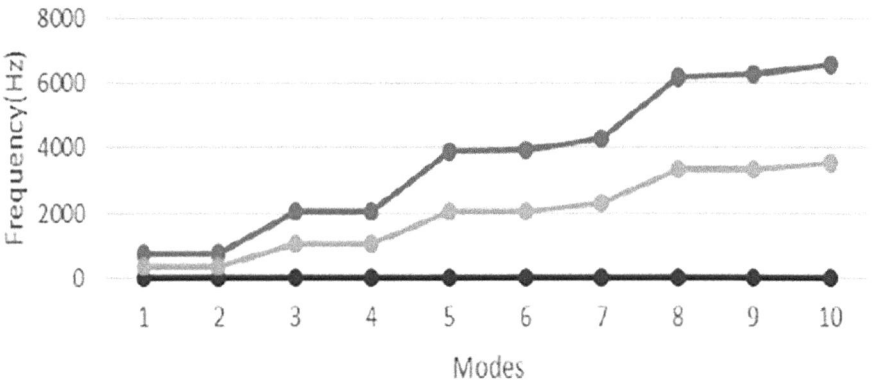

FIGURE 14.8   Frequency variation plot for natural frequency of the scale-down model.

Table 14.3 shows that the first natural frequency under fixed-fixed conditions for scaling down model 0.85 is 757.08 Hz. For the free-free condition, the first and second natural frequency is 0 Hz. The third boundary condition one side fixed and one side free has been introduced. The first natural frequency is 71.189 Hz. The lowest frequency has been identified for one side fixed and one side free conditions. The results match with those of Khalili et al. [9].

The frequency variations of two geometries (scale up and scale down) for three different boundary conditions: first for both side free, second for both side fixed, and third for one side fixed and one side free, are compared and are shown in Figure 14.8. The figure shows the variation in the frequency of both the geometries under three boundary conditions.

Figure 14.8 shows two different frequency variation plots for two different scales. The first scale is 0.85, and the second is 1.5. This graph represents frequency variation for two different scales but for the same boundary condition (fixed-fixed condition). The range of scale-up frequency is low compared to scale down; it varies from 384.85 to 3561.9 Hz. The range of scale-down frequency is high; it varies from 757.08 to 6563.9 Hz. From Figure 14.8, it can be concluded that the modal frequencies of scale 1.5 are in the range of experimental range. So it is a suitable design.

14.6 FRACTURE ANALYSIS OF HUMERUS BONE

A deformation at first geometry is studied to identify the crack initiation point. The analysis has been performed for fixed-fixed boundary conditions. The deformation result for geometry is already shown in the above slides. We can conclude that the crack initiation point will lie at the middle of the shaft. After studying the crack phenomenon and the types of crack, we have designed a crack at the center of the shaft. Crack dimension is taken as: length = 4.2 mm and crack angle = 7°. The different load applied to the geometry varies from 2500 to 4000 N. The applied loads are given in Table 14.4. Figure 14.9 shows the crack generated in the geometry. The mode shape results calculated for the crack profile are also shown in Table 14.5.

From Table 14.4, the four different loads are applied to the crack geometry to study its behavior. The loads applied are 2500, 3000, 3500, and 4000 N. Compressive load is applied to the bone geometry. The load applied to the bone profile with crack

TABLE 14.4
Forces and Their Magnitude

Forces	Magnitude (N)
Force1	2500
Force2	3000
Force3	3500
Force4	4000

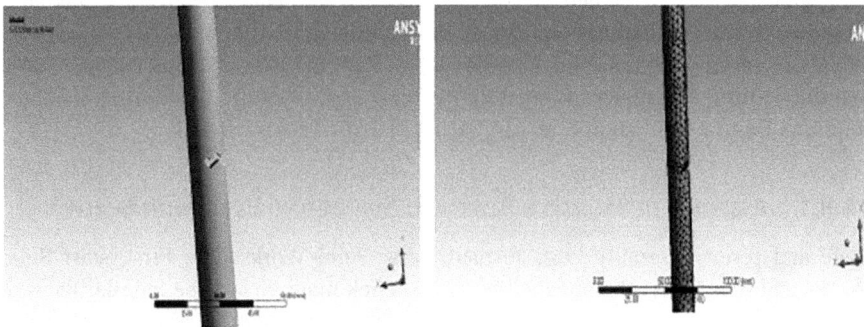

FIGURE 14.9   Crack geometry.

TABLE 14.5
Modal Analysis for Cracked
Humerus Bone

Modes	Frequency [Hz]
1	51.48
2	56.165
3	383.86
4	433.43
5	510.15
6	1204.1
7	1257.8
8	1692.6
9	2300.4
10	2341.3

is shown in Figure 14.10. The mode shape results generated for the first ten modes are shown in Figure 14.11.

14.7 STATIC STRUCTURAL ANALYSIS

Structural analysis was performed for strength determination of bone. A static structural analysis determines the displacements, stresses, strains, and forces in structures or components caused by loads. Figure 14.12 gives the comparison for all four forces. Structural analysis was performed to check the strength of bone and find the value of damage under different loading conditions. To support the damaged bone for strengthening purpose, titanium-based supporting plates were fixed with a bone to enhance the load-carrying capacity.

14.8 SUPPORTING PLATE AND SCREW DESIGN

Plate and screw are designed in Solid Works [21]. The plate dimension is taken as length = 90 mm and thickness = 1.5 mm. We have designed 8 screw holes on the plate. The diameter of each hole is 3 mm. The screw dimension is taken as length = 9 mm and dia = 3 mm. The materials used for the plate and screw are of stainless steel and titanium. Figure 14.13 shows the supporting plate and screw model.

14.8.1 ASSEMBLY OF HUMERUS BONE AND SUPPORTING PLATE WITH SCREW

Plate and screw assembly is performed using Solid Works [21]. First, start Solid Works and then insert the attached parts and click mate. Select the circular faces to move the screw away from the plate. Under mechanical mates, click screw and select distance (pitch) and input value. Figure 14.14 shows the assembly of a cracked bone with a supporting plate and screw.

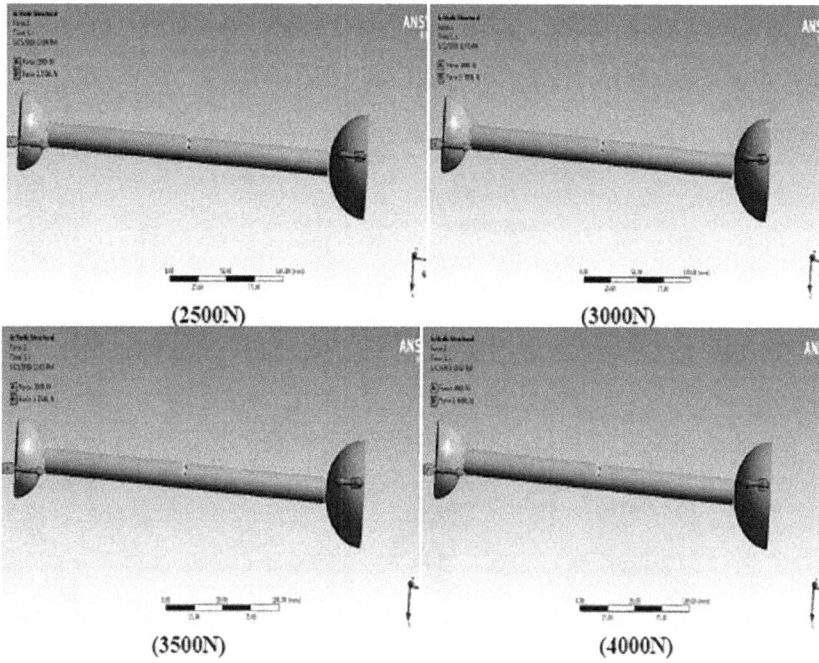

FIGURE 14.10 Load applications on humerus bone geometry.

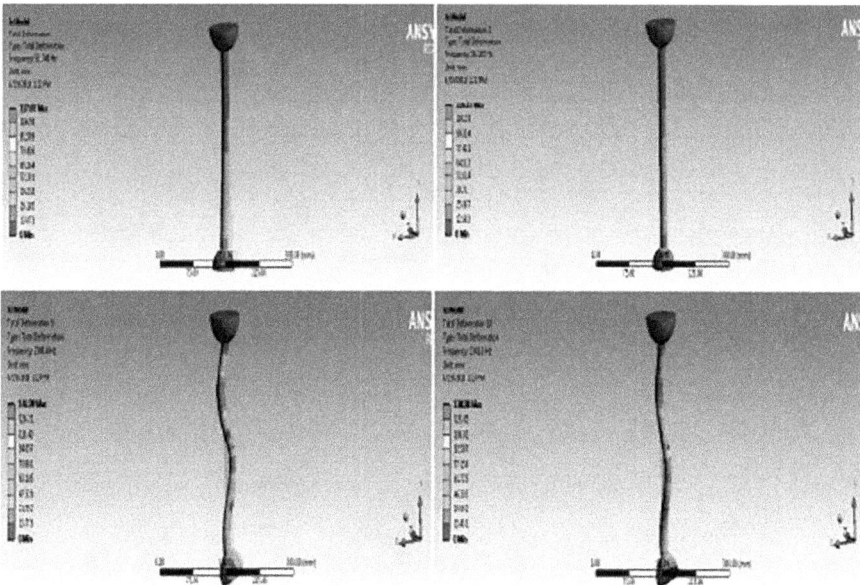

FIGURE 14.11 Different mode shapes for load with crack-generated bone.

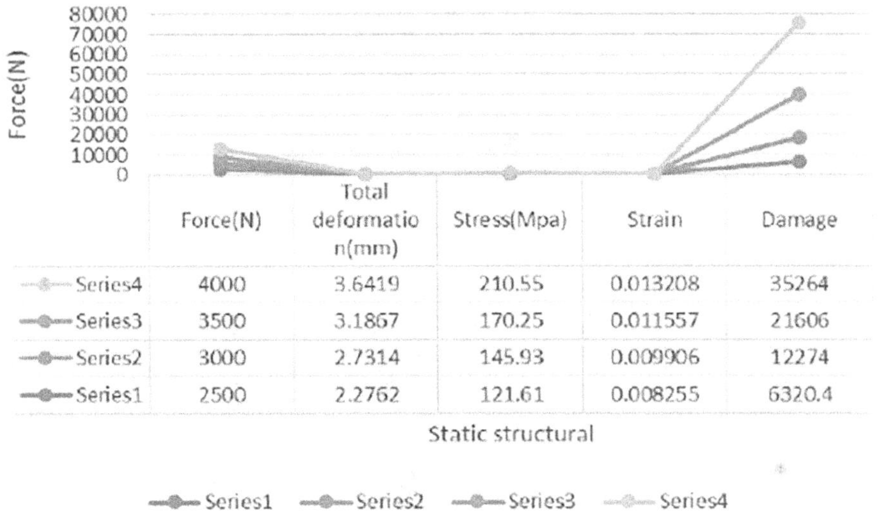

	Force(N)	Total deformation(mm)	Stress(Mpa)	Strain	Damage
Series4	4000	3.6419	210.55	0.013208	35264
Series3	3500	3.1867	170.25	0.011557	21606
Series2	3000	2.7314	145.93	0.009906	12274
Series1	2500	2.2762	121.61	0.008255	6320.4

Static structural

Series1 Series2 Series3 Series4

FIGURE 14.12 Comparison of forces (2500, 3000, 3500, and 4000N) effect on different parameters.

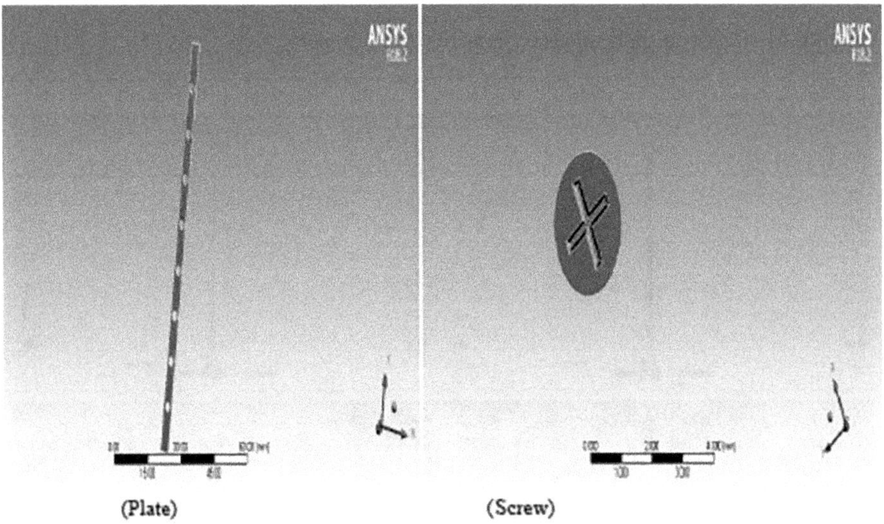

(Plate)   (Screw)

FIGURE 14.13 Solid model of supporting plate and screw design for cracked bone.

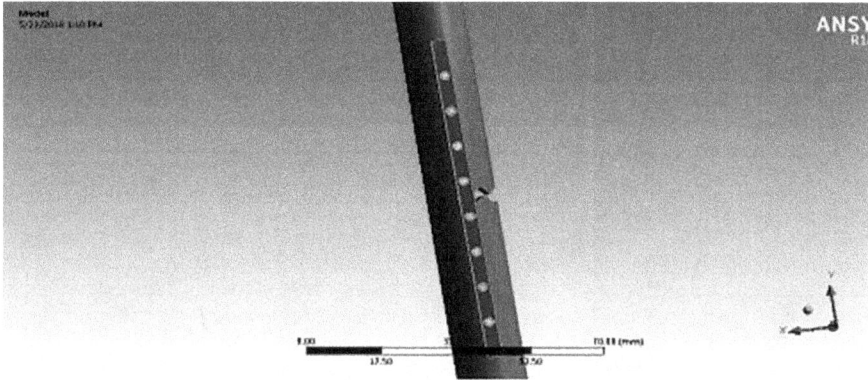

FIGURE 14.14   Assembly of cracked humerus bone with supporting plate and screw.

TABLE 14.6
Stainless Steel Properties of Supported Plate and Screw

Property	Stainless Steel Properties	Titanium Properties
Density	8.00 g/cm³	4.506 g/cm³
Young's modulus	205 GPa	116 GPa
Poisson's ratio	0.275	0.32
Thermal expansion	15.9×10^{-6}/k	8.9×10^{-6}/k
Melting point	1400°C	1668°C
Electrical resistivity	0.074×10^{-6} Ω/m	420 Ω/m
Thermal conductivity	16.3 W/m.k	21.9 W/m.k
Modulus of elasticity	193 GPa	44 GPa

14.8.2   MATERIAL PROPERTIES OF SUPPORTING PLATE AND SCREW

Two different materials, stainless steel and titanium, have been selected for supporting plate and screw to be assembled with cracked bone. Table 14.6 gives the material property of stainless steel and the material property of titanium. Stainless steel has been selected due to its highest resistance against corrosion. Its toughness is high, and it has a higher strength to sustain against loading. The tensile and yield strength are also high. Titanium has been selected due to its highest strength against loading. Its toughness is high, and it has a good hardening rate. The tensile and yield strength are also high. Table 14.7 shows frequency variation analysis of stainless steel-supported humerus bone.

The assembly of crack geometry and supporting plates (stainless steel and titanium plate) is analyzed for modal analysis (Figures 14.15 and 14.17). The resonance frequency calculated for the assembly is shown in Table 14.8. Figure 14.16 shows the

TABLE 14.7
Stainless Steel-Supported Plate
Assembly Frequency Variation of Bone

Modes	Frequency (Hz)
1	67.353
2	71.557
3	393.36
4	480.4
5	584
6	1261.5
7	1335.8
8	1800.8
9	2330.1
10	2561.5

fixing of the titanium plate and humerus bone and the healing method of fractured humerus bone was analyzed.

14.9   CONCLUSIONS

A detailed analysis of humerus bone was performed using FEA. It was observed that continuous vibration is harmful to bone and sudden loading may cause damage or fracture of the humerus bone. The results of this chapter show that the chances of bone fracture are through a bone shaft and joint. The following results have been obtained during analysis of humerus bone:

- FEA-based frequency analysis was performed for humerus bone. The natural frequency for both side free conditions was (0–805.9 Hz); for fixed-fixed boundary conditions, it was (565.47–5321.2 Hz), and for one side fixed and one side free, it is (53.13–2229.5 Hz).
- Scaling 0.85 of the original geometry was performed to check the dimension variation and natural frequency variation. For this, the natural frequency varies (71.189–6563.3 Hz) for three different boundary conditions.
- Humerus bone fractured condition modal analysis was performed with natural frequency in the range of (51.48–2341.3 Hz).
- For minimum load, 2500 N deformation is 2.27 mm and for maximum loads, 4000 N deformation is 3.6419 mm. As the load varies (2500–4000 N), the deformation variation increases (2.27–3.64 mm).
- Natural frequency of a stainless steel-supported plate varies (67.35–2561.5 Hz) and that of a titanium fitted bone is (66.81–2543.2 Hz).

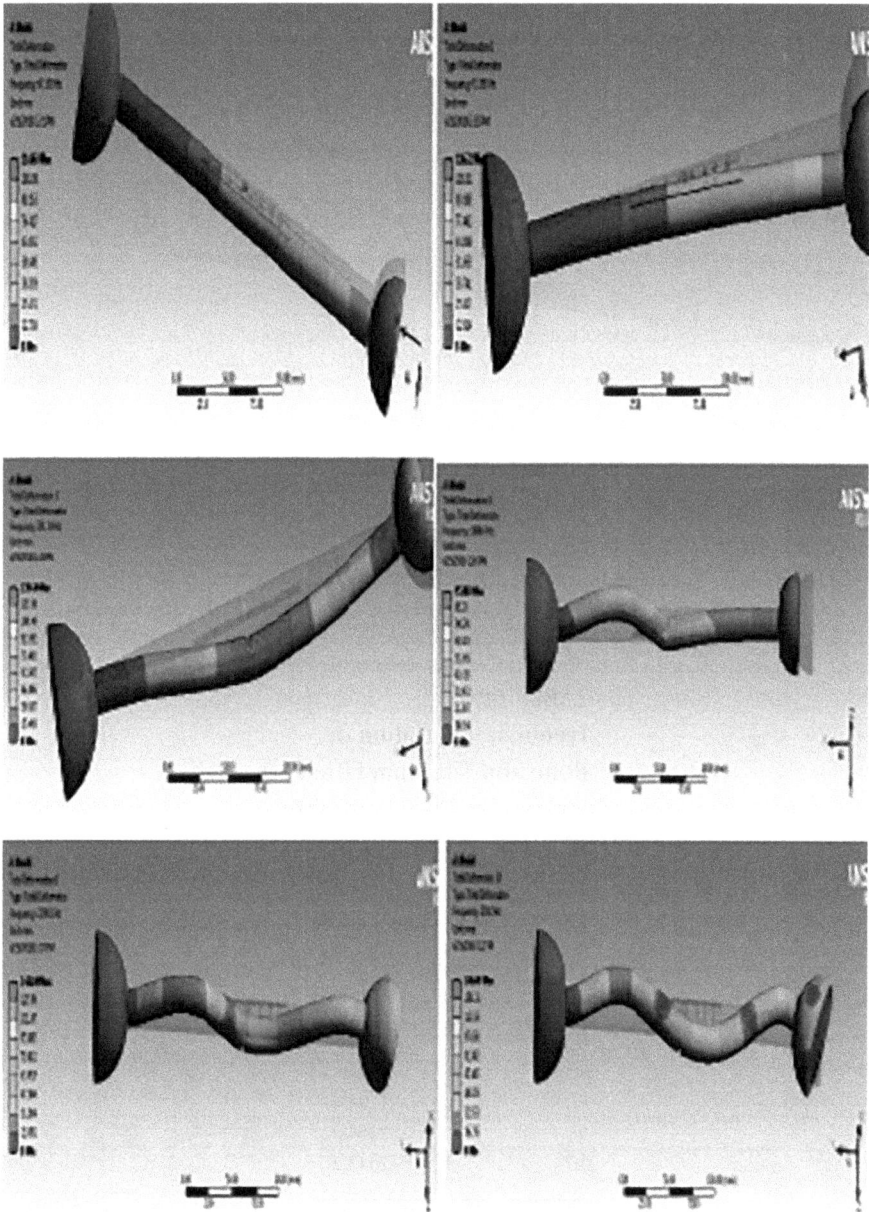

FIGURE 14.15 Different mode shapes of cracked humerus bone fitted with stainless steel supporting plate and screw.

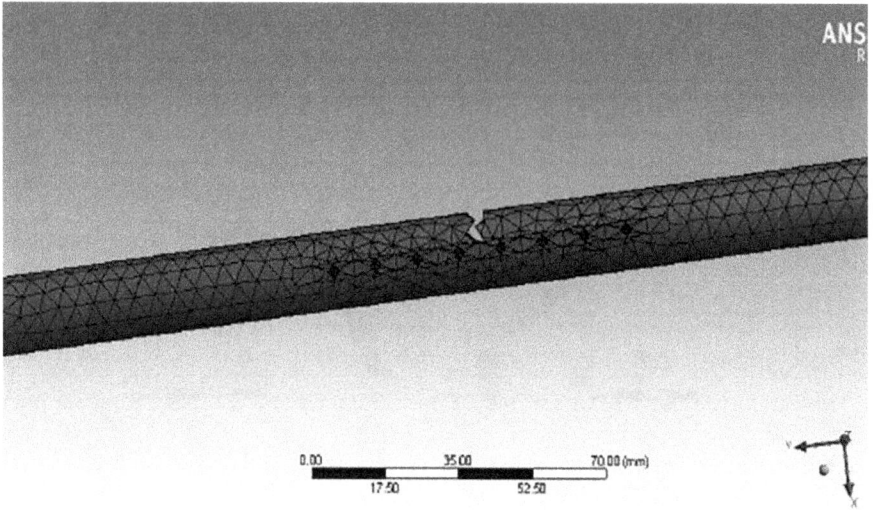

FIGURE 14.16   Titanium supporting plate fitted with cracked bone.

TABLE 14.8
Frequency Variation of Bone and Titanium Fitted Supporting Plate Assembly

Modes	Frequency (Hz)
1	66.815
2	70.645
3	400.47
4	477.2
5	586.37
6	1267.1
7	1339.2
8	1794.4
9	2364.2
10	2543.2

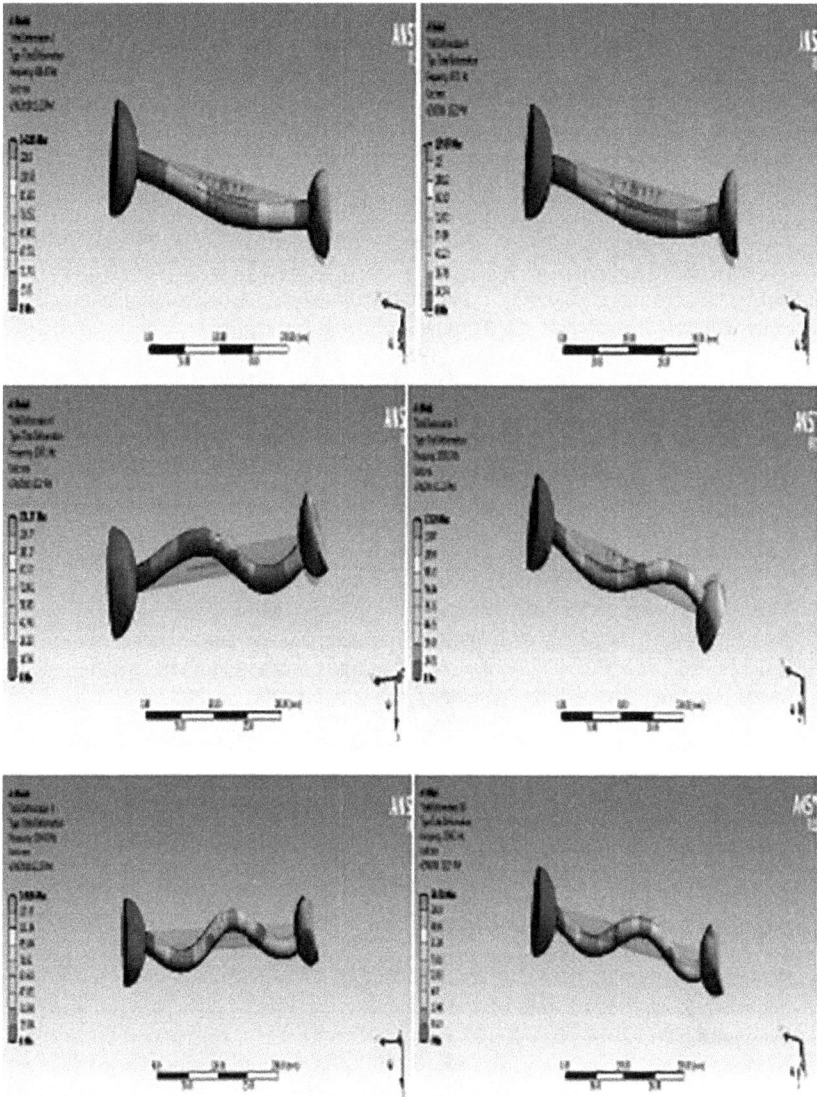

FIGURE 14.17 Different mode shapes of cracked humerus bone fitted with titanium supporting plate and screw.

REFERENCES

1. ANSYS 16.2. Academic, structural analysis Guide.
2. Zadpoor, A.A (2006). Finite element method analysis of human hand arm vibration. *International Journal of Science and Research* 16, pp. 391–395.
3. Wirtz, D.C. (2000). Critical evaluation of known bone material properties to realize anisotropic FE simulation of the proximal femur. *Journal of Biomechanics* 33, pp. 1325–1330.

4. Ingólfsson, E.T., Georgakis, C.T., Jönsson, J. (2012) Pedestrian-induced lateral vibrations of footbridges: A literature review. *Journal of Engineering Structures* 45, pp. 21–52.

5. Paddan, G.S., Griffin, M.J. (1998) A review of the transmission of translational seat vibration to the head. *Journal of Sound and Vibration* 215, pp. 863–882.

6. Hight T.K., Piziali, R.L., Nagel, D.a. (1980) Natural frequency analysis of a human tibia. *Journal of Biomechanics* 13, pp. 139–147.

7. Tiemessen, I. J., Carel, T.J., Monique, H.W. (2007) An overview of strategies to reduce whole-body vibration exposure on drivers: A systematic review. *International Journal of Industrial Ergonomics* 37, pp. 245–256.

8. Misra, J.C., Samanta, S. (1988) A mathematical analysis of the vibration characteristics of human tibia. *Computers and Mathematics with Applications* 16, pp. 1017–1026.

9. Khalil T.B., Viano, D.C., Taber, L.A. (1981) Vibrational characteristics of the embalmed human femur. *Journal of Sound and Vibration* 75, pp. 417–436.

10. Oliver, M., Conrad, L., Jack, R.J., Dickey, J.P., Eger, T. (2012) Improving WBV attenuation through field vibration tested heavy equipment seat retrofitting – A field to lab to field case study. *Proceedings of the Fourth American Conference on Human Vibration.*

11. Pelker, R.R., Saha, S. (1983). Stress wave propagation in bone. *Journal of Biomechanics* 16, pp. 481–489.

12. Holmlund, P., Lundstrok, R.M, Lindberg, L. (2000). Mechanical impedance of the human body in vertical direction. *Journal of Applied Ergonomics* 31, pp. 415–422.

13. Valentini, P.P. (2012) Modeling human spine using dynamic spline approach for vibrational simulation. *Journal of Sound and Vibration* 331, pp. 5895–5909.

14. Huiskes, R., Chao, E.Y.S. (1983) A survey of finite element analysis in orthopedic biomechanics: The first decade. *Journal of Biomechanics* 16, pp. 385–409.

15. Dong, R.G., Mcdowell, T.W., Welcome, D.E. (2005) Biodynamic response at the palm of the human hand subjected to a random vibration. *Industrial Health* 43, pp. 241–255.

16. Dong, R.G., Schopper, A.W., McDowell, T.W., Welcome, D.E., Wu, J.Z., Smutz, W.P., Warren, C., Rakheja, S. (2004) Vibration energy absorption (VEA) in human fingers-hand-arm system. *Medical Engineering & Physics* 26, pp. 483–492.

17. Kumar, A., Mamgain, D.P., Jaiswal, H., Patil, P. (2015) Modal analysis of hand arm vibration (humerus bone) for biodynamic response using varying boundary conditions based on FEA. *Advances in Intelligent Systems and Computing*, 308, pp. 169–176. doi: 10.1007/978-81-322-2012-1_18.

18. Kumar, A., Behmad, S.I., Patil, P. (2014) Vibration characterization and static analysis of cortical bone fracture based on finite element analysis. *Engineering and Automation Problems*, No 3–2014, pp. 115–119. UDC–621.

19. Kumar, A., Jaiswal, H., Garg, T., Patil, P. (2014) Free vibration modes analysis of femur bone fracture using varying boundary conditions based on FEA. *Procedia Materials Science*, 6, pp. 1593–1599. doi: 10.1016/j. mspro.2014.07.142.

20. Gangwar, A.K.S., Rao, P.S., Kumar, A. (2021) Bio-mechanical design and analysis of femur bone. *Materials Today: Proceedings* 44, Part 1, pp. 2179–2187, ISSN 2214-7853. Doi: 10.1016/j.matpr.2020.12.282.

21. Solid works, structural design guide.

22. Kumar, A., Rana, S., Gori, Y., Sharma, N. K. (Eds.) (2021) Thermal contact conductance prediction using FEM based computational techniques. In *Advanced Computational Methods in Mechanical and Materials Engineering*, pp. 183–220. DOI: 10.1201/-9781003202233-13, ISBN: 9781032052915.

23. Gangwar, A. K. S., Rao, P. S., Kumar, A., Patil, P. P. (2019) Design and analysis of femur bone: BioMechanical aspects. *Journal of Critical Reviews* 6(4), pp. 133–139, ISSN-2394-5125.

15 Design of Energy Harvesting Mechanism for Walking Applications

Ankit Meena and T. Jagadeesha
National Institute of Technology Calicut

Manoj Nikam
BV College of Engineering Navi Mumbai

Seung-Bok Choi
The State University of New York Korea

Vikram G. Kamble
Technical University Dresden

CONTENTS

DOI: 10.1201/9781003286806-15

15.1   INTRODUCTION

In today's world where the pace of life has significantly accelerated, amputations are no exceptions. The development of sensors and actuators significantly decreases the energy utilization of small electronic items, and in the upcoming age, devices are self-sustaining from the energy point of view; these gadgets must be issued with definite power collecting device, which should be able to collect power from environment origins (solar, wind, water and vibration). There are various mechanisms like electromagnetic, electrostatic, electrochemical and piezoelectric to transform these available energies into electrical energy. Piezoelectric technique has led among all due to high-normalized energy density that assembles it perfect for small-scale application devices.

The piezoelectric generators do not need any voltage origin to collect power, but they are further tough to combine toward microsystems [1]. Electrostatic generators are not difficult to combine toward microsystems, still need a different voltage origin to work. Electromagnetic generators need no voltage to work, still, they yield a comparatively small amount of voltages. A thorough study of all three power transformation techniques is introduced and further opinions are made [2]. It is established that the greatest technology requires to be chosen to build upon the ambient situations and the material restriction of the system. Piezoelectric generators generate excessive voltages and little currents. In both piezoelectric and electrostatic generators, current production is reduced by decreasing the dimension of the gadgets. Electromagnetic generators normally generate little voltages and the output voltage is reduced on decreasing the dimensions of the gadgets. It is inferred that electromagnetic transformation is most acceptable for huge structures in the huge energy collecting gadget. Electrostatic generators are most acceptable for especially little structures because of the little gap needed among plates of a capacitor. Piezoelectric transformers should be able to collect power among all dimension extents [3]. It is deduced that a piezoelectric structure provides an excessive energy density, manufacturing it interesting in micro-scale implementations, and electromagnetic structures are more acceptable in macro-scale implementations.

The kind of piezoelectric substance picked for energy collecting implementation can have a crucial impact on the harvester's compatibility and production. The most commonly used piezoelectric substance used in energy harvesting units is PZT (lead zirconate titanate). The PZT (piezoceramic) especially breakable character gives rise to restrictions in the strain that it can carefully soak up free from being harmed. PZT substances are working broadly on a power harvesting basis. The energy due to vibration is transformed to electrical energy composition (like beams and plates) implanted with PZT patches. A beam composition is commonly utilized because of its clarity and dimensions. The acceptance of PZT is due to the fact that it is one of the best well-organized and cost-affordable substances. In current times, the energy extracting systems below parametric and direct excitation are considerably investigated. In direct excitation, the force and displacement are in the same manner while in parametric excitation, both of them are perpendicular. The resonance in the case of direct excitation takes place when the exterior excitation frequency is equal to the original frequency of structure while in parametric excitation, resonance occurs when the frequency of excitation becomes twice that of the original frequency of the structure [4–8].

Daqaq et al. [9] calculated power collecting under parametric excitation in which the active feedback of the structure was explored utilizing a lumped parameter pattern. Energy collecting utilizing linear vibration has been explored broadly, and clear declarations for perfect parameters are obtainable [3]. The other constructive method to enhance the output power is to stack a great number of narrow piezoceramic wafers simultaneously, called stack arrangement, with an electric field appealed next to the length of the stack. It is deduced that both output voltage and the complementing resistive load are much better achievable in a PZT stack than in a monolithic arrangement for the same geometry, thus building the stack a better functional alternative. A comparison among rectangular and triangular shaped cantilever beam by keeping the large end attached and small end free was studied in literature. It is shown that if we assume the base and height dimensions of a triangular-shaped beam equal to the base and length dimensions of a rectangular beam, then the triangular beam will have a higher strain and maximum deformation. So, a triangular-shaped beam will give better energy than a rectangular beam [10].

A piezoelectric energy harvester has two basic parts. The first one is the mechanical component, which gives rise to electrical power, and the second one is the electrical component, which contains an electrical circuit that changes and corrects the generated voltage. So, the efficacy of the power harvester is based on both the piezoelectric transducer and its incorporation with an electrical circuit.

In the present work, a vertical cantilever beam-based PEH (piezoelectric energy harvester) structure is explored under parametric excitation. A mass is attached at a random position along with a PZT patch (PZT-5H). The governing equation of motion is derived with the help of Hamilton's principle, Galerkin's approximation and method of multiple scales. Several analyses (like static, dynamic and kinematic) are done for theoretical exploration on the harvester. The different characteristic curves are analyzed using MATLAB®. The frequency and voltage response (and their fast Fourier transform) are compared by selecting different materials. A PID control mechanism for the motor is designed and tuned to control the system and its varying parameters. The tuning of the controller is done to prevent overshoot and account for the steady-state errors.

15.1.1 Electromechanical Equations of Cantilever Beam-Based Piezoelectric Energy Harvesters

Let us consider a unimorph energy harvester shown in Figure 15.1 involving the PZT patch layer attached over it. Generally, there are two types of harvesters – unimorph and bimorph. When there is only a single layer of PZT over the substructure layer,

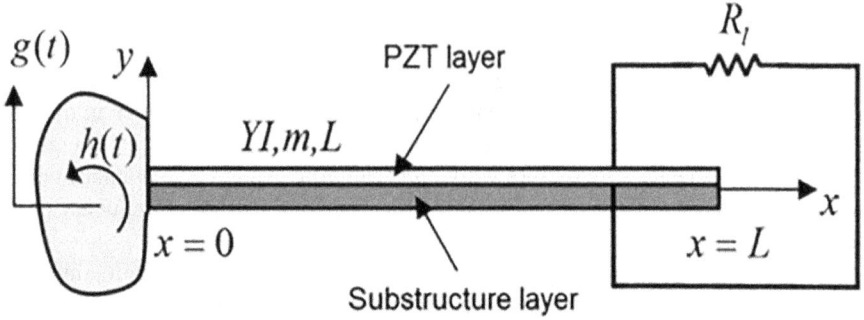

FIGURE 15.1   Unimorph energy harvester.

then it is termed as unimorph and when there are two layers of PZT (i.e.in both sides) over the substructure layer, it is termed as bimorph harvester.

From the above figure, the base motion

$$u_b(x,t) = g(t) + u_b x h(t) \tag{15.1}$$

the basic governing equation of motion that we use,

$$\frac{\partial^2 M(x,t)}{\partial x^2} + c_s I \frac{\partial^5 u_{rel}(x,t)}{\partial x^4 \partial t} + c_a \frac{\partial u_{rel}(x,t)}{\partial t} + m \frac{\partial^2 u_{rel}(x,t)}{\partial t^2}$$
$$= -m \frac{\partial^2 u_b(x,t)}{\partial t^2} - c_a \frac{\partial u_b(x,t)}{\partial t} \tag{15.2}$$

where

$u_{rel}(x,t)$ = deflection in perpendicular direction with respect to the base

$M(x,t)$ = moment

csI = damping due to structural visco-elasticity

c_a = damping due to air

m = mass of beam per unit length.

The strain rate damping truly shows itself as an internal moment in the resulting equation of motion and that can be written as

$$(M_s = c_s I \partial^3 u_{rel} / \partial x^2 \partial t)$$

The piezoelectric constitutes relations for substructure and PZT layer are given below:

$$T_1^s = Y_s S_1^s \tag{15.3}$$

$$T_1^p = Y_p\left(S_1^p - d_{31} E_3\right) \tag{15.4}$$

where

T = stress

S = strain

$Y=$ Younf's modulus
$D=$ piezoelectric constant
$E=$ electric field
The relation used to derive the above expression

$$\left(S_{11} = s_{11}^E T_{11} + d_{31}E_3\right)$$

where
$s_{11}^E=$ elastic conformance

$$Yp = 1/s_{11}^E$$

Here subscripts s and p are used for the substructure layer and PZT layer, respectively; directions 1 (axial direction) and 3 (polarization direction) are coincide with x and y, respectively. The internal moment will be

$$M(x,t) = -\int_{h_a}^{h_b} T_1^s b y\, dy - \int_{h_b}^{h_c} T_1^p b y\, dy \qquad (15.5)$$

where
$b=$ width of the beam
$h_a=$ distance from the neutral axis to the bottom of substructure layer
$h_b=$ distance from the neutral axis to the bottom of 3PZT layer
$h_c=$ distance from neutral axis to the top of PZT layer
Employing equations (15.3) and (15.4) in equation (15.5), we get

$$M(x,t) = \int_{h_b}^{h_a} Y_s b \frac{\partial^2 u_{\text{rel}}(x,t)}{\partial x^2} y^2 dy + \int_{h_b}^{h_a} Y_p b \frac{\partial^2 u_{\text{rel}}(x,t)}{\partial x^2} y^2 dy - \int_{h_b}^{h_c} v(t) Y_p b \frac{d_{31}}{h_p} y\, dy \qquad (15.6)$$

Since the electric field component can be written in terms of thickness and voltage as

$$E_3(t) = \frac{-v(T)}{h_p}$$

The above moment equation can be further reduced to

$$M(x,t) = \text{YI} \frac{\partial^2 u_{\text{rel}}(x,t)}{\partial x^2} + \upsilon v(t) \qquad (15.7)$$

where
$\text{YI}=$ bending stiffness of the structure

$$\text{YI} = b \left[\frac{Y_s\left(h_b^3 - h_a^3\right) + Y_p\left(h_c^3 - h_b^3\right)}{3} \right] \qquad (15.8)$$

The coupling term is given by

$$\upsilon = -\frac{Y_p d_{31} b}{2h_p}\left(h_c^2 - h_b^2\right) \qquad (15.9)$$

Since in our case we assume that the patch layer shields the whole length as shown in the figure initially, we can rewrite equation (15.7) as

$$M(x,t) = YI\frac{\partial^2 u_{rel}(x,t)}{\partial x^2} + \upsilon v(t)[H(x) - H(x-L)]$$ (15.10)

where

L = length of the beam

$H(x)$ = heaviside function

By using equations (15.10) and (15.2), we get

$$YI\frac{\partial^4 u_{rel}(x,t)}{\partial x^4} + c_s I\frac{\partial^5 u_{rel}(x,t)}{\partial x^4 \partial t} + c_a\frac{\partial u_{rel}(x,t)}{\partial t} + m\frac{\partial^2 u_{rel}(x,t)}{\partial t^2}$$

$$+ \upsilon v(t) \times \left[\frac{d\delta(x)}{dx} - \frac{d\delta(x-L)}{dx}\right] \qquad = -m\frac{\partial^2 u_b(x,t)}{\partial t^2} - c_a\frac{\partial u_b(x,t)}{\partial t}$$ (15.11)

where $\delta(x)$ is the Dirac delta function and it satisfies

$$\int_{-\infty}^{\infty} \frac{d^{(n)}\delta(x - x_0)}{dx^{(n)}} f(x)dx = (-1)^n \frac{df^{(n)}(x_0)}{dx^{(n)}}$$ (15.12)

To obtain the equation for the electrical circuit, we have to use the following piezo-electric relation:

$$D_3 = d_{31}T_1 + \varepsilon_{33}^T E_3$$ (15.13)

where

D_3 = electric displacement and

e_{33}^t = permittivity at constant stress.

The permittivity at constant strain is given by

$$(e_{33}^S = e_{33}{}^T - d^2 33, Yp)$$

Then equation (15.13) can be rewritten as

$$D_3(x,t) = d_{31}Y_p S_1(x,t) - \varepsilon_{33}^s \frac{v(t)}{h_p}$$ (15.14)

The average bending strain is given by

$$S_1(x,t) = -h_{pc}\frac{\partial^2 u_{rel}(x,t)}{\partial x^2}$$ (15.15)

and equation (15.14) becomes

$$D_3(x,t) = -d_{31}Y_p h_{pc}\frac{\partial^2 u_{rel}(x,t)}{\partial x^2} - \varepsilon_{33}^s \frac{v(t)}{h_p}$$ (15.16)

The charge q(t) evolved in the patch will be

$$q(t) = \int_A D.ndA = -\int_{x=0}^{L} \left(d_{31} Y_p h_{pc} b \frac{\partial^2 u_{rel}(x,t)}{\partial x^2} + \varepsilon_{33}^s b \frac{v(t)}{h_p} \right) dx \qquad (15.17)$$

where

D = vector of electrical displacement

N = unit outward normal

The current developed in the PZT patch can be obtained by using the above expression as

$$i(t) = \frac{dq(t)}{dt} = -\int_{x=0}^{L} d_{31} Y_p h_{pc} b \frac{\partial^3 u_{rel}(x,t)}{\partial x^2 \partial t} dx - \frac{\varepsilon_{33}^s bL}{h_p} \frac{dv(t)}{dt} \qquad (15.18)$$

The first component of the above current expression shows the vibratory motion of the beam, and the second term shows voltage evolved over the patch layer.

The voltage produced over load resistance is obtained by using the above expression as

$$v(t) = R_l i(t) = -R_l \left[\int_{x=0}^{L} d_{31} Y_p h_{pc} b \frac{\partial^3 u_{rel}(x,t)}{\partial x^2 \partial t} dx + \frac{\varepsilon_{33}^s bL}{h_p} \frac{dv(t)}{dt} \right] \qquad (15.19)$$

or we can write the above equation as

$$\frac{\varepsilon_{33}^s bL}{h_p} \frac{dv(t)}{dt} + \frac{v(t)}{R_l} + \frac{v(t)}{R_l} = -\int_{x=0}^{L} d_{31} Y_p h_{pc} b \frac{\partial^3 u_{rel}(x,t)}{\partial x^2 \partial t} dx \qquad (15.20)$$

15.1.2 PERTURBATION ANALYSIS

This analysis is performed to determine the approximate analytical solution of the electromechanical equation. For that, let us consider the case in which the beam is held in a vertical manner having length L, a small mass 'm' is added on that at a distance 'd' and also a patch (PZT) is attached to it close to the base. The schematic diagrammatical representation is shown in Figure 15.2. The electrodes are connected to an external resistance by using an electric circuit. This will help us to determine the output power from the energy harvester. The longitudinal and transverse motion of the cantilever beam is represented by $u(\xi,t)$ and $v(\xi,t)$ respectively where ξ represents the curvilinear co-ordinates along the direction of the length of the beam. We found the voltage and current expression in mathematical modeling for a cantilever beam placed in horizontal manner. Similarly, calculations are done for vertical position, where the gravity effect is put up into the dynamics of the system.

Then the circuit equation obtained in this case will be

$$Cp \cdot \frac{dV(t)}{dt} + \frac{V}{2R_l} - i(t) = 0 \qquad (15.21)$$

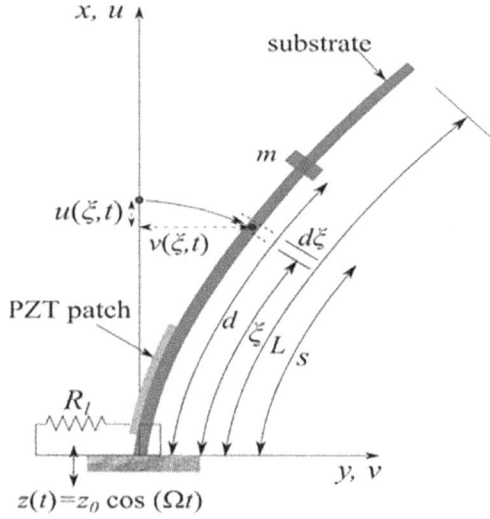

FIGURE 15.2   Schematic diagram of a PEH system with parametric excitation.

$$i(t) = -d_{31}Y_p b_p h_{pc} \int\limits_{x=L_1}^{x=L_2} \left(\frac{D^3 V}{Ds^2 \cdot Dt} \right) ds \tag{15.22}$$

$$Cp = \frac{e_{33}^s b_p L_p}{h_p} \tag{15.23}$$

The boundary conditions that we use in a given case are

$$V(0,t) = 0 \quad \frac{Dv}{Ds}\Big|(0,t) = 0 \tag{15.24}$$

$$\frac{D^2 v}{Ds^2}\Big|(0,t) = 0 \quad \frac{D^3 v}{Ds^3}\Big|(0,t) = 0$$

By using the Galerkin approximation method, the displacement in the transverse direction can be written as

$$v(s,t) = rN(s)m(t) \tag{15.25}$$

The nonlinear electromechanical governing equation of motion can be written as

$$\ddot{m} + 2c\tau\dot{m} + m + c\alpha m^3 + c\beta m\dot{m}^2 + c\gamma m^2 \ddot{m} + c\eta V = c\overline{mf}\cos(\varnothing t) \tag{15.26}$$

$$\dot{V} + XV + \Theta\dot{m} = 0 \tag{15.27}$$

The dependence of time is indicated by using a method of multiple scales as

$$T_n = c^n t \tag{15.28}$$

and time derivatives are expressed as

$$\frac{d}{dt} = D_0 + cD_1 + O(c^2)$$

$$\frac{d}{dt^2} = D_0^2 + 2cD_0D_1 + O(c^2) \tag{15.29}$$

The system solution (m, V) enlarged in a series form like

$$m(t,c) = m_0(T_0, T_1) + cm_1(T_0, T_1) + O(c^2) \tag{15.30}$$

$$V(t,c) = V_0(T_0, T_1) + cV_1(T_0, T_1) + O(c^2) \tag{15.31}$$

By substituting equations (15.30) and (15.31) in equations (15.26) and (15.27) and equating the coefficients of c^0 & c^1 to zero, we obtain

$$D_0^2 m_0 + m_0 = 0 \tag{15.32a}$$

$$D_0 V_0 + X V_0 + D_0 m_0 = 0 \tag{15.32b}$$

$$D_0^2 m_1 + m_1 - 2\tau D_0 m_0 - 2D_0 D_1 m_0 + m_0 \overline{f} \cos(\emptyset t)$$
$$-\eta V_0 - \alpha m_0^3 - \beta m_0 (D_0 m_0)^2 - \gamma m_0^2 D_0^2 m_0 \tag{15.33a}$$

$$D_0 + V_1 + X V_1 = -D_0 V_0 - (D_0 m_1 + D_1 m_0) \tag{15.33b}$$

The solution of equations (15.32a) and (15.32b) will become

$$m_0 = C(T_1)e^{iT_0} + cc$$

$$V_0 = -ZC(T_1)e^{iT_0} + cc \tag{15.34}$$

where
Cc = complex conjugate of preceding terms
$C(T_1)$ = unknown complex function
By substituting equation (15.34) in (15.33a), the temporal term and near temporal term are obtained as

$$\frac{\overline{f}}{2} \overline{c} \, e^{(iT_0\emptyset - iT_0)} - (3\alpha + 3\beta - 3\gamma)\overline{c}c^2 e^{iT_0} - 2i(c^1 + \tau c)e^{iT_0} - \eta Zce^{iT_0} = 0 \quad (15.35)$$

To indicate the closeness of $\emptyset$ to that of 2 (principal parametric resonance), the parameter μ is established as

$$\emptyset = 2 + \in \mu$$

The function $C(T_1)$ is written in polar form as

$$C(T_1) = \frac{1}{2}C(T_1)e^{iv(T_1)}$$

where the amplitudes of $C(T_1)$ and phase $v(T_1)$ are diversifying functions of time scale T_1.

By using the above written polar form of $C(T_1)$ in equation (15.29) and eliminating the coefficient of e^{iT_o}, we obtained the following reduced equation

$$c^1 = T_{\text{eff}}a + aF_{\text{eff}}\sin(\delta) \qquad (15.36)$$

$$\frac{1}{2}a\delta^1 = \frac{1}{2}\mu_{\text{eff}}a - R_{\text{eff}}a^3 + aF_{\text{eff}}\cos(\delta) \qquad (15.37)$$

where

$$R_{\text{eff}} = \frac{3\alpha}{8} + \frac{\beta}{8} + \frac{3\gamma}{8}$$

$$T_{\text{eff}} = -\tau + \tau_e - \tau_a$$

$$\mu_{\text{eff}} = \mu + \mu_e$$

$$F_{\text{eff}} = \frac{\overline{f}}{4}\tau_e = \frac{\eta X}{2(X^2+1)}$$

$$\mu_e = \frac{\eta}{(X^2+1)}$$

$$\delta = \mu T_1 - 2v$$

$$\tau_a = \frac{4a}{3\pi}u_a$$

τ = internal material damping
τ_e = damping caused by an electric circuit
τ_a = aerodynamic damping
μ_e = shifts in system frequency
R_{eff} = total effects due to cubic and nonlinear term in the equation of motion
The natural frequency response can be calculated as

$$\mu = 2R_{\text{eff}}a^2 - \mu_e \pm 2\sqrt{F_{\text{eff}}^2 - \tau_{\text{eff}}^2} \qquad (15.38)$$

Steady-state displacement, output voltage and power are obtained by using

$$v(s,t) = rN(s)a\cos(\omega t + v) \qquad (15.39)$$

$$V(t) = r_v \frac{1}{\sqrt{X^2+1}} a\cos(\omega t + v + \varnothing) \qquad (15.40)$$

$$P = \frac{a^2}{R_l} \left(r_v \frac{1}{\sqrt{X^2+1}} \right)^2 \qquad (15.41)$$

where $\varnothing = \tan^{-1}(X)$.

15.1.3 FINITE ELEMENT MODELING

Before discussing the section, we will know about certain steps and atmosphere that we use for doing this approach. It includes

1. Forces and moments can only be applied at nodes of the beam element.
2. Forces are static in nature.
3. The cross-section area and moment of inertia will be constant for the beam element.
4. The cross-section of the beam is symmetric about the plane of bending.
5. The beam element material is homogeneous in nature.

Steps in Finite Element Analysis
1. Discretization of structure
2. Numbering of nodes and elements
3. Selection of displacement function
4. Formation of elemental and global stiffness matrix and then load vector also
5. Apply boundary conditions
6. Analysis and interpretation of results

The schematic diagram is shown in Figure 15.3.

Here in this, we measure that 'L' is the length of the cantilever beam, 'B' is the width of the cantilever beam and the origin was presumed to be the middle line of

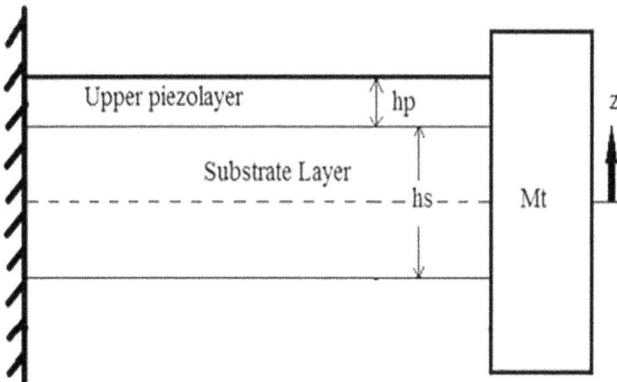

FIGURE 15.3   Schematic diagram of unimorph PEH.

the harvester. In this figure, 'z' is the coordinate through the direction of thickness, h_s represents the thickness of the structure layer, h_p represents the thickness of the upper piezolayer and M_t represents the tip mass.

Figure 15.4 is for one discretized beam element in which element and node are represented by 'i' and 'j', respectively. For each element 'i', there will be two nodes 'j' and 'j+1'.

Generally, there will be three forces present at each node, i.e. axial force, transverse force and rotational force. But for our calculation, we neglect the axial force (i.e. axial force = 0) and assume that there will be two degrees of freedom present for each node, i.e. transverse degree of freedom 'w_i' and rotational degree of freedom 'ψ_j'. For each element, we can equate the force expression and the generalized equation obtained using Hamilton's principle can be written as

$$M_{ij}^e \times \left[\ddot{\Delta}\right]_j^e + C_{ij}^e \times \left[\dot{\Delta}\right]_j^e + K_{ij}^e \times \Delta_{ij}^e - \theta_i^e \times v(t) = F_i^e \tag{15.42}$$

$$C_p \times \frac{dv}{dt} + \frac{v}{R_1} + \left([\theta]^G\right)^T \times \left[\dot{\Delta}\right]^G = 0 \tag{15.43}$$

For our simplification in calculation, we assume that the damping term is neglected and then displacement matrix Δ will be written as follows:

$$\Delta = \left\{W_j \ \Phi_j \ W_{j+1} \ \Phi_{j+1}\right\}^T$$

Here we will see only transverse and rotational components and equations using which we can find out the equivalent mass matrix and equivalent stiffness matrix:

$$M_{ij}^e = \int_0^{l_i} \left(D_p \frac{d\psi_i}{dx} \frac{d\psi_i}{dx}\right) dx$$

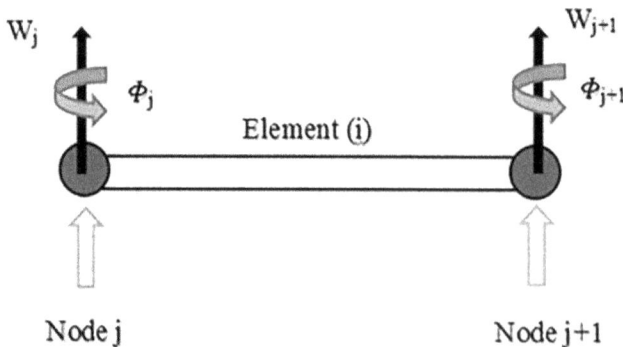

FIGURE 15.4 Force representation in one discretized beam element at both nodes.

$$K_{ij}^e = \int_0^L \left(D_p \frac{d^2\psi_i}{dx^2} \frac{d^2\psi_j}{dx^2} \right) dx$$

where ψ_i and ψ_j are Hermitian shape functions and the term D_p can be obtained by using the expression given below:

$$D_p = \rho \times \frac{h_p^3}{3}$$

where ρ is the equivalent density of a substrate and a piezo layer and h_p is the thickness of the piezo layer.

To find out the equivalent stiffness matrix, we consider a cantilever beam element and consider all the forces (i.e. axial forces, rotational forces and transverse forces) that exist on both the nodes of the beam element. We assume the displacement in the axial direction, transverse direction and slope at the ends due to rotational force and finally use the expression

$$[F] = [K][X]$$

where
  $[F]$ = force matrix
  $[K]$ = stiffness matrix
  $[X]$ = displacement matrix

$$
\begin{bmatrix} F_1 \\ S_1 \\ Q_1 \\ F_2 \\ S_2 \\ Q_2 \end{bmatrix}
=
\begin{bmatrix}
\frac{AE}{L} & 0 & 0 & -\frac{AE}{L} & 0 & 0 \\
0 & \frac{12EI}{L^3} & \frac{6EI}{L^2} & 0 & -\frac{12EI}{L^3} & \frac{6EI}{L^2} \\
0 & \frac{6EI}{L^2} & \frac{4EI}{L} & 0 & -\frac{6EI}{L^2} & \frac{2EI}{L} \\
-\frac{AE}{L} & 0 & 0 & \frac{AE}{L} & 0 & 0 \\
0 & -\frac{12EI}{L^3} & -\frac{6EI}{L^2} & 0 & \frac{12EI}{L^3} & -\frac{6EI}{L^2} \\
0 & \frac{6EI}{L^2} & \frac{2EI}{L} & 0 & -\frac{6EI}{L^2} & \frac{4EI}{L}
\end{bmatrix}
\begin{bmatrix} u_1 \\ v_1 \\ \Phi_1 \\ u_2 \\ v_2 \\ \Phi_2 \end{bmatrix}
$$

Then we use our boundary conditions according to our assumption and an equivalent stiffness matrix can be obtained as

$$K_{ij}^e = \frac{(YI)}{l^3}
\begin{bmatrix}
12 & 6l & -12 & 6l \\
6l & 4l^2 & -6l & 2l^2 \\
-12 & -6l & 12 & -6l \\
6l & 2l^2 & -6l & 4l^2
\end{bmatrix}$$

Similarly, an equivalent mass matrix can be obtained as

$$
M_{ij}^e = \frac{(\rho A)l}{420}
\begin{bmatrix}
156 & 22l & 54 & -13l \\
22l & 4l^2 & 13l & -3l^2 \\
54 & 13l & 156 & -22l \\
-13l & -3l^2 & -22l & 4l^2
\end{bmatrix}
$$

In equations (15.42) and (15.43), coupling term Q_i^e can be defined as

$$
\Theta_i^e = \frac{1}{v} \times \{0 \; -B_e E_3 \; 0 \; B_e E_3\}
$$

and capacitance C_p will be

$$
C_p = \frac{A_e L}{4h_p^2}
$$

Here, $E_3 = \dfrac{-v}{h_p}$ (electric field component).

Terms B_e and A_e in coupling term expression can be obtained as

$$
B_e = \int B \times e_{31} \times z\,dz
$$

$$
A_e = \int B \times e_{33} \times z\,dz
$$

where e_{31} = piezoelectric stress constant and e_{33} = permittivity constant.

The equivalent forcing term when the beam vibrates in the transverse direction,

$$
F_i = F_{oi} \times \frac{d^2 w_b}{dt^2}
$$

where F_{oi} can be obtained by using the below expression:

$$
F_{oi} = \int \left[m + M_t \delta (x - L) \right] \times \psi_i dx
$$

where m = mass per unit length.

   M_t = tip mass attached at cantilever beam

$$
\frac{d^2 w_B}{dt^2} = \text{Base acceleration}
$$

All the above equations which are discussed can be calculated from equations (15.42) to (15.43) and the global forms of mechanical and electrical components are obtained as in equations (15.44) and (15.45):

$$[M]^G * \left[\ddot{\Delta}\right] + [K]^G * [\Delta] - [\theta]^G * v(t) = [F]^G \qquad (15.44)$$

$$C_p * \frac{dv}{dt} + \frac{v}{R_1} + \left([\theta]^G\right)^T * \left[\dot{\Delta}\right]^G = 0 \qquad (15.45)$$

where

$[M]^G$ = global mass matrix

$[K]^G$ = stiffness matrix

$[F]^G$ = force vector

$[Q]^G$ = global coupling term

All the above equations can be analytically simulated in MATLAB software and can be solved, and finally transverse displacement and equivalent induced voltage can be calculated.

15.2 MODELING OF ENERGY HARVESTER

15.2.1 DESIGNING THE ROUGH MODEL

The basic characteristics on which the design is based are the stroke length or amplitude, the frequency of excitation of the specimen, its dimensions and corresponding weight.

The specimen in consideration, cantilever beam, is made of stainless steel and is vertical in orientation, having dimensions of 300 mm × 25.5 mm × 5.1 mm. A piezo-electric patch has attached dimensions of 50 mm × 25 mm × 0.5 mm, closed to the fixed end of the beam.

The attached mass is fixed at a random distance 'd' from the fixed end of a cantilever beam. The material used are neodymium magnets (rectangular in shape with dimensions of 25 mm × 10 mm × 1 mm and a weight of 4.5 g each).

The mechanism chosen is a slider-crank mechanism to transform rotational motion to translation motion. Here the DC motor will provide a rotational motion to its base plate and the slider crank will convert it to a translation motion, which will be transferred to the holder of the cantilever beam. Electronics are used to control the speed of the motor and hence the frequency of vibration. The CAD model is shown in Figure 15.5.

15.2.2 STATIC ANALYSIS ON CRANK AND CONNECTING ROD

The static analysis has been done in Ansys. The material chosen is stainless steel (modulus of elasticity 193–200 GPa, tensile yield strength 215 MPa). The force on the parts is supposed to be 25 N (calculated from the natural frequency of the specimen). The von-Mises stress and total deformation on the crank and connecting rod are shown in Figures 15.6 and 15.7.

15.2.3 KINEMATIC ANALYSIS ON THE SLIDER-CRANK MECHANISM

The stroke length of the slider crank is assumed to be between 13 and 22 mm and the energy harvester is excited under the principal parametric resonance condition,

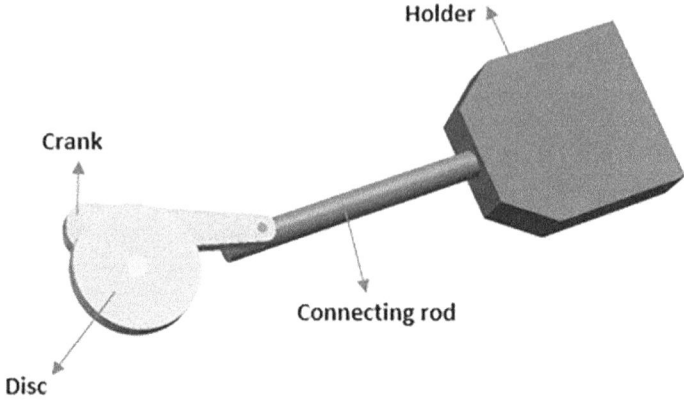

FIGURE 15.5 Design of rough model.

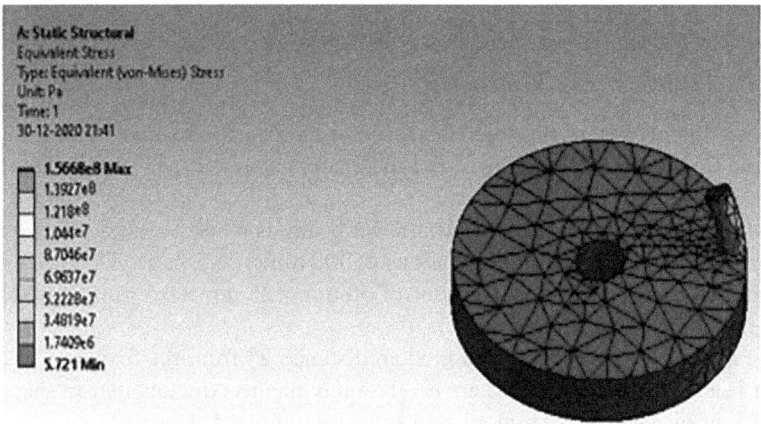

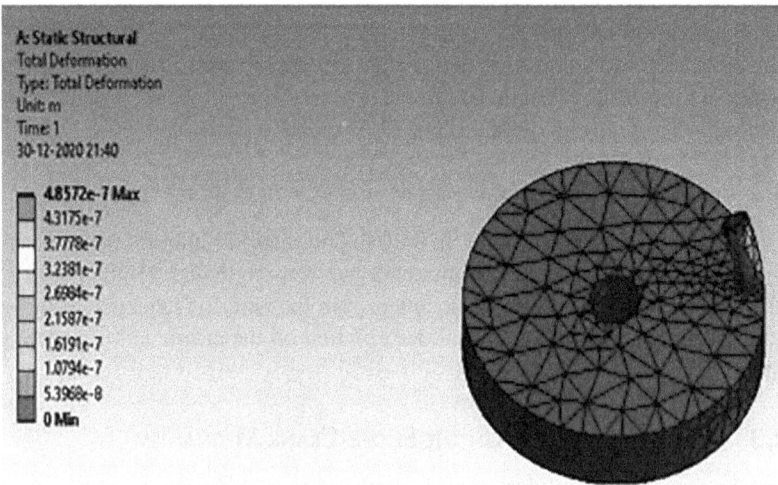

FIGURE 15.6 von-Mises (top) and total deformation (bottom) of the crank on the application of forces corresponding to movement and weight.

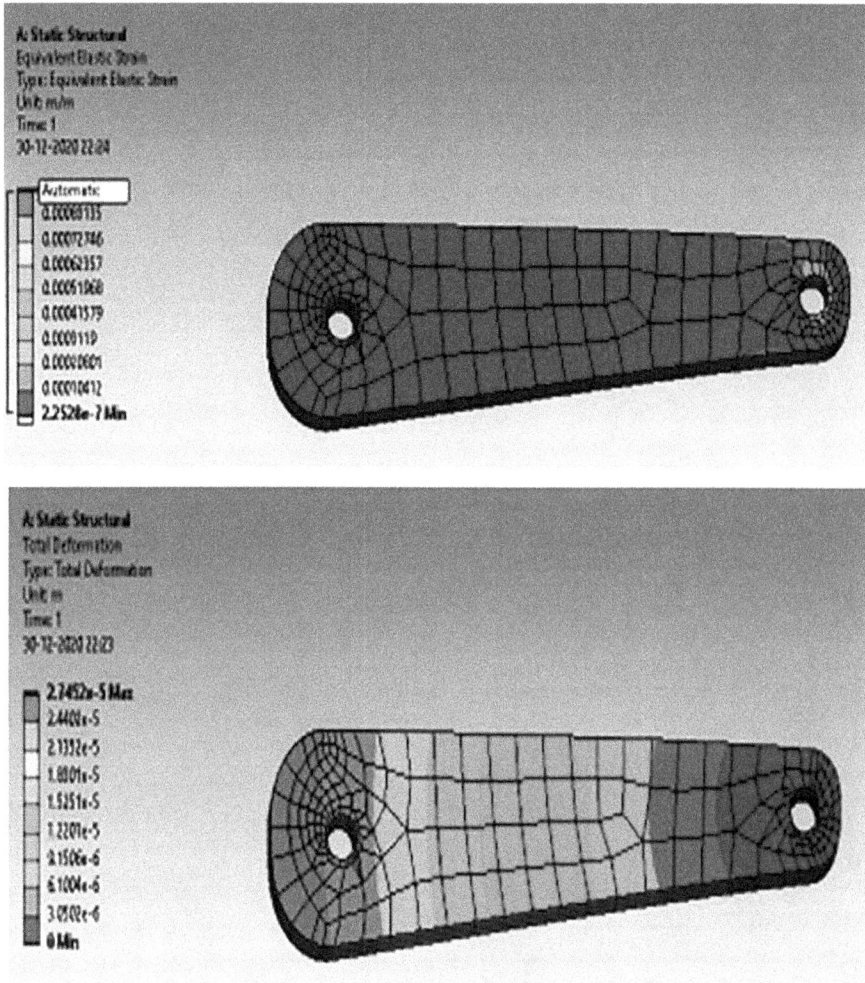

A: Static Structural
Equivalent Elastic Strain
Type: Equivalent Elastic Strain
Unit: m/m
Time: 1
30-12-2020 22:24

Automatic
0.000083133
0.000072746
0.000062357
0.000051968
0.000041579
0.00009119
0.000020801
0.000010412
2.2528e-7 Min

A: Static Structural
Total Deformation
Type: Total Deformation
Unit: m
Time: 1
30-12-2020 22:23

2.7452e-5 Max
2.4401e-5
2.1352e-5
1.8301e-5
1.5251e-5
1.2201e-5
9.1506e-6
6.1004e-6
3.0502e-6
0 Min

FIGURE 15.7 von-Mises (top) and total deformation (bottom) of the connecting rod on the application of forces corresponding to movement and weight.

which results in a maximum frequency of 25 Hz (1500 rpm). Since the length of stroke is assumed to be between 13 and 22 mm, the crank developed will be a circular disk with a radius of 12 mm. The shaft of the DC motor and crank is attached. A guided extension rod is tuck into the coupling rod at a point using a bolt in a perpendicular manner. A holder is put above the rod to fix a beam. After several optimizations, the weight of the components is determined for the material chosen, stainless steel. Details are given in Table 15.1.

Motion analysis of the cantilever beam holder is found out so that it will resemble the motion characteristics of the cantilever beam as shown in Figure 15.8. The linear displacement, velocity and acceleration are shown in Figures 15.9, 15.10 and 15.11, respectively.

TABLE 15.1

Details of Motion Path Holder

Components	Weight (g)
Crank with a connecting rod	45
Slider with holder	131
Cantilever beam	62 (approx.)
Others(screw)	10
Total	248

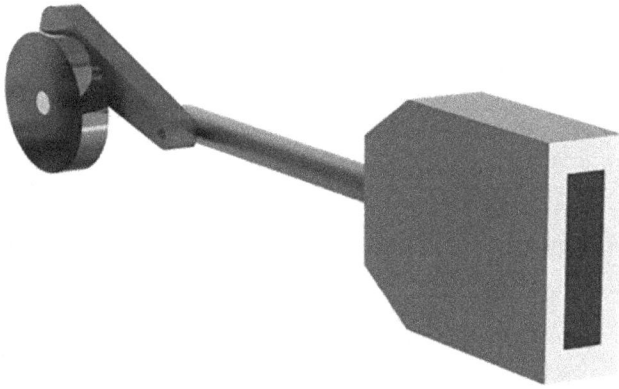

FIGURE 15.8   Motion path of holder.

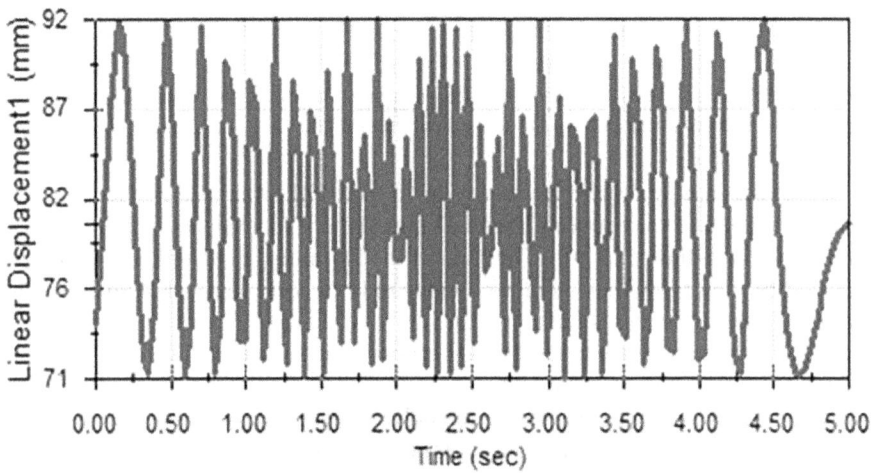

FIGURE 15.9   Linear displacement (mm) of holder vs time (s).

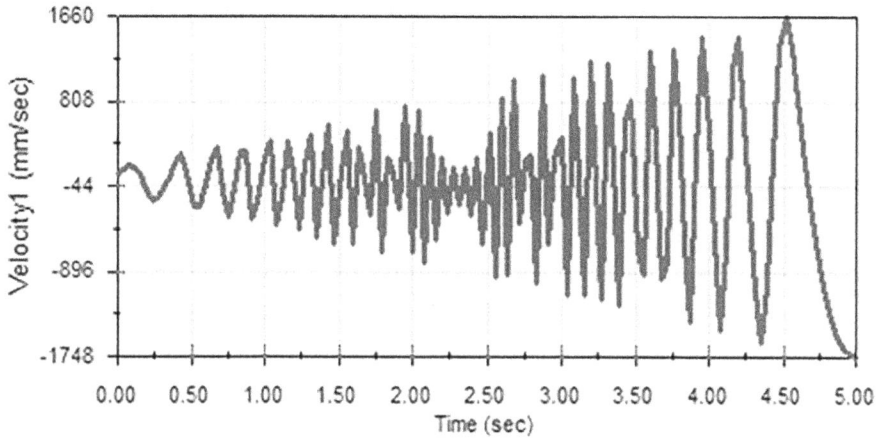

FIGURE 15.10 Velocity (mm/s) of holder vs time (s).

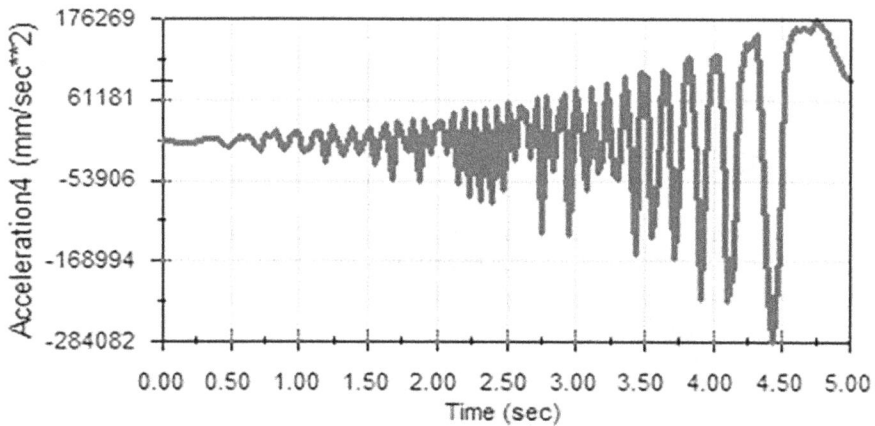

FIGURE 15.11 Acceleration of holder (mm/s²) vs time (s).

15.2.4 DYNAMIC ANALYSIS ON THE SLIDER-CRANK MECHANISM

To find out the torque required to excite the system, dynamic analysis of the system is performed and the torque characteristics are found out:

$$\tau_r = \left(m_s r^2 \omega^2 \left(\cos\theta + \frac{\cos 2\theta}{n} \right) + m_s g r \right) \times \left(\sin\theta + \frac{\sin 2\theta}{2\sqrt{n^2 - \sin^2\theta}} \right)$$

where r=radius of crank, m=mass of system, ω = angular velocity, θ = crank angle (in radian), g=acceleration due to gravity and n=ratio of connecting rod length to the radius of crank. Taking $m=0.248$ kg, $r=0.012$ m, $lc=0.05$ m, $n=lc/r$, $N=1500$ rpm and $g=9.8$ m/s², the variation of the torque with the crank angle is shown in Figure 15.12.

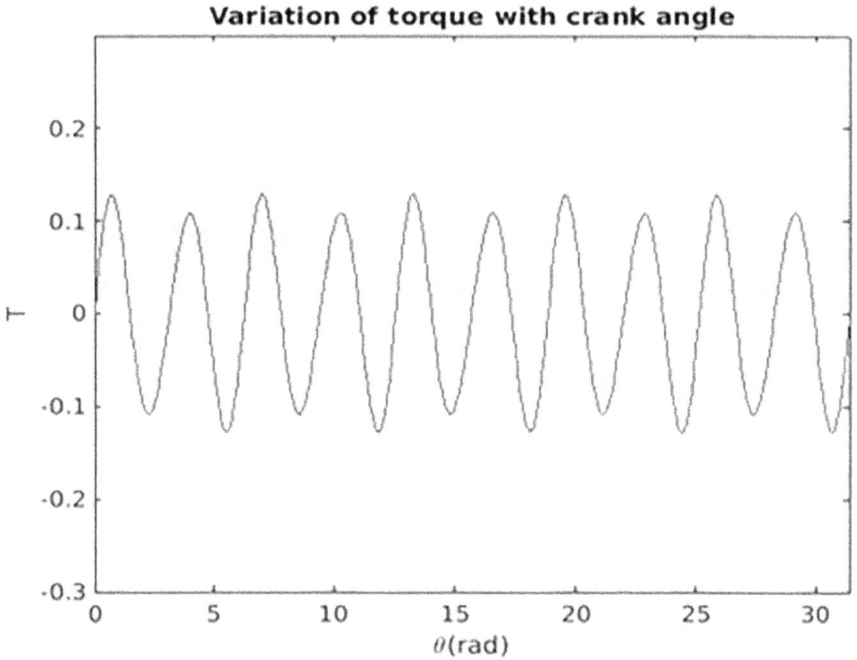

FIGURE 15.12   Torque vs crank angle.

Torque calculation helps us in selecting a range of the motor to be used and a 24 V DC motor is chosen which has the capability of developing 6000 rpm. Though, a 12 V supply is used to develop a speed of 3000 rpm. The natural frequency of the cantilever beam is the parameter that will decide the operating range of motor speed.

15.3   RESULTS AND DISCUSSION

15.3.1   Variation of Torque with Crank Angle

A simulation is performed to calculate the torque required to be generated by the DC motor. This helps the manufacturer buy the right motor to manufacture the device. The expression for torque required by the motor is calculated as follows:

$$\tau_r = \left(m_s r^2 w^2 \left(\cos\theta + \frac{\cos 2\theta}{n} \right) + m_s gr \right) \times \left(\sin\theta + \frac{\sin 2\theta}{2\sqrt{n^2 - \sin^2\theta}} \right)$$

$m_s = 0.225$ kg, $r = 0.0065$ m, $l_c = 0.05$ m, $n = \frac{l_c}{r}$, $N = 1500$ rpm, and $g = 9.8$ m / s^2.

The simulated results are shown in Figure 15.13.

The maximum value of torque was found to be 0.129 Nm. The DC motor should be selected such that it can provide at least this much torque for the device to work.

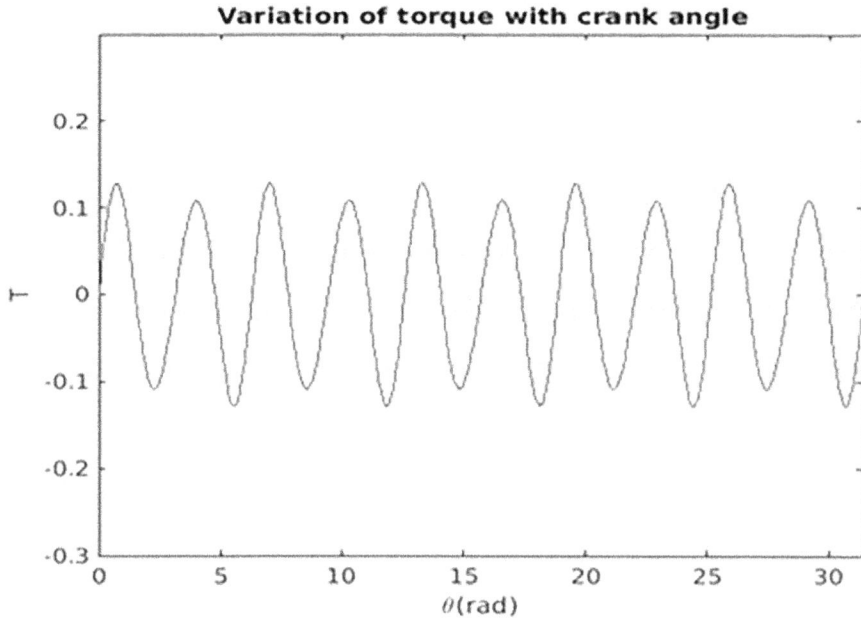

FIGURE 15.13   Variation of torque with crank angle.

15.3.2   TIME DOMAIN REPRESENTATION OF GENERATED VOLTAGE

Through the analytical work done in [1], the expression for voltage induced by the device was obtained as

$$v(t) = r_v \frac{1}{\sqrt{\chi^2 + 1}} a \cos(\omega t + \upsilon + \phi), \quad \text{where} \quad \chi = \frac{1}{C_p \omega R_l} \quad \text{and} \quad \phi = \tan^{-1} \chi$$

A sinusoidal signal with a frequency of 7.18 Hz is shown in Figure 15.14.

15.3.3   VARIATION OF POWER WITH FREQUENCY OF EXCITATION

Through the analytical work done in [1], the expression for determining the variation of power with frequency is obtained as

$$P = \frac{a^2}{R_l} \left(r_v \frac{1}{\sqrt{\chi^2 + 1}} \right)^2$$

The simulated power vs frequency curve is shown in Figure 15.15.

The power is seen to increase with an increase in excitation frequency. This makes sense as it requires more power to rotate the DC motor faster.

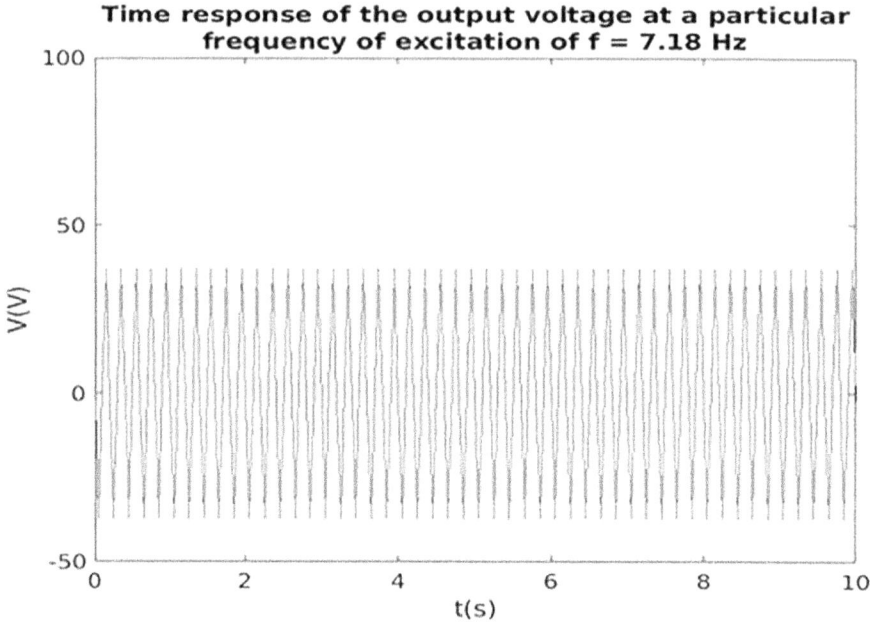

FIGURE 15.14   Time response of the output voltage at a particular frequency.

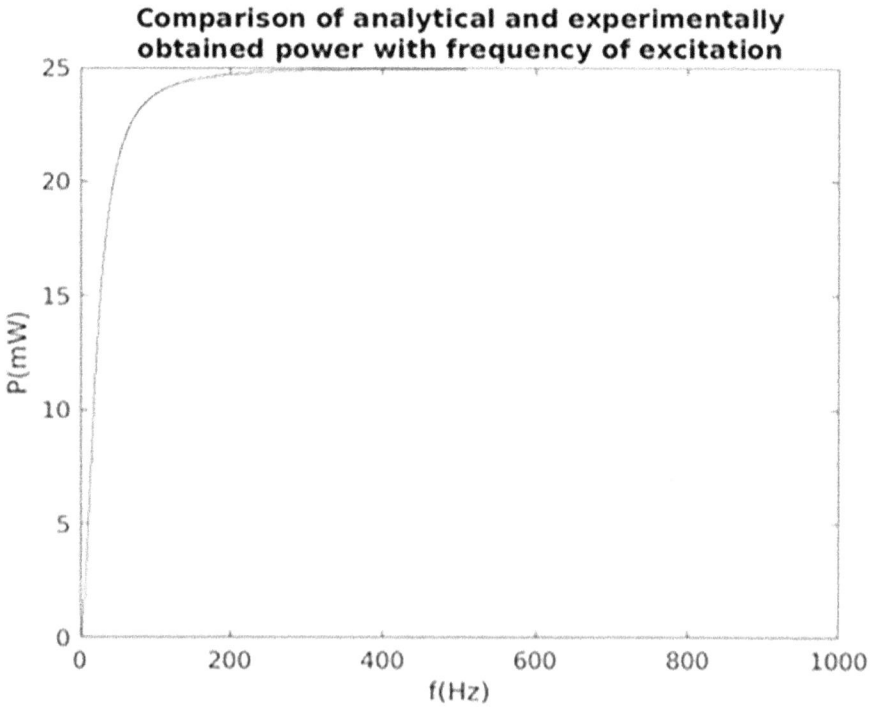

FIGURE 15.15   Power vs frequency curve.

15.3.4 Voltage–Time Response of the System when Just Tapping the Top Edge of the Beam

This is achieved by first disconnecting the DC motor from the microcontroller. When the top edge of the beam is just tapped, the beam begins to oscillate. But since energy is not continuously supplied to the system, the magnitude of oscillation decreases with time. The expression for the voltage–time response in this case is given as

$$v(t) = -R_l\left[\int_{x=0}^{L} d_{31}Y_p h_{pc}b\frac{\partial^3 u_{rel}(x,t)}{\partial x^2 \partial t}dx + \frac{\int_{33}^{s} bL}{h_p}\frac{dv(t)}{dt}\right]$$

where $u_{rel}(x,t) = e^{-at}A\cos(\omega t)$.

The voltage–time expression can be simplified to

$$v(t) = Me^{-at}\sin(kL - \omega t + \phi) + Ne^{-at}\sin(-\omega t + \phi)$$

On plotting this, a damped sinusoidal signal is obtained as shown in Figure 15.16 (Figure 15.17).

15.3.5 Effect of Beam Material on Induced Voltage in a Piezoelectric Energy Harvester

The specifications of the materials used in this experiment are shown in Table 15.2.

A load resistance (R_l) of 100 kΩ is used. The simulated graph of induced voltages and their frequency responses is shown in Figure 15.18. All substrates have

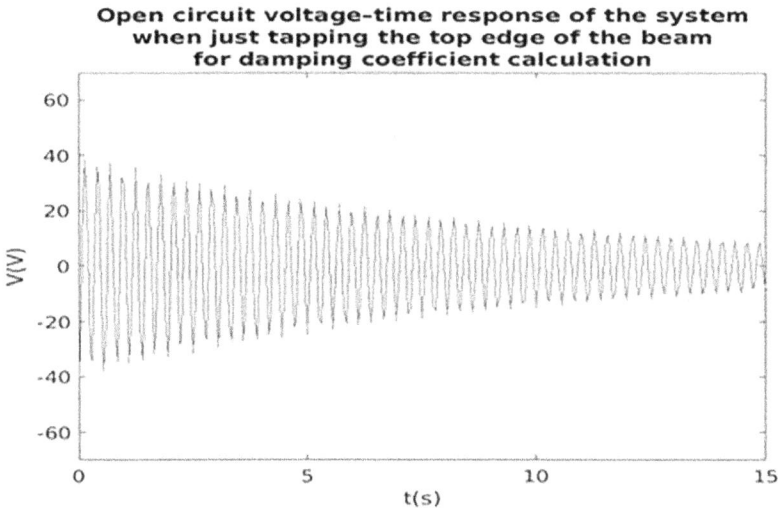

FIGURE 15.16 Open circuit voltage–time response of the system.

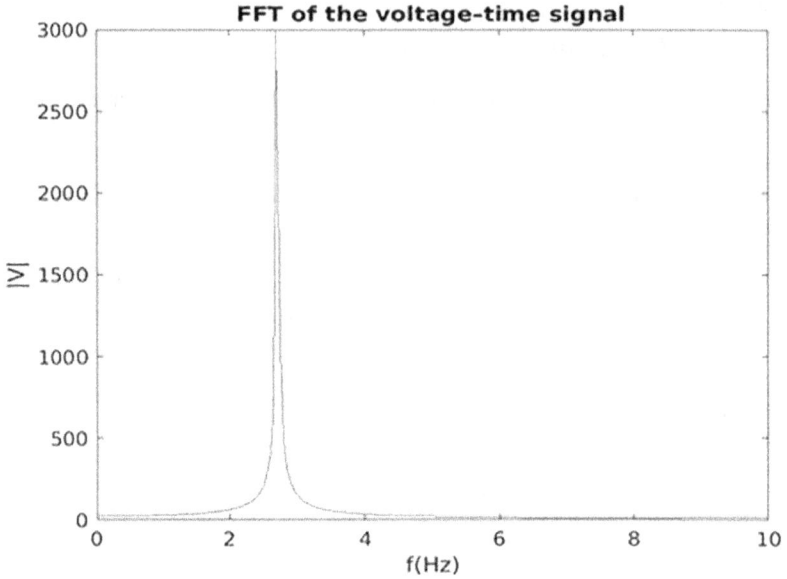

FIGURE 15.17 FFT of the voltage–time signal.

TABLE 15.2
Specification of the Substrate and PZT Materials

Property	PZT Patch	Steel Substrate	Aluminum Substrate	Copper Substrate
Young's modulus (GPa)	66.7	190	70	120
Density (kg/m³)	7500	7800	2700	8940
Length (mm)	50	300	291	300
Width (mm)	25	25.5	25.5	25.5
Height (mm)	0.5	0.51	0.51	0.65
Capacitance (nF)	71.3			
Mass (g)	5	30.4	10.2	44.5

approximately the same dimensions. Due to their differences in densities and Young's modulus, cantilever beams made of these materials have a different natural frequency. The natural frequencies of the beams made of these materials can be seen from the frequency response. Copper beam induces a higher amplitude voltage, but it has a lower frequency. Aluminum induces a lower amplitude but a higher frequency voltage. Steel has moderate values for both. This result makes sense as aluminum has the lowest density and Young's modulus. This means that the molecules are held together by weaker bonds and can move more freely. This makes it more flexible and gives it a higher natural frequency. The natural frequencies of copper, steel and aluminum beams were found to be 563, 577 and 619 Hz, respectively.

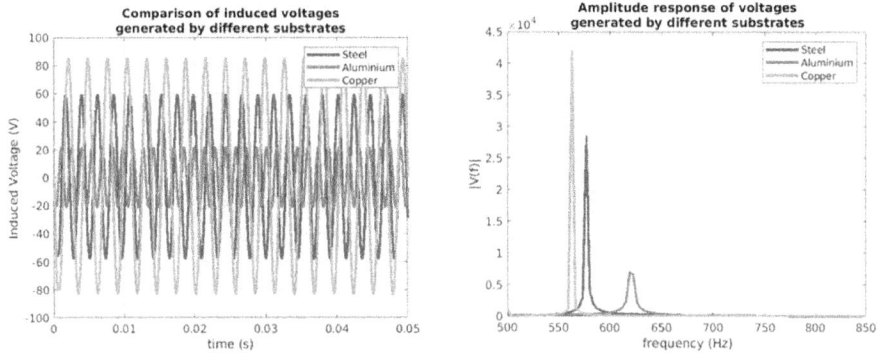

FIGURE 15.18 Comparison of induced voltages generated by different substrates and their frequency response.

15.4 DEVELOPMENT OF CONTROL STRATEGIES

15.4.1 CHOICE OF CONTROL STRATEGIES

To vibrate the beam at different frequencies, we need to control the speed of the motor used. In this case, a DC motor is used to rotate the slider-crank mechanism connected to the cantilever beam. A PID control mechanism was chosen. An initial circuit was made using LabVIEW. The inbuilt PID algorithm was used and the motor was represented by a transfer function. A standard transfer function was used where the input was the voltage and the output was the angular speed:

$$\frac{\Phi(s)}{V(s)} = \frac{\dfrac{K}{JL}}{s^2 + \left(\dfrac{JR+BL}{JL}\right)s + \dfrac{BR+K^2}{JL}}$$

$\Phi(s)$ = angular velocity (rad/s)
$V(s)$ = applied voltage (V)
J = rotor inertia (9.64E-6)
R = rotor resistance (3.3 Ω)
K = torque constant (0.028 N.m\A)
L = inductance (4.64E-3 H)
B = friction torque constant (1.8E-6 N.m.s)

If we replace the variables with the standard values specified, the equation obtained is

$$G(s) = \frac{3.5276 * 10^6}{s^2 + 1591.46s + 109,711}$$

Using the equation that represents the transfer function, a block diagram was built to represent the circuit, as shown in Figure 15.19.

The tuning of the controller was done to prevent overshoot and account for the steady-state errors, by using an XY chart shown in Figure 15.20.

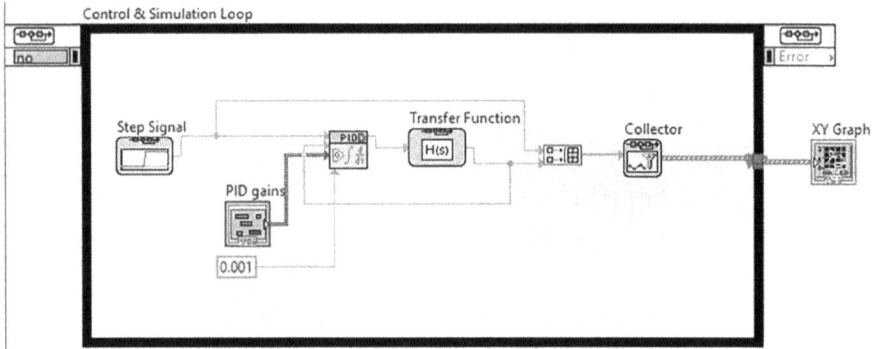

FIGURE 15.19 Block diagram developed for an initial PID controller.

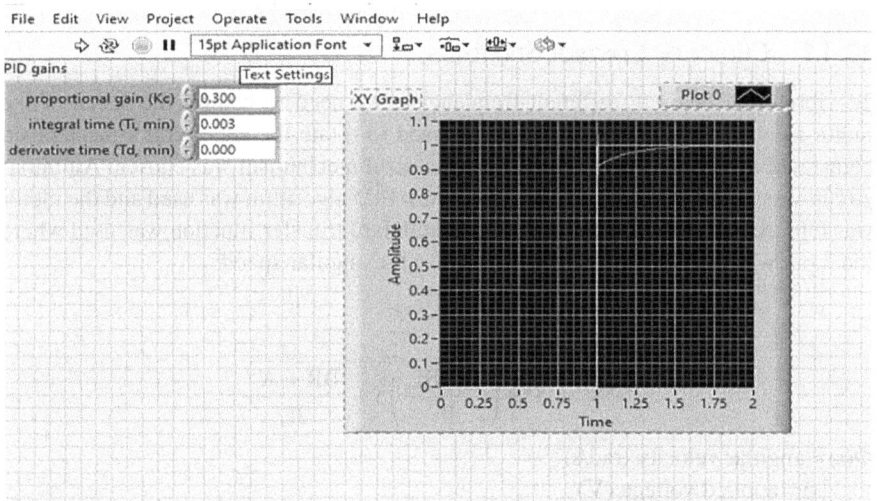

FIGURE 15.20 Simulation of results with given constants.

15.4.2 Development and Tuning of PID Using MATLAB

To tune the PID controller with the variation of speed and to use the motor of our requirements, a circuit was created in Simulink using MATLAB, as shown in Figure 15.21. The PID controller was tuned for different speeds within the range, as shown in Figure 15.22.

The values for a particular setting are shown in Figure 15.22, where the PID controller was tuned for a speed of 1500 rpm.

The PID controller was tuned for different speeds within the range, and the graph of the desired speed vs estimated speed is shown in Figure 15.23 for a desired speed of 1500 rpm. The overshoot and the steady-state error were accounted for using the inbuilt PID tuner in Simulink.

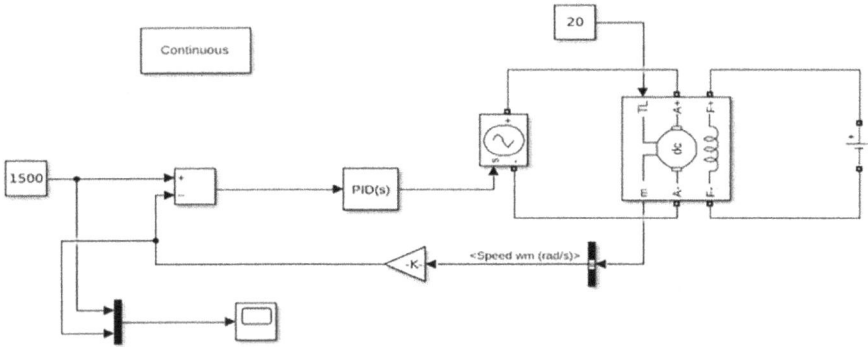

FIGURE 15.21 Circuit diagram for the control strategy developed.

Source: internal

Proportional (P): 0.214596036046498

Integral (I): 5.26646706519129

Derivative (D): 0.00216589040036506

FIGURE 15.22 PID control values for speed at 1500 rpm.

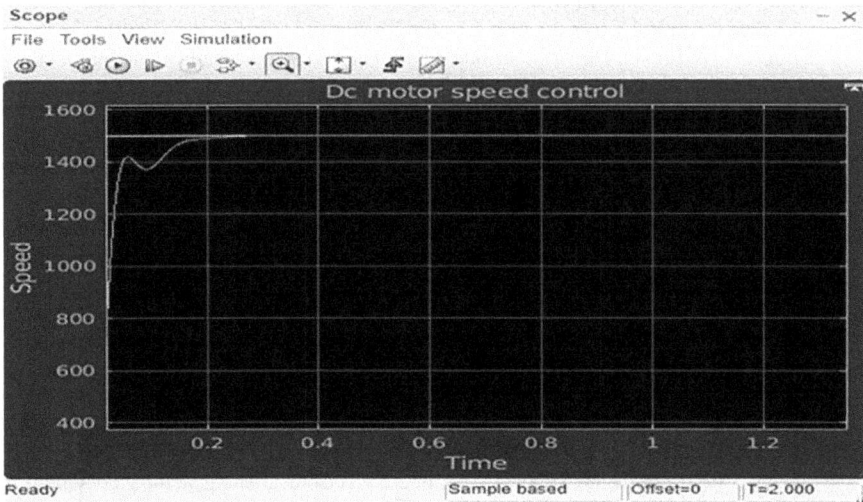

FIGURE 15.23 Speed vs time graph for comparing the desired speed and the estimated speed.

15.5 CONCLUSION

1. A vertical cantilever beam system based on a PEH is simulated and investigated theoretically in our present work under parametric excitation.
2. A model of the low-cost shaker is developed. Material and dimensional properties of the setup are determined during motion analysis. Motion characteristics of the beam are obtained, where value and operational range and maximum values are determined and used for calculation in mathematical modeling.
3. Simulation is carried out on the optimized model. The theoretical analysis and the simulation results seem to be in good agreement. It is noticed that a vertically oriented cantilever beam produced more output voltage than a horizontally oriented beam of similar configurations because the effect of gravity is put up into the dynamics of the system.
4. The simulated graph of induced voltages and frequency responses for three different substrates is plotted above.
5. A control strategy is developed where a PID controller is used. The block diagram of the control strategy is developed and simulated. The PID parameters are tuned and an efficient control mechanism is obtained with minimum error. Such a strategy can be used for the experimental setup of the model developed.

REFERENCES

1. Abdelkefi, A., Nayfeh, A.H., & Hajj, M.R., "Global nonlinear distributed-parameter model of parametrically excited piezoelectric energy harvesters", *Nonlinear Dynamics*, Vol.67/2, pp. 1147–1160, (2012).
2. Garg, A. & Dwivedy, S.K. "Piezoelectric energy harvester under parametric excitation: A theoretical and experimental investigation", *Journal of Intelligent Materials Systems and Structures*, Vol. 31(4), pp. 612–631, (2020). doi:10.1177/1045389X19891523
3. Erturk, A., & Inman, D.J. "A distributed parameter electromechanical model for cantilevered piezoelectric energy harvesters", *Journal of Vibration and Acoustics*, Vol. 130/4, p. 041002, (2008).
4. Friswell, M.I., Ali, S.F., & Bilgen, O, "Non-linear piezoelectric vibration energy harvesting from a vertical cantilever beam with tip mass", *Journal of Intelligent Material Systems and Structures*, Vol. 23/13, pp. 1505–1521, (2012).
5. Garg, A., & Dwivedy, S. K., "Non-linear dynamics of parametrically excited piezoelectric energy harvester with 1:3 internal resonance", *International Journal of Non-Linear Mechanics*, Vol. 111, pp.82–94, (2019).
6. Kar, R.C., & Dwivedy S K. "Non-linear dynamics of a slender beam carrying a lumped mass with principal parametric and internal resonances", *International Journal of Non-Linear Mechanics*, Vol. 34/3, pp.515–529, (1999).
7. Anderson, T.J., Nayfeh, A.H., & Balachandran B," Experimental verification of the importance of the nonlinear curvature in the response of a cantilever beam", *Journal of Vibration and Acoustics*, Vol. 118/1, pp.21–27, (1996).
8. Beeby, S.P., Torah, R., & Tudor, M, "A micro electromagnetic generator for vibration energy harvesting", *Journal of Micromechanics and Microengineering*, Vol. 17/7, pp.1257–1265, (2007).

9. Daqaq, M.F., Stabler, C., & Qaroush Y, "Investigation of power harvesting via parametric excitations", *Journal of Intelligent Material Systems and Structures*, Vol.20/5, pp.545–557, (2009).

10. Dwivedy, S.K., & Kar, R.C, "Simultaneous combination, principal parametric and internal resonances in a slender beam with a lumped mass: Three-mode interactions", *Journal of Sound and Vibration*, Vol. 242/1, pp.27–46, (2001).

Index

303

For Product Safety Concerns and Information please contact our EU
representative GPSR@taylorandfrancis.com
Taylor & Francis Verlag GmbH, Kaufingerstraße 24, 80331 München, Germany

www.ingramcontent.com/pod-product-compliance
Lightning Source LLC
Chambersburg PA
CBHW060815220326
41598CB00022B/2618